Observe how all things are continually being born of change; teach yourself to see that Nature's highest happiness lies in changing the things that are, and forming new things after their kind. Whatever is, is in some sense the seed of what is to emerge from it. Nothing can become a philosopher less than to imagine that seed can only be something that is planted in the earth or the womb.

Marcus Aurelius

Contents

Preface

'What is the use of a book', thought Alice, 'without pictures or conversations'.

Lewis Carroll

Any artist will tell you that in drawing objects, you cannot ignore the spaces in between. The picture ceases to exist when only one aspect is viewed in isolation. Musical pieces composed entirely of notes and without pauses would be nothing more than noise and an irritation. Yet when it comes to teaching, we ignore this fact and fail to put our own speciality into the context of the whole curriculum.

Recently there has been a trend towards a more integrated approach to medical education. We are delighted that such an approach, which we have used in our teaching for the last 7 years, is now adopted widely in the UK and abroad.

Our aim has been to create a tutorial on the mechanisms of disease over a background of history, science and clinical relevance. The goal is to give the students a sense of belonging to a movement – the movement from past to present and from laboratory to the patient.

The synoptic approach to learning has a great many advantages, but sometimes it can be helpful to take a step back and assess just what it is one has learned. We have produced colour-coded theme maps (see page 279–285), which outline the main constituents of the four traditional pathology disciplines – **histopathology**, haematology, immunology and microbiology. We have added two 'overview' themes – science and disease and patient and disease. Coloured dots to match the theme maps are used in the chapter headings for each of the four parts of this book.

This book has been written in the hope that students will read the text fully and at leisure. This not only contains details about the disease processes but also historical anecdotes and clinical scenarios. The cartoons are intended to amuse as well as illustrate the importance of certain topics, and we sincerely hope that students reading the book will be able to shed the dull, dreary image of histopathology that they all seem to be born with. Pathology is one of the most fascinating and fun subjects students are likely to encounter during their undergraduate training.

At the end of each section we include a small number of questions. These are not intended as a revision guide for exams but aim to highlight the most important topics covered, i.e. those that you should remember for life.

Many of the tables and lists have logos attached to them. These are:

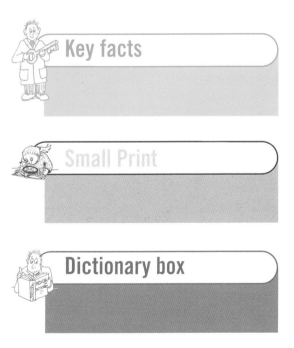

Although the book is primarily intended for undergraduate medical students, we hope that it will also be amusing and useful to students of dentistry, human biology and some paramedical specialities. Postgraduate students studying for pathology or surgical examinations may also wish to consult the book.

Acknowledgements

When we set out over 10 years ago to write a textbook in which we would take the students on a journey, from past to present and from patient to the cell and back again, the phrase 'integrated curriculum' was not in common usage. Today, every medical school in the country has had to switch to the new style curriculum in which pathology is supposedly taught as an integrated subject with other disciplines. We have always believed that pathology should be taught in context of the clinical situation and hope that this has been reflected by the content of this and the previous editions. It would be a shame, however, if pathology rather than being integrated with clinical work was lost because it was not deemed as important as clinical training for the new generation of doctors, nurses and disciplines allied to medicine.

Pathology is the study of the mechanism of disease. It has therefore been, and hopefully will remain, at the heart of anybody's desire to understand and manage disease.

Our endeavours to produce this third edition have been considerably aided by help, comments and constructive criticism from a number of people and we would like to acknowledge their time and effort. They include Prof. Philip Butcher, Prof. Mike Davies (deceased) and Dr Grant Robinson, who helped us with the second edition and whose efforts are still included in the current work. We would like to acknowledge the work that Drs Laura Fulford and Jorge Reis-Filho, both clinical research fellows at The Breakthrough Toby Robins Breast Cancer Research Centre, have put in to read and review the current literature on genetics and cancer. The staff in the molecular pathology laboratory headed by SRL has also directly or indirectly contributed to ideas or material for the book and we are grateful to Sophie Johnson for administrative help. CJF would also like to thank Dr Jo Sheldon, Dr Sandra Gibson, Dr Gerald Levin and Dr Barry Newell.

We would like to make a special acknowledgement to Prof. John P. Sloane who sadly died two years ago. Three of us (SRL, SAD and CJF) trained and worked very closely with him over a number of years and there is little doubt in our minds that we were greatly influenced by him in our professional and personal lives.

Finally and most importantly, we would like to thank our families for their encouragement and support. But for their understanding, it would be difficult to get away with the disproportionate amount of time that such projects consume.

SRL, SAD, CJF, AD
May 2003

PART 1
Introduction – What is a Disease?

Prologue: Definition of disease

You have just opened a book entitled *Basic Pathology – An Introduction to the Mechanisms of Disease*, is it fair to face you with an enormous challenge in the opening paragraph by asking 'What is a disease'? Although you might expect the authors to offer you a definition, we would prefer you to think it through with friends and colleagues because there is no simple answer.

This book will adopt a strongly biomedical concept of disease. This is a mechanistic model that regards the body as a machine with repairable or replaceable parts. It looks for specific underlying biological causes and places a high emphasis on the scientific evidence-base for untangling cause and effect in both the disease and its treatment, because this is important for patient care and prognosis. However, it is important that you appreciate that the definition of diseases is fraught with problems. Disease definitions change with time and across cultures and social classes. Naming a condition can create a spurious impression of understanding and inhibit further patient investigation or research. Measuring biochemical changes in the blood can provide an early warning of the onset of disease, but does a person have the disease before the symptoms appear? Do you, in fact, need to suffer from a disease as part of the definition? If you do not, then where do you draw the line in deciding who has a disease when the 'marker' follows a normal pattern of distribution within the population? For example, is hypertension a disease defined by a particular level of blood pressure? Alternatively, should we talk of cardiovascular disease and define that through the symptoms of strokes and heart attacks? Then the 'marker' of raised blood pressure is but one consideration in a complex multifactorial process. In psychiatric practice, doctors have no problems in dissecting the symptoms from the 'disease' or 'illness'. A person presenting with a phobia today almost certainly started their mental 'illness/disease' many years previously.*

Although it is sometimes said that 'health' should not be defined as merely the absence of disease, as pathologists we might argue that disease is best defined as a reduction in health – then it embraces almost everything. This also reflects the origin of the word 'disease' from the French: *des* = from, *aise* = ease.

With all those caveats, we shall offer a biomedical definition of disease. 'Disease is a consequence of a failure of homeostasis', where homeostasis is the concept of equilibrium within the body despite changes in the internal or external environment. If you accept this definition then understanding the mechanisms of disease will involve understanding the processes for maintaining homeostasis, identifying the agents and events that disrupt homeostasis, trying to determine why homeostatic mechanisms fail and whether any intervention can prevent or correct this sequence that results in a disease. Rather arbitrarily, we shall decide that a disease should have the potential to produce some impairment of function, but may be detected and defined while asymptomatic. It may also be treated or healed through the body's normal processes so that no permanent damage is produced.

---

*Although this book is concerned with cell and tissue manifestations of disease, it is not unreasonable for students to broaden their knowledge of 'disease' by considering mental illness, for example by reading *The Road Less Travelled* by M. Scott Peck.

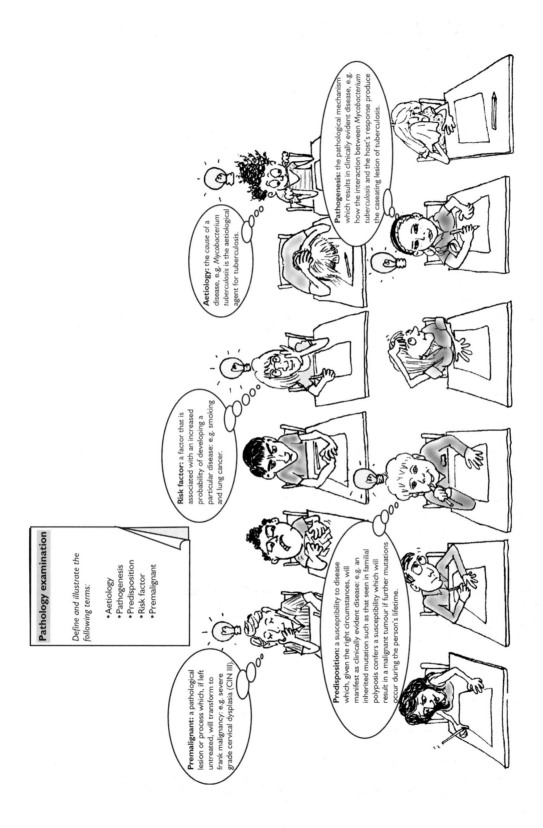

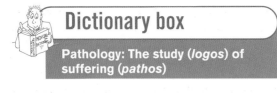

Dictionary box

Pathology: The study (*logos*) of suffering (*pathos*)

Medicine, to produce health, has to examine disease.

Plutarch (c.46–120)
Greek biographer and essayist

Diseases have causes (aetiology) and mechanisms (pathogenesis). They may result in symptoms (experienced by the patient) and signs (elicited by the physician). There may be structural changes that are visible to the naked eye (gross or macroscopical appearances) or only detectable down a microscope (microscopical appearances). Functional changes may be detectable by an ever increasing range of clinical and laboratory techniques. All of this is pathology, and pathology is the study (*logos*) of suffering (*pathos*).

Although we adopt a mechanistic model here, it is a complex model with multiple parts that interconnect. A change in one area is likely to affect another. Thus maintaining homeostasis is not a simple single feedback loop and it is perfectly acceptable that a new equilibrium is achieved under a new set of circumstances, a new baseline; you do not have to return to the original state. Let us take the example of lobar pneumonia (page 90) and introduce a diagram that helps to illustrate the various components of the disease process (Figs 1 and 2).

In its simplest form, an intrinsic or external factor (the cause) acts on a cell, tissue, organ or whole person to produce structural or functional changes and a response. If an adaptive response is 100 per cent successful, then homeostasis is maintained and no symptoms or signs result. If unsuccessful, then the disease manifests and the structural and functional changes may have an impact on another cell, tissue or organ to produce another set of reactions. Thus

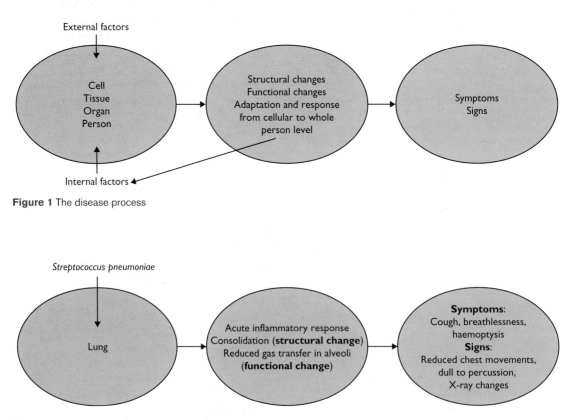

Figure 1 The disease process

Figure 2 Lobar pneumonia: primary mechanism

in lobar pneumonia, the extrinsic cause is the bacterium *Streptococcus pneumoniae*, which affects the lung. This stimulates an acute inflammatory response that can produce the structural changes of consolidation and functional changes of reduced gas transfer in alveoli.

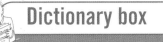

Dictionary box

Consolidation: The process by which the tissue becomes solid; process of solidification.

The patient suffers from cough, breathlessness and even haemoptysis (coughing up blood). The physician may detect the signs of reduced chest movements, an area that is dull to percussion and X-ray opacity reflecting the solidification. However, that is not the end of the story. We can produce another 'disease sequence' in which the reduced gas transfer results in hypoxia (reduced oxygen saturation in the blood); this acts as an intrinsic factor that leads to the heart responding with an increased heart rate (tachycardia). More blood is pumped through the part of the lung that is not consolidated, so increasing gas transfer, and this may successfully compensate so that the hypoxia is corrected, i.e. a new equilibrium is achieved (Fig. 3). But before you

relax, look at page 103 and Fig. 4.19, where we explain about pyrogens that may accompany the inflammatory response to bacteria and the effect that they may have on the heart. Yes, that is another route for producing a tachycardia and so our diagram could become almost infinitely complex as we add the different pathways. This complexity is not unique to pathology or the human body but is true of almost everything as our knowledge and understanding increases. In order to avoid being confused, you need to appreciate and accept the 'interconnectedness'. It is important not to divide the phenomena into different pieces, as in a jigsaw, but to think of them as interlacing connections. In any one situation, it is the unique combination of these connections that produces the final picture.

The idea that it is connections rather than individual objects that are important is well recognized in atomic physics. As Heisenberg (of Heisenberg's uncertainty principle) said:

> (In modern physics), one has now divided the world not into different groups of objects but into different groups of connections. What can be distinguished is the kind of connection which is primarily important in a certain phenomenon ... The world thus appears as a complicated tissue of events, in which connections of different kinds alternate or overlap or combine and thereby determine the texture of the whole.

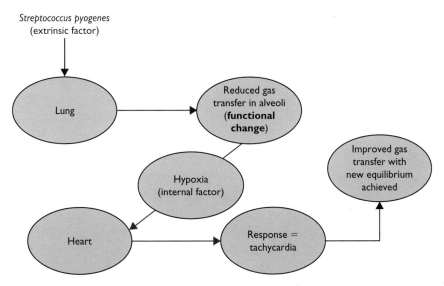

Figure 3 Lobar pneumonia: additional secondary mechanism

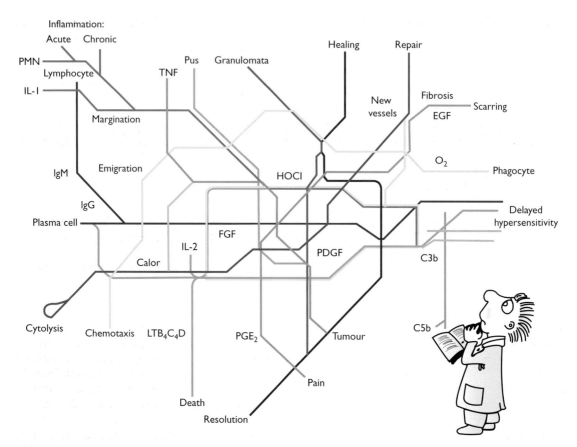

Figure 4 The disease process can be viewed as being made up of many interlacing connections – rather like a metro map

CHAPTER 1

Causes and mechanisms – general principles

Those who are enamoured of practice without science are like a pilot who goes into a ship without rudder or compass and never has any certainty where he is going. Practice should always be based upon a sound knowledge of theory.

Leonardo da Vinci (1452–1519)

Almost anything can cause 'disease' if the conditions are right. For example, water is essential for life but if taken in extreme excess or given intravenously, particularly in a patient with kidney failure, it can cause problems. In this situation, the body is unable to respond adequately so homeostasis is not maintained and a 'disease state' occurs. What may be harmless to one person may cause disease in another. A sudden drop in oxygen during a flight may not affect most of the passengers but could be potentially serious to a person with sickle cell disease (page 64). Thus there is interplay between the potential causes of disease and the potential victim.

Factors that predispose an individual to disease may occur at many levels. They may be genetic and inherited from parents, such as a predisposition to cancer or Huntington's chorea (a neurological disorder), congenital, i.e. present from birth but not necessarily genetic and perhaps acquired during fetal life because of conditions in the uterus, or acquired during life. Such factors often combine with others to produce disease.

Life is fairly simple when a single cause produces a clearly defined and easily recognized disease, especially if that disease is uncommon (e.g. abnormally short limbs due to the drug thalidomide). It is much more difficult to disentangle 'cause and effect' from 'associated with' for most health problems and it is important to appreciate how new causes of disease may be identified.

Often the starting point is information gathered by epidemiologists. On page 73, we describe how

John Snow came up with the idea that cholera was spread via water before bacteria had been identified. He tested his hypothesis by mapping the positions of the cholera cases and the water pumps. Thus, he established an association and some ideas about a mechanism. From this first clue that a disease state and a potential causative agent are 'associated', it is important to try to establish a mechanism whereby an agent could produce the necessary changes. The precise approach will depend on the agent and the disease but this is a crucial step, not only for establishing causation but also for identifying possible methods of treatment. This is why a basic understanding of the principles of the mechanisms of disease (the subject of this book) is so important. Details of specific diseases and treatments can be learnt or looked up later, when required, but an understanding of the mechanisms will allow you to identify new diseases or develop new treatments. Think big – someone has to win the Nobel prizes!

WHAT ARE THE MOST COMMON MECHANISMS?

Here we view diseases from a biomedical standpoint that regards the body as a machine and sees disease as some impairment of function. That impairment of function or homeostasis can affect the whole person, a particular tissue or a cell, and this will influence the symptoms. The common building blocks for most parts of the body are cells and these have a common

Autopsy report

Name: I B Ede
Age: 60 years
Date of admission: 24.7.02
Date of death: 24.7.02
Date of autopsy: 25.7.02

External findings:
The body was that of a Caucasian male. A central venous line in the right jugular vein and peripheral cannula in the left arm were present. There was bruising on the chest related to resuscitation attempts. No other abnormalities seen.

Internal examination:
Cardiovascular system – There was marked atheroma within the aorta and large vessels. The left coronary artery and the left anterior descending (LAD) artery both showed atheroma with 90 per cent occlusion. In addition, there was a fresh thrombus at the origin of the LAD. The right coronary artery showed 50 per cent occlusion. There was no macroscopical evidence of an infarction, however, staining with NBTZ confirmed a full-thickness anterior infarct.
Respiratory system – Both lungs showed evidence of pulmonary oedema.
Renal system – The kidneys showed evidence of ischaemic scarring.
Central nervous system – There was marked atheroma in the carotids and cerebral vessels but no evidence of a cerebral infarction.

Cause of death:
        1a Myocardial infarction
due to 1b Coronary artery thrombosis
due to 1c Coronary artery atheroma

genetic code and a broadly similar set of metabolic pathways, though each will express different pathways dependent on its specialized function. Almost always, something goes wrong at a cellular level leading to dysfunction within the tissue or organ. The ramifications may be quite complex and impact on many other areas of the body.

Thus we will work through the common mechanisms by considering the cell as the key building block. Let us take the most extreme example first of complete failure of cell function, either due to cell damage or cell death: what are the biochemical changes that occur in an injured cell and what distinguishes reversible from irreversible damage? Rather than discuss this exclusively as a cellular problem, let us consider its clinical importance by using the example of heart muscle cells suddenly being deprived of oxygen and nutrients (also known as ischaemia) because a coronary artery is blocked with thrombus (i.e. a heart attack).

CLINICAL CASE – MYOCARDIAL INFARCTION

A 60-year-old man complained of sudden onset of chest pain which had started 2 hours previously. It radiated down his left arm. He was found to be in shock with a blood pressure of 90/50 mmHg and his electrocardiogram (ECG) showed evidence of an anterior myocardial infarction. He also had bilateral pulmonary oedema. The serum cardiac enzymes were elevated, including the creatinine kinase MB isoenzyme. Before he could be transferred to the coronary care unit, he developed ventricular fibrillation and, despite resuscitation attempts, died.

The following day, an autopsy was carried out and part of the report is illustrated below.

Let us use this example to consider the changes that take place in myocardial cells following an ischaemic insult. We know that the final outcome is dependent on a number of variables. These include the severity and duration of the ischaemia and the volume of heart muscle affected. It will also be influenced by any collateral circulation (page 158) and the metabolic demands of the myocardial cells at the time of the insult. Hence, the extent of cell damage and death and whether the injury is reversible or irreversible depends on a number of factors and may be altered by medical intervention. The changes in the heart following ischaemia also vary with time.

Macroscopic appearance

Although biochemical changes may take place very quickly after infarction, the gross appearance of the myocardium is generally entirely normal for the first 6–12 hours. The NBTZ test can be used to highlight the area of infarction in this early period (page 190) and this is what was done in the patient described above. After about 18 hours, the myocardium generally appears slightly pale but may look red-blue due to the entrapped red blood cells within the area of infarction. Each day that follows makes the area of infarction a little more defined, paler and softer. By the end of the first week, there is usually a rim of hyperaemia surrounding the pale yellow-brown area of infarction. This is due to the ingrowth of richly vascularized connective tissue that will be involved in the healing and repair process. As time goes by, the dead myocardial cell debris is removed and a pale firm fibrous scar laid down; a process which is complete by 6 weeks.

Microscopic appearance

As with the gross appearance, the light microscopic changes lag behind the biochemical changes. The earliest change (4–12 hours) is mild oedema and separation of the muscle fibres. The cells adjacent to the area of infarction may also show small droplets within the cytoplasm and this phenomenon is called vacuolar degeneration. By 24 hours, neutrophil polymorphs infiltrate the area of necrosis and the necrotic myocytes undergo cytoplasmic and nuclear changes typical of necrosis. The cytoplasm appears more pink (eosinophilic) and the nuclei become pyknotic. Later the nuclei are lost and the cross-striations disappear. By day 3, the infiltrate of neutrophils is heavy and, by the end of the week, the cellular debris from dead cells is being removed by macrophages. The fibrovascular connective tissue, which gives the hyperaemia seen macroscopically, is also evident. Examination at later stages shows the varying amounts of fibrous scar tissue seen on gross inspection.

Figure 1.1 summarizes the main findings on gross and microscopical examination of the myocardium at different times following the ischaemic episode.

BIOCHEMICAL CHANGES IN THE CELLS

There are two important questions to consider:

- What are the biochemical changes that occur in an injured cell?
- What distinguishes reversible from irreversible injury?

There are four sites within the cell that are of paramount importance in cell damage and death. These are the:

- mitochondria
- plasma membrane
- ionic channels in cell membranes
- cytoskeleton.

The first effect of ischaemia is to reduce the production of adenosine triphosphate (ATP) by the mitochondrial oxidative phosphorylation system. If the production of energy slows down or stops, then the cells cannot function; in the case of heart muscle, the cell cannot contract – as simple as that! Obviously, if the ischaemic cells cannot partake in aerobic metabolism, then they will switch over to anaerobic metabolism to derive energy from stored glycogen. The enzyme creatine kinase, which is present in the myocardial cells, is also used to produce energy from the anaerobic metabolism of creatinine phosphate. The net effect of these mechanisms is to deplete the cells of glycogen and to produce acidosis within the cells by the production of lactic acid and inorganic phosphates. This further inhibits the normal function of the myocardial cells. The acidosis within the cells is thought to be responsible for one of the observed histological hallmarks of cell damage – the clumping of the nuclear chromatin and pyknosis of the nuclei.

Ischaemia also has profound effects on the plasma membranes and on the ionic channels within the membranes. These are vital in maintaining the normal ionic gradients across the cell membranes, with sodium and calcium at low concentrations inside the cells and potassium lower in the extracellular space. These concentrations are maintained by pumps that are energy-dependent; hence it is not difficult to see that the loss of oxidative phosphorylation and any direct damage to the membranes will disrupt the function of these pumps. So what is the effect?

First, the failure of the pumps will result in the leakage of sodium into the cells and potassium out of the cells. Sodium has a larger hydration shell than potassium so more water moves into the cell, in association with sodium ions, than exits with the potassium. Additional water enters because the acidosis and raised intracellular concentrations of high-molecular-weight phosphates increases the osmotic pressure inside the cell. The result is acute swelling of the cell due to cellular oedema. The endoplasmic reticulum also swells, the ribosomes detach from the endoplasmic reticulum, the mitochondria become swollen and blebs begin to appear on the cell surface.

This last phenomenon is intriguing as the changes in cell shape and surface blebbing imply alterations in the cytoskeleton of the cell. Changes in the microfilaments of the cytoskeleton are believed to be caused by the increased concentration of calcium, which also results from the failure of the membrane pumps. Calcium is a very important ion in cell death and we will see why in a minute.

You might find it difficult to believe, but all the changes described so far are reversible! If the oxygen supply is restored, the cells still have the capacity to

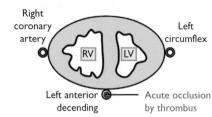

0–12 hours: *Potentially reversible*

Gross: Nil, but NBTZ positive 2–8 hrs
Light microscopy (LM): Nuclear pyknosis, vague loss of striations, scanty polymorph (PMN) infiltrate 8–12 hrs

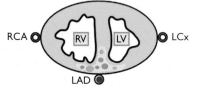

12–24 hours: *Ischaemic damage*

Gross: Blotchy, pale, slightly soft
LM: Increase in PMN's, obvious loss of striations, coagulative necrosis of myocytes

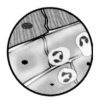

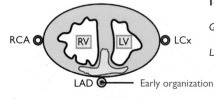

1–3 days: *Necrosis & inflammation*

Gross: Mottled pale infarct, red hyperaemic border
LM: As above, more marked mainly PMN infiltrate and early capillary ingrowth, particularly at periphery

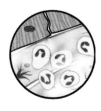

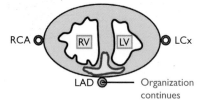

4–7 days: *Removal of debris, early organization*

Gross: Depressed, soft, yellow infarct, prominent hyperaemic edge
LM: As before, with increased macrophages phagocytosing debris from dead myocytes, peripheral granulation tissue formation

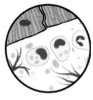

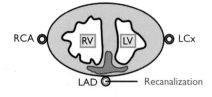

7–14 days: *Organization*

Gross: 'Bruised' look: red/purple colour, increasingly firm as granulation tissue forms
LM: Decreased inflammation as dead tissue is cleared, granulation tissue replaces damaged area

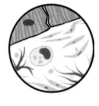

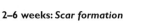

2–6 weeks: *Scar formation*

Gross: Infarct becomes firm and white and eventually contracts, the LV wall is thinned
LM: Capillaries and fibroblasts are replaced by acellular fibrous scar tissue

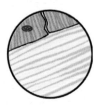

Figure 1.1 Myocardial infarction: changes with time

return to their normal state and the ability of the myocardial cells to contract is restored. So what are the changes that finally tip the cell beyond the point of no return?

The morphological hallmarks are a severe disruption of the mitochondrial membranes with deposition of matrix lipoproteins, disruption of the plasma membranes and rupture of lysosomes with release of enzymes. Calcium is thought to play a central role in this final progression to irreversible cell death. In the normal cell, the concentration of calcium is tightly controlled by the calcium pump in the cell membrane. Inside the cell, it binds to two important proteins, troponin and calmodulin. Troponin has a role in muscle contraction and calcium binding to calmodulin is a switch to turn on phosphorylation of important enzyme systems inside the cell. Ischaemia disrupts oxidative phosphorylation, so affecting the energy-dependent calcium pump, leading to a rapid influx of calcium and saturation of the calcium-regulating proteins. High levels of calcium are toxic to the cell, leading to changes in the cytoskeleton, cell surface blebbing, and damage to the mitochondria, the lysosomal membranes and cell membranes. The calcium also binds to phosphates within the cell, leading to a precipitation of hydroxyapatite crystals which can be observed in the mitochondria. The release of enzymes from the ruptured lysosomes also contributes to the final destruction of the cellular components (see Fig. 1.3).

The biochemistry of cell damage and death is a complex process, with many systems interacting. In summary, ischaemia decreases the energy production by the oxidative phosphorylation system in mitochondria, which leads to loss of integrity of the plasma membrane, loss of function of the Na^+/K^+ and Ca^{2+} pumps and severe injury to the mitochondria, nucleus, cytoskeleton and lysosomes. Experimental evidence suggests that calcium has a pivotal role in pushing the cell into irreversible cell damage and death.

CLINICAL RELEVANCE OF THE CELL CHANGES

So much for science. Do these biochemical and microscopical changes help us to understand any of the clinical manifestations of our patient with myocardial infarction, chest pain and cardiac failure? We know that ischaemia leads to a decrease in

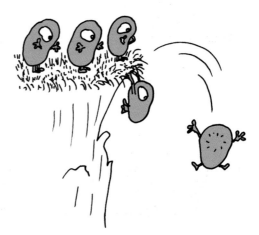

Figure 1.2 Reversible and irreversible changes

![Key facts]

Key facts

Features of reversible and irreversible cell damage

Reversible

Cell swelling
Mitochondrial swelling
Endoplasmic reticulum swelling
Detachment of ribosomes
'Myelin' figures
Loss of microvilli
Surface blebs
Clumping of nuclear chromatin
Lipid deposition

Irreversible

Release of lysosomal enzymes
Protein digestion
Loss of basophilia
Membrane disruption
Leakage of cell enzymes and proteins
Nuclear changes: pyknosis, karyorrhexis, karyolysis

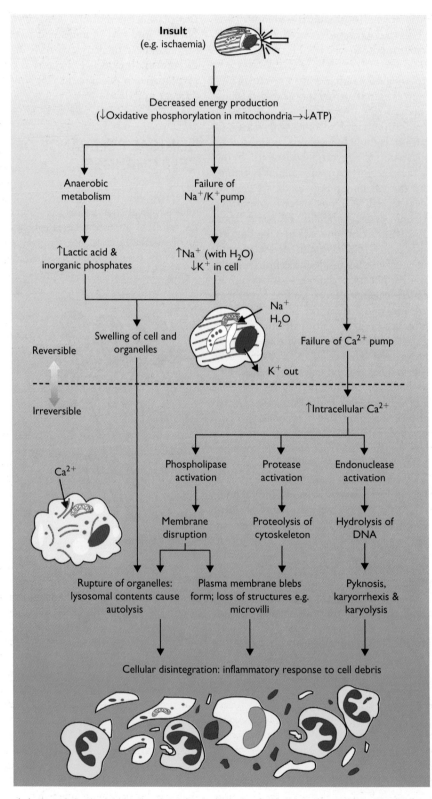

Figure 1.3 Necrosis is the culmination of a series of events, the first phases of which are reversible. The failure of the calcium pump marks the onset of irreversible change

mitochondrial function and, hence, a decrease in ATP formation so that the cells stop contracting. What is absolutely staggering is that an ischaemic episode lasting only one minute can produce this change!

The cellular damage may be reversible but the changes still profoundly affect the function of the organ. If the area of ischaemia is large, enough cells stop contracting to reduce the pumping power of the heart and cause cardiac failure. Any arrhythmia will exacerbate the cardiac failure. You will know that the rhythmic contraction of the heart is due to the passage of electrical impulses down the specialized conduction pathways and within the myocardium. Abnormal conduction can occur if there is damage to the sinoatrial or atrioventricular nodes, the conduction bundles or the myocardium. Conduction of electrical impulses requires an intact cell membrane and functioning ionic channels within the membrane. Ischaemia interferes with membrane and ionic channel function and produces abnormal conduction.

The right coronary artery supplies the atrioventricular node in 85 per cent of people; hence right coronary artery occlusion can produce complete heart block as well as inferior infarction. If the area of ischaemia involves the specialized bundles, the bundles may be selectively affected, resulting in either a right bundle branch block or a left bundle branch block. Occlusion of the left anterior descending artery produces an anterior infarction which may be complicated by blockage of both conduction bundles. This is frequently fatal, not purely because of the conduction problem, but because it is associated with a large area of infarction. Finally, the myocardium itself may affect the passage of impulses. An infarcted area of myocardium may not only slow down or stop the passage of electrical current, but may also generate an arrhythmia.

An ECG is a standard investigation for these patients. It will detect disorders of cardiac rhythm and can give information about the approximate position and size of the infarction. The 12-lead ECG essentially produces a three-dimensional electrical picture of the heart. When part of the myocardium is damaged by ischaemia, the normal path of the electrical wave is impeded and the impulse has to travel via an alternative route. Consequently, the ECG pattern is altered and the type of change on the tracing helps to identify the area and the approximate size of the infarction (Fig. 1.4).

Our patient had elevated levels of cardiac enzymes in the blood. Many enzymes are common to a variety of cells but other enzymes are associated with the cell's specialist functions and will be restricted to only a few cell types. Cardiac muscle cells contain creatine kinase (CK), aspartate aminotransferase (AST) and lactate dehydrogenase (LDH). Ischaemic damage to the myocardial cells disrupts the cell membranes, allowing leakage of these enzymes. If it is suspected that a patient has suffered a myocardial infarction, then serial measurements of these 'cardiac enzymes' can be helpful to confirm the diagnosis and give a rough indication of the size of the damage. In recent years, troponins have been found to be the most sensitive and specific indicators of myocardial infarction.

You can see how knowledge of the cellular events helps us to understand the gross and histological appearances as well as the clinical measurements that are useful in diagnosis and management of the patient. Since mild reversible injury to cells is probably more common than irreversible injury we will examine the histological patterns of reversible sublethal injury before going on to look at types of necrosis.

SUBLETHAL CELL INJURY

The changes of reversible, sublethal injury are often difficult to demonstrate in human tissues. There are two patterns that can be identified in tissues using light microscopy: cloudy swelling and fatty change.

Cloudy swelling

This has already been mentioned when considering myocardial ischaemia. The insult affects membrane ion-exchange mechanisms, altering the ionic gradients and leading to increased intracellular sodium and water. This produces acute cellular oedema or 'cloudy swelling'. At the light microscopic level, this appears as expansion of the cell and a pale granular look to the cytoplasm. Vesicles may also appear due to the distension of the endoplasmic reticulum. This picture of cellular oedema is also referred to as hydropic or vacuolar degeneration. Remember that a whole range of insults may precipitate cellular oedema and that it is not specific to ischaemia. Chemical toxins, infections and radiation can all induce similar changes. Remember also that cellular oedema is reversible.

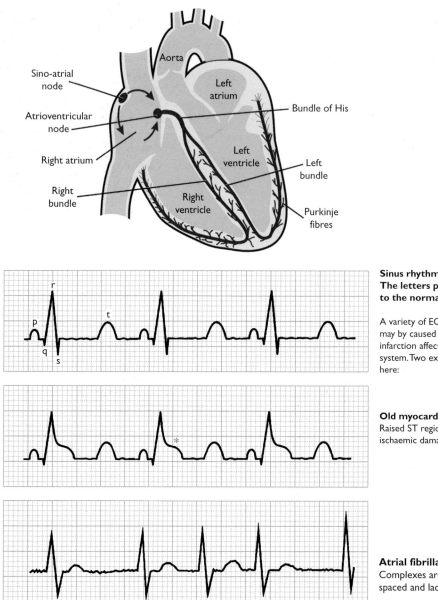

Sinus rhythm (normal)
The letters p q r s t are assigned to the normal waves in the ECG

A variety of ECG changes may by caused by myocardial infarction affecting the conducting system. Two examples are shown here:

Old myocardial infarction
Raised ST region*, indicating ischaemic damage

Atrial fibrillation
Complexes are irregularly spaced and lack 'p' waves

Figure 1.4 Conduction system of the heart and ECG patterns in ischaemic change

Fatty change

This refers to an excess of intracellular lipid which appears as vacuoles of varying size within the cytoplasm. Like cellular oedema, it is entirely reversible and is a non-specific reaction to a variety of insults. Sometimes it is present adjacent to tissues that are more severely damaged or show frank evidence of necrosis. Fatty change can occur in any organ but is most frequent in the liver, which is not surprising since the liver is the major site of lipid metabolism. For this reason, we will use the liver as an example to discuss the pathogenesis of fatty change.

Figure 1.7 illustrates the fate of fatty acids after uptake by the liver and the possible sites at which alteration may lead to an increased accumulation of lipid within the liver cells. Very simply, adipose tissue releases fat as free fatty acids. These enter the

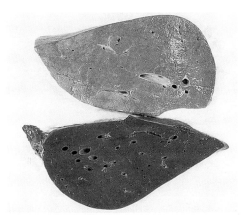

Figure 1.5 Normal and fatty liver (pale)

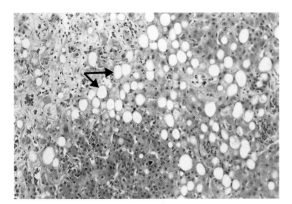

Figure 1.6 Photomicrograph of liver showing fatty change (vacuoles, arrowed)

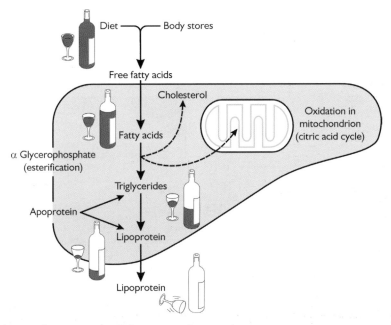

Figure 1.7 Alcohol causes fat to accumulate in hepatocytes for several reasons:
Increase in production of fatty acids:
- Increased release of fatty acids by tissues
- Increased triglyceride synthesis in the liver because of increased smooth endoplasmic reticulum induced by alcohol metabolism

Accumulation of triglyceride in liver:
- Decreased utilization by liver mitochondria
- Decreased protein available for conjugation with fatty acids, thus decreased export of lipoprotein from liver

hepatocytes where they are converted to triglycerides and, to a smaller extent, cholesterol. Triglycerides are complexed with apoproteins to form lipoproteins, which are then secreted into the blood. Changes at any of the illustrated sites will lead to lipid accumulation within the hepatocytes.

This is not just a hypothetical model derived from experimental systems but a common problem in people who abuse alcohol. Alcohol is a hepatotoxin that has wide-ranging effects on fatty acid metabolism. It increases peripheral tissue release of fatty acids so that more is delivered to the liver

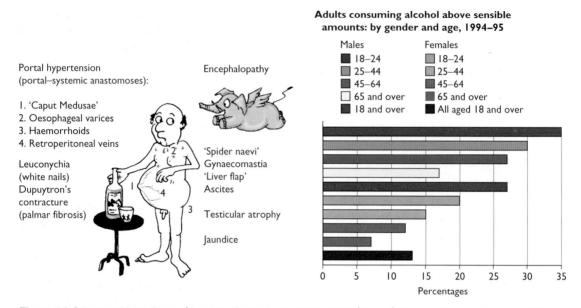

Portal hypertension
(portal–systemic anastomoses):

1. 'Caput Medusae'
2. Oesophageal varices
3. Haemorrhoids
4. Retroperitoneal veins

Leuconychia
(white nails)
Dupuytron's
contracture
(palmar fibrosis)

Encephalopathy

'Spider naevi'
Gynaecomastia
'Liver flap'
Ascites

Testicular atrophy

Jaundice

Figure 1.8 Stigmata of liver disease (data from Social Trends 1994–1995 (Alcohol), General Household Survey, Office for National Statistics, Crown Copyright 1997)

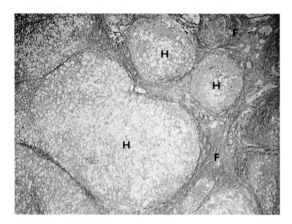

Figure 1.9 Photomicrograph of liver with cirrhosis showing nodules of hepatocytes (H) separated by fibrous bands (F). The hepatocytes are distended with fat

Figure 1.10 Cirrhosis of liver. The irregular nodular pattern is also visible to the naked eye

and, within the liver, it is implicated in increasing fatty acid synthesis, in decreasing the utilization of triglycerides, decreasing fatty acid oxidation and blocking lipoprotein excretion. Thus, it is common for the causative agent to interfere with a variety of biochemical pathways. Malnutrition particularly affects two steps. It increases the release of fatty acids from peripheral tissue and protein deficiency reduces the cell's ability to combine the triglycerides with apoprotein. Carbon tetrachloride also exerts its effect through reducing the availability of apoprotein. Disordered carbohydrate metabolism

in uncontrolled diabetes leads to excessive peripheral release of fatty acids.

Gross examination of the organs affected by fatty change will show that they are enlarged, yellow and tend to be greasy to touch. Microscopically, the characteristic finding is of vacuoles within the cytoplasm. These may begin as small vacuoles but if the fatty accumulation continues, the vacuoles will coalesce to form larger vacuoles or 'fatty cysts'.

To reiterate, this type of change is entirely reversible if the insult is withdrawn. A binge in the medical school bar on a Friday night may produce

Key facts

Causes of fatty change in the liver

- Alcohol
- Protein malnutrition
- Diabetes
- Acute fatty liver of pregnancy
- Congestive cardiac failure
- Ischaemia/anaemia
- Drugs: steroids, methotrexate, intravenous tetracyclins
- Carbon tetrachloride
- Obesity

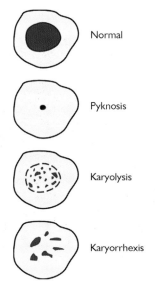

Normal

Pyknosis

Karyolysis

Karyorrhexis

Figure 1.11 Nuclear changes in cell death

fatty change but this will disappear if one is able to abstain for a few days afterwards! Chronic abuse of alcohol may produce sufficient fatty change to interfere with the normal function of the hepatocytes and, in the long term, excessive alcohol consumption will lead to cell death, scarring and cirrhosis, which is not reversible.

There comes a stage at which reversible damage becomes irreversible and cell damage becomes cell death. The cells die or are killed in many ways

(though each cell dies only once!). However in each case the final events follow one of two distinct processes: 'necrosis' or 'apoptosis' (page 21).

NECROSIS

Necrosis is cell death due to lethal injury. Unlike apoptosis, the cell death is not an energy-dependent active process but is a consequence of sudden changes in the microenvironment abolishing cell function. The changes seen in the tissues are a consequence of the denaturation of proteins and the release of digestive enzymes which destroy the tissue.

In general terms, the microscopic changes include eosinophilia (red staining on the haematoxylin and eosin stain) of the cytoplasm, pyknosis and disintegration of the nuclei (karyorrhexis) and, finally, complete dissolution of the nucleus (karyolysis). However, there are different morphological patterns of necrosis under different circumstances. The principal types are:

- coagulative
- colliquative or liquefactive
- caseous.

Coagulative necrosis

If you consider Figs 1.12 and 1.13, you will see that one is a photomicrograph of normal kidney with normal glomeruli and tubules; the other is from a kidney that has suffered an ischaemic insult and is showing coagulative necrosis. Spot the difference?

The second picture is essentially the ghost outline of the first! The difference between the two is that the damaged kidney shows loss of nuclei from the cells and the cytoplasm stains a little darker pink. This pattern of necrosis is the most common type and occurs in many solid organs like the heart and kidney. The necrosis following a myocardial infarction is therefore of the coagulative type. Strange isn't it? Why should the basic architecture and cellular outline be preserved if the cells are dead?

Perhaps the offending injury not only destroys the vital structural proteins within the membrane, cytoplasm and nucleus but also destroys the enzymes within the lysosomes that would otherwise degrade the cellular and extracellular components. The tissue,

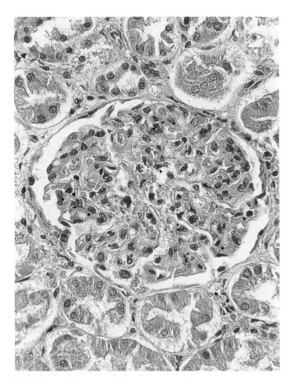

Figure 1.12 Normal kidney

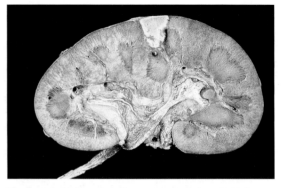

Figure 1.14 Kidney, showing wedge-shaped cortical infarct

of course, does not remain in that state forever. If you remember the example of myocardial infarction, we stated that polymorphs move in within 24 hours of infarction. These inflammatory cells release enzymes that digest the cellular components and the resulting debris will be removed by phagocytic cells such as the macrophages. It should be clear from this that the appearance of an area of coagulative necrosis will change with time.

Colliquative or liquefactive necrosis

The hallmark of this type of necrosis is the release of powerful hydrolytic enzymes that degrade cellular components and extracellular material to produce a proteinaceous soup. Characteristically, it occurs in the brain, where it produces a cystic cavity containing fluid and necrotic debris.

Liquefaction may also be encountered in tissues when there is a superadded bacterial infection. Then, enzymes are released from both the bacteria

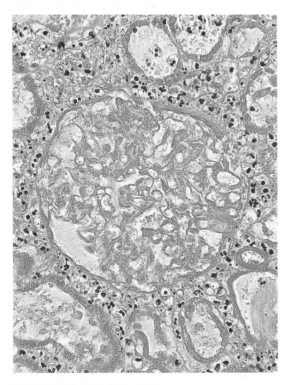

Figure 1.13 Coagulative necrosis

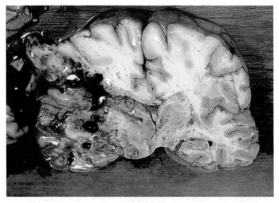

Figure 1.15 Brain with cerebral infarction

and the inflammatory cells that have been recruited to fight the infection.

Caseous necrosis

Caseous necrosis typically occurs in tuberculosis and is so-called because of a resemblance to soft crumbly cheese! The necrotic area is not quite liquid but neither is the outline of the tissue retained as in coagulative necrosis. On microscopic sections stained with haematoxylin and eosin (H&E) (Fig. 1.16), the necrotic area appears homogeneously pink (eosinophilic) with a surrounding inflammatory response involving multinucleate giant cells, macrophages and lymphocytes (see granulomatous inflammation, page 106).

It is believed that lipopolysaccharides in the capsules of the mycobacterium which causes tuberculosis may be responsible for this peculiar reaction but the mechanism is unclear.

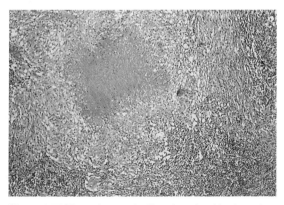

Figure 1.16 Photomicrograph of lymph node with tuberculous granuloma and caseous necrosis

Other types of necrosis

Although these are the main types of necrosis, for completeness, we should briefly mention four others: fat necrosis, gangrene, fibrinoid necrosis and autolysis.

FAT NECROSIS

This type of necrosis is peculiar to fatty tissue and is most commonly encountered in the breast following trauma and within the peritoneal fat due to pancreatitis. Within the breast, trauma may lead to the rupture of adipocytes and release of fatty acids. This will elicit an inflammatory response and the area will become firm due to scarring and forms a palpable lump. Clinically, the lump may be mistaken for a carcinoma and excision and microscopical examination may be required to determine the diagnosis.

In pancreatitis, damage to the pancreatic acini results in the release of proteolytic and lipolytic enzymes, which denature fat cells in the peritoneum and lead to an inflammatory reaction. Calcium is also deposited in the tissues in combination with fatty acids to form calcium soaps. This is a form of dystrophic calcification and we will consider calcification again in the section on tissue response to necrosis.

GANGRENE

This does not represent a distinctive type of necrosis but is a term used in clinical practice to describe black, dead tissue. It is most commonly seen in the lower limb in patients with severe atherosclerosis, which often causes irreversible ischaemic damage to the most peripheral tissues in the body. If the pattern of necrosis is mainly of the coagulative type, it is referred to as dry gangrene, while the presence of infection with Gram-negative bacteria converts it into a liquefactive type of necrosis, called wet gangrene. It will be apparent from the preceding discussion that the type of necrosis encountered depends on a number of factors, including the type of tissue involved and the nature of the offending agent. Gas gangrene is the disastrous complication that follows infection of tissue by the Gram-positive organism *Clostridium welchii*, found in soil. The bacterium releases a toxin and also produces gas, which can be felt as crepitation when the affected area is pressed.

Fibrinoid necrosis or fibrinoid change refers to the microscopical appearance seen when an area loses its normal structure and resembles fibrin. It does not have any distinctive gross appearance and most commonly occurs in arteries.

Autolytic change is completely different from the others as it refers to cell death occurring after the person has died. Obviously, the heart stops pumping and all the tissues become irreversibly ischaemic. Enzymes leaking from the cells digest adjacent structures but there is no inflammatory response because the inflammatory system is dead!

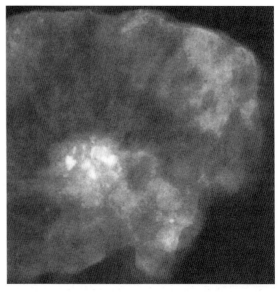

Figure 1.17 X-ray of breast tissue (mammogram) showing a circumscribed abnormality, which is radio-opaque because of dystrophic calcification

Calcification in necrotic tissue

Necrotic tissue may become calcified. When a cell undergoes necrosis, large amounts of calcium enter the cell and this combines with phosphates within the mitochondria to produce hydroxyapatite crystals. Extracellular calcification can also occur, the crystals forming in membrane-bound vesicles derived from degenerating cells. This is the initiation phase. There is then propagation of crystal formation, depending on the local concentration of calcium and phosphate and the amount of collagen present (this enhances calcification). Usually such dystrophic calcification is not a problem to the body, but if it affects an important site, such as heart valves, it may affect function. Dystrophic calcification may be useful, as in the microcalcification observed on mammograms – this can alert the radiologist to an early breast cancer.

Dystrophic should be distinguished from metastatic calcification, which affects normal tissues and occurs when serum calcium levels are high. Causes include hyperparathyroidism (increased parathyroid hormone secretion mobilizes calcium from the bones), or excess vitamin D ingestion (increased calcium absorption from the gut). Metastatic carcinoma within bones may liberate calcium and result in metastatic calcification – the term metastatic referring to the widespread and scattered nature of the lesions encountered rather than inferring a similar mechanism.

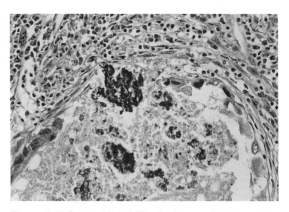

Figure 1.18 Dystrophic calcification in necrotic tumour

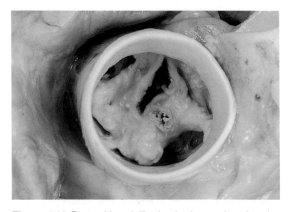

Figure 1.19 Dystrophic calcification in damaged aortic valve, producing stenosis

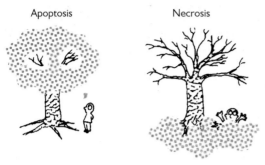

Figure 1.20 The word 'apoptosis' comes from the Greek meaning 'a falling off'.

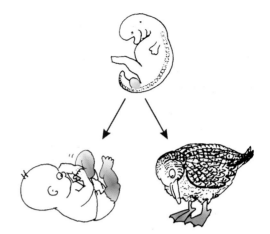

Figure 1.21 Apoptosis at the embryonic stage allows limbs to develop appropriately

APOPTOSIS

The word apoptosis is derived from Greek and was originally used to describe individual leaves falling from a tree. In pathology, apoptosis is a specific type of cell death that involves single cells or small groups of cells in a tissue where the other cells are functioning normally. A similar pattern of cell death is also encountered in plants and invertebrates and is called programmed cell deletion. The term programmed cell death may be more appropriate than apoptosis as it emphasizes that programmed cell death appears to be under physiological and genetic control, whereas cell necrosis is due to injury. Genetic control of death! That is quite a statement to make for it implies that our own genes, selected by the pressures for survival, are also involved in causing cell death! Can death be a necessary part of life? The philosophers and gardeners amongst you will have no difficulty with this concept; after all, a good rose garden requires a certain amount of pruning.

Can cell death be useful?

The importance of programmed cell death is evident from the earliest stages of the embryo through to the involutional changes of the menopause. Let us consider the production of a limb with its five digits. To achieve this, tissue growth has to occur by cell division but it is also necessary to produce interdigital cell death – otherwise you will end up with a duck's foot! This type of cell death is genetically controlled.

Similarly there are the stages of metamorphosis that take place to turn a tadpole into a frog. Metamorphosis requires not only mitotic activity and tissue growth but also a large amount of programmed cell death. When a tadpole turns into a frog, the most obvious change is that limbs are formed and the tail is resorbed. During the process of resorption, there is an increase in thyroxine which appears to lead to the activation of collagenases and, hence, destruction of the tail. Here we have an example of how programmed cell death may depend on the production of a hormone with activation of protein enzyme systems to assist the process.

Hormonal effects on cell death are also important in the maturation of the human reproductive system. The reproductive system has an early indifferent phase when it is neither male nor female. The Wolffian duct will differentiate into the epididymis and vas deferens in the male, while the Müllerian duct forms the uterus and Fallopian tubes in the female. We know from experimental observations that administration of oestrogens at a critical time will feminize the male, while administration of testosterone will masculinize the female. In order for that to happen, there has to be regression of the primitive Wolffian or Müllerian structures and this occurs via programmed cell death.

The development of the nervous system is also dependent on programmed cell death. There is an excess of neurons and only those that produce the correct synaptic connections with their target cells survive. The rest, up to 50 per cent of the neurons, die as a result of apoptosis.

The thymus is large in the fetus and infant but atrophies before adulthood. This involution occurs via cell death which is thought to be steroid sensitive. The steroid hormones are produced in the adrenal gland so that, in this case, one organ is responsible for

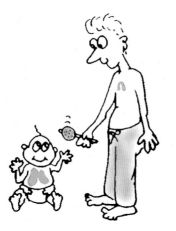

Figure 1.22 The thymus is comparatively large in the infant but atrophies during childhood

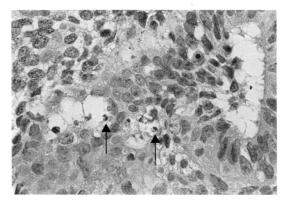

Figure 1.23 Apoptosis in the endometrial glands

the involution of another via its secreted product. This observation is useful in perinatal autopsies for deciding whether the death of a newborn baby is a sudden event or whether it follows several days of problems *in utero*. If the baby has been stressed *in utero*, adrenal steroids will cause premature involution of the thymus so that it is less than half of its normal size. If the baby has been normal *in utero* but has suffered a problem during delivery (e.g. birth asphyxia), then the thymus will be of normal size. There is some recent evidence that this steroid-sensitivity is under the control of a single gene and the same gene may be involved in apoptosis caused by cytotoxic T lymphocytes.

The endometrium is a hormone-dependent tissue that undergoes cyclical changes during the reproductive period as well as involutional changes after the menopause. The oestrogens secreted by the ovary in the early part of the menstrual cycle induce endometrial proliferation and, if pregnancy does not occur, there is programmed cell destruction that results in menstrual shedding. If pregnancy occurs, then there is hyperplasia of the breast in preparation for lactation, which will be followed by physiological atrophy involving apoptosis after weaning. This atrophy is not only due to cell loss but also results from a reduction in cell size and loss of extracellular material. Following the menopause, the withdrawal of the hormonal influence results in involution of the uterus and ovaries.

Apoptosis plays an important role in the immune system. It is necessary for the selection of specific subpopulations of both T and B lymphocytes and is also important in the destruction of target cells by cytotoxic T cells. For example, in a liver infected by hepatitis B virus, a liver biopsy will reveal many individual apoptotic cells and this is due to the immune cells attacking hepatocytes bearing the antigens of hepatitis B. It appears that cytotoxic T cells and natural killer cells are capable of directing a target cell to commence apoptosis, i.e. to commit suicide.

Structural changes in apoptosis

The original term for apoptosis was 'shrinkage necrosis' because apoptotic cells tend to shrink while necrotic cells initially swell. Apoptotic cells lose their contact with neighbouring cells early on. After 1–2 hours the nuclear chromatin condenses on the nuclear membrane and then the membrane 'packages' these small aggregates of nuclear material to give membrane-bound nuclear fragments. The cytoplasm shrinks and the cell's organelles also become parcelled into membrane-bound vesicles. These are called apoptotic bodies and they contain morphologically intact mitochondria, lysosomes, ribosomes, etc. Finally, these apoptotic bodies are phagocytosed by neighbouring cells or by macrophages. Experimental evidence suggests that an apoptotic cell acquires molecules on its surface which allow neighbouring cells and macrophages to identify it as having committed suicide and hence leads to clearing of the fragments.

A crucial feature of apoptosis is that the cell's contents are not allowed to leak into the extracellular space, where enzymes may digest adjacent structures, or proteins may stimulate an immune response. Instead, the cell packages itself into small membrane-bound vesicles, which contain functioning mitochondria and other cell organelles. These survive long enough to be phagocytosed by macrophages which can degrade the components in secondary lysosomes. This mechanism is essential for allowing cell death without secondary inflammation and scarring.

Biochemical changes in apoptosis

The orderly packaging of cells into membrane-bound parcels, visible on light microscopy of apoptotic cells, comes about through a mixture of cleavage and cross-linkage of protein. These parcels are then phagocytosed.

Protein is cleaved by hydrolysis by a series of enzymes called caspases, whose action is mediated by the Bcl-2 family of proteins (Fig. 1.24). DNA is broken down into large pieces by endonucleases. Nuclear fragments, together with cell proteins are wrapped in a lipid membrane, which is then marked 'for disposal' by specific markers, such as phosphatidylserine or thrombospondin. These residues can be recognized by macrophages and adjacent epithelial cells, which are then stimulated to phagocytose them. Thus no messy acute inflammatory process is initiated. However, this process requires the expenditure of energy – as with any good garbage disposal system!

Genetic events in apoptosis

Our knowledge has advanced somewhat since the first genetic events in apoptosis were elucidated by the study of the nematode *Caenorhabitis elegans*. We now know that a variety of initiating events can trigger apoptosis, via a final common pathway of caspase activation, leading to endonuclease-mediated cleavage of nuclear DNA and catabolism of the cytoskeleton. In some instances, such as via the action of cytotoxic T cells, the caspases can be activated more or less directly; there is also a so-called 'death-receptor' on the cell surface (otherwise known as the Fas receptor or CD95), which can stimulate the caspases once activated, for example, by tumour necrosis factor.

Apoptosis can be initiated by cell injury, for instance by radiation, toxins or free radicals. This mechanism is largely brought about by the product of the *p53* gene, which is responsible for checking the integrity of the cell's genome before mitosis occurs. Apoptosis can be initiated if there is an absence of cellular growth factors (a pathway that

is important in embryogenesis). The effects of these last two groups of agents are mediated by the Bcl-2 family of proteins. As with so much that goes on in the body, the Bcl-2 family includes some proteins that promote caspase activation and thus apoptosis and some that inhibit the process. Most prominent in the inhibition stakes is Bcl-2 itself, whereas the chief promoter is Bax. Thus, in the majority of cells that undergo apoptosis the effects are mediated either by Bcl-2 (inhibits apoptosis) or p53 (initiates apoptosis).

To summarize, apoptosis is initiated by a signal, it is regulated by positive and negative influences, it is executed by a final common pathway of caspase activation and the resultant debris is phagocytosed by macrophages and adjacent cells.

Apoptosis and disease

It follows from the previous discussion that a lack of balance in initiating or suppressing apoptosis can lead to problems.

Apoptosis is an important host-defence mechanism against viral infection. When viruses infect cells, they attempt to take over the cell's replication machinery in order to proliferate and spread. Viral antigens are expressed on the host cell membrane and (in concert with CD4$^+$ lymphocytes) CD8$^+$ lymphocytes bind to this and secrete a pore-forming protein called perforin, lysing the affected cell. Alternatively, natural killer (NK) cells recognize the viral antigen and initiate cell lysis. Viruses can sometimes get round this with anti-apoptotic mechanisms, which come into play when breaks occur in DNA strands as the viral genome incorporates itself into the cell's DNA. Many viruses code for proteins that block apoptosis. Examples include the inactivation of *p53* by human papillomavirus type 16 (HPV-16) and Epstein–Barr virus (EBV), which produce molecules that either stimulate Bcl-2 production or block molecules related to the TNF/CD40 pathway.

Excess apoptosis may be seen if the effector mechanisms malfunction, as in the acquired immune deficiency syndrome (AIDS), when infection of T cells by human immunodeficiency virus (HIV) leads to deletion of the CD4$^+$ population of T cells, wreaking havoc in the immune system due to the loss of its most crucial regulatory cell. HIV expresses a protein called gp120, which activates the Fas ligand on CD4$^+$ cells and leads to apoptosis. CD4$^+$ cells are essential for the generation

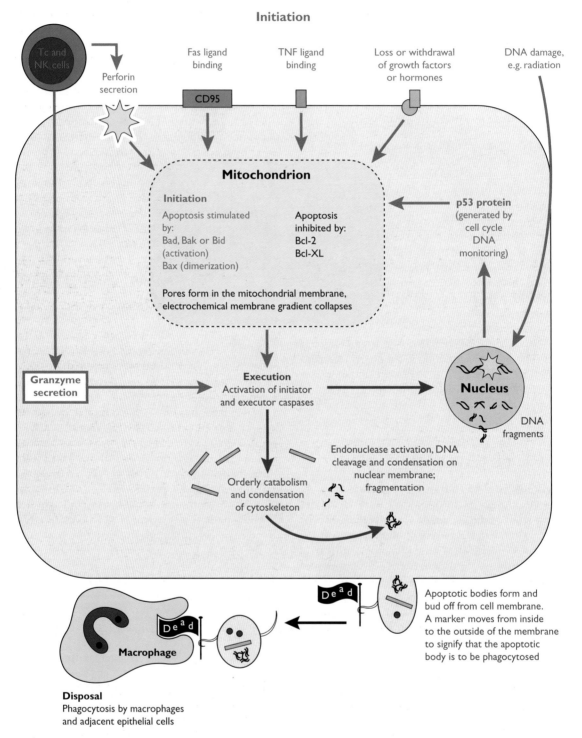

Figure 1.24 Apoptosis is an ordered and energy-requiring process that can be stimulated by diverse agents. Once initiated, the process is irreversible. There is no associated inflammation. It can be thought of in three stages: initiation, execution and disposal

of memory to intercurrent and opportunistic infections.

It has become clear that apoptosis (or the lack of it) has a role in the development of tumours. The inactivation of the cell cycle regulatory genes (which act as 'quality control officers' on the integrity of the DNA) permits mutations to be passed to daughter cells by allowing cell replication to take place; usually such cells would be directed to undergo apoptosis. See page 255 for more information on the role of anti-apoptosis mechanisms in tumour formation.

APOPTOSIS VERSUS NECROSIS

It is clear that apoptosis is the result of the planned, ordered, death of individual cells and is a process requiring energy input from the targeted cell. The packaged, membrane-bound bundles that are produced are quickly tidied away by nearby cells. On the other hand, necrosis is the result of accidental damage of various types, invariably involves groups of cells and usually generates an inflammatory reaction, tissue damage and often scarring.

TREATING DISEASES BY INTERFERING WITH CELL DEATH

The study of cell death and apoptosis has raised important therapeutic issues, none more so than in the field of oncology. It is now generally accepted

that tumour growth is a result of the fine and precarious balance that exists between cell proliferation and cell loss. Tumours that grow fast do so not only by proliferating rapidly but also by keeping cell death to a minimum.

Cancer treatment involves surgery, radiation and chemotherapy. The latter two act by changing the rate of cell proliferation, and are successful in many types of cancer. The first reported cure with radiotherapy was in 1899 on a basal cell carcinoma of the skin. Therapeutic radiation damages cells by generating ions in the tissue, the most common of which are the oxygen free radicals derived from water. These are the same as those involved in bacterial killing in inflammation (page 99). Indirect biochemical damage includes the peroxidation of molecules (especially lipids), interference with oxidative phosphorylation, changes in membrane permeability and the inhibition of some enzymes. All of these produce necrosis and generate a tissue response to the damage, and of course normal as well as tumour cells are affected. In addition, radiation damages DNA (as we shall discuss on pages 236 and 253), producing breaks in the strands. These are normally repaired promptly but there may on occasions be errors in the repair, leading to cell death.

There are numerous chemotherapeutic agents with a variety of modes of action. Alkylating agents (e.g. cyclophosphamide and melphalan) form covalent links with certain molecules, the most important of which is the guanine base in DNA. This leads to breaks in the DNA and faulty transcription. Antimetabolites (e.g. cytarabine and methotrexate) resemble naturally occurring substances but are

Key facts

Differences between necrosis and apoptosis

Necrosis	Apoptosis
Group of cells affected	Single or few cells selected
Caused by injurious agent/event	Programmed death
Reversible events precede irreversible	Irreversible once initiated
Energy deprivation causes changes	Events are energy-driven
Cells swell due to influx of water	Cells shrink as cytoskeleton is disassembled
Haphazard destruction of organelles and nuclear material by enzymes from ruptured lysosomes	Orderly packaging of organelles and nuclear fragments in membrane-bound vesicles
Cellular debris stimulates inflammatory cell response	New molecules expressed on vesicle membranes stimulate phagocytosis; no inflammatory response

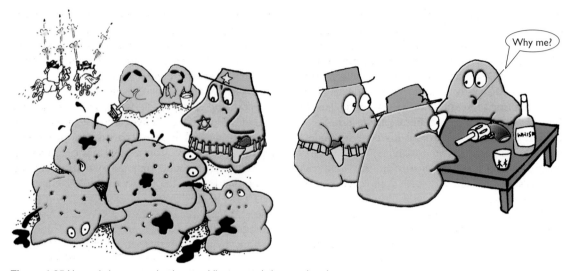

Figure 1.25 Necrosis is a messy business, while apoptosis is an ordered event.

subtly different so that they block an enzyme pathway or damage the macromolecular structure in which they are incorporated. Many are analogues of purine or pyrimidine bases and affect nucleic acid synthesis, while methotrexate interferes with folic acid metabolism, thus blocking DNA and RNA synthesis. Antibiotics useful in chemotherapy (e.g. adriamycin and daunorubicin) often produce a local distortion of the DNA helix that interferes with the function of DNA and RNA polymerases. The vinca alkaloids (e.g. vinblastine) act in a completely different manner and bind to tubulin in the microtubules of the mitotic spindle to block division. The hallmark of both radiotherapy and chemotherapy is that the cell's metabolism becomes irreversibly damaged and the proliferating cell is most likely to perish, i.e. undergo necrosis.

What about apoptosis? Does that have any therapeutic potential? The answer is 'yes'. We are still at an early stage but there is considerable interest in the various cytokines that might be able to promote apoptotic tumour cell death. Cytokines are proteins produced by lymphocytes and macrophages following stimulation and, besides modifying the immune response, they may act directly to cause death of tumour cells.

Tumour necrosis factor (TNF or cachectin) is produced by activated macrophages, and its action on tumour cells takes place via various distinct mechanisms. It has a role in inflammation that alters endothelial cells, promoting thrombosis and thus causing ischaemic cell necrosis in the tumour.

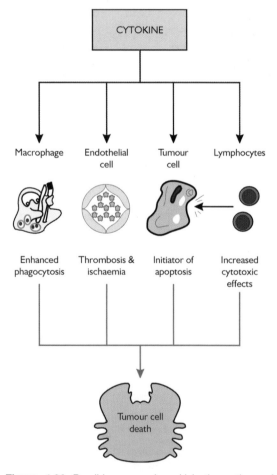

Figure 1.26 Possible means by which the actions of cytokines may inhibit tumour growth

Although the death of cells in a tumour is rather complex, ischaemia playing a major role, there is evidence that at least some of the cells die as a result of attack by lymphocytes. In experimental models, TNF also causes an increase in apoptotic cell death, which appears to be a direct effect as there is an early rise in the synthesis of RNA in the affected cell. We have already mentioned the interaction of the TNF pathway with the Fas receptor. Various interleukins appear to produce tumour cell death secondary to stimulation of cytotoxic T cells and NK cells, which then act on the tumour cells to initiate apoptosis.

Interferons, on the other hand, appear to exert their effects by acting in synergy with the above factors. They have been shown to enhance the cytotoxicity of T lymphocytes and NK cells, and they also increase the phagocytic activities of macrophages on tumour cells. They are known (in combination with TNF) to reduce the rate of tumour cell multiplication.

The study of mediators and mechanisms of cell death has caused tremendous excitement in clinical oncology. With the advent of genetic engineering it is possible to produce the quantities of cytokines necessary for cancer treatment. The initial euphoria was dampened a little when it was discovered that some cytokine treatment is rather toxic, but important advances continue to be made in both the biology and the clinical regimens.

As Lewis Thomas says, cell death is indeed a natural marvel! It seems to be such an integral part of life, yet until recently we paid little attention to it. The study of cell death is assuming an increasingly important role in the understanding of such diverse processes as embryogenesis, infections and neoplasia.

> It is a natural marvel. All of the life on earth dies, all of the time, in the same volume as the new life that dazzles us each morning, each spring. All we see of this is the odd stump, the fly struggling on the porch floor of the summer house in October, the fragment on the highway. I have lived all my life with an embarrassment of squirrels in my backyard, they are all over the place, all year long, and I have never seen, anywhere, a dead squirrel.
>
> *Lewis Thomas, Professor Emeritus, Memorial Sloan-Kettering Cancer Centre (1988)*

CHAPTER 2

What is a cause?

> In the post-mortem room we witness the final result of disease, the failure of the body to solve its problems and there is an obvious limit to what one can learn about normal business transactions from even a daily visit to the bankruptcy court.
>
> *Walter Russell Brain (1895–1966)*

If you look back at page 8, the autopsy report on our patient gave the cause of death as 'myocardial infarction due to coronary artery thrombosis due to coronary artery atheroma'. But what caused the atheroma? Was it diet or smoking or lack of exercise or genes or a combination? In many situations it is a combination of factors and the person's response that determines any symptoms or signs. Thus, we could list a variety of factors that have contributed to this man's heart attack and could call them 'causes'. Just as we have chosen a definition for 'disease', we should choose a definition for 'cause', though remembering that there is no correct answer. Our definition will be 'the cause of a disease is a factor that is clearly associated with the occurrence of the disease and that plays an identifiable role in the initiation of a mechanism(s) that significantly contributes to the manifestation of that disease'. Since multiple mechanisms operate in most diseases, there will be multiple factors involved in causation.

We shall leave the body's response to later sections and concentrate now on a way of classifying the range of causes of diseases. This is inevitably arbitrary but should provide a useful checklist of the broad categories and some specific examples. In simple terms, it is 'intrinsic' versus 'extrinsic'; that is, which factors are personal to the individual and which are acquired from the environment? A classification of the extrinsic agents is fairly straightforward because we are used to listing them under particular headings (Table 2.1). The 'intrinsic' factors are less simple because our ideas have changed enormously over the last decade as the human genome has been

sequenced. It is tempting now to imagine that every 'intrinsic' factor could be listed under the category of genetic, just as every idea in this book is composed of letters clustered as words and arranged in sentences. However, a book would not be defined as a collection of letters. The science of gene expression and the steps between genotype and phenotype have some gaps left so we shall subdivide the intrinsic factors into genetic, metabolic, cellular and structural. The intrinsic ones will include mechanisms that involve an abnormal response to an extrinsic agent, e.g. the abnormal lymphocyte response in a hypersensitivity reaction is an 'intrinsic cellular' cause that also involves an external factor.

Let us consider the possible mechanisms involved in these varied causes of cell injury and death, bearing in mind that it is not always possible to define the exact site of action of the initial insult. Since the cell membrane, oxidative phosphorylation and DNA are vital to the cell, it is very likely that these will be involved. You will also recall from our earlier consideration of a patient with a myocardial infarct that the final outcome is dependent on the severity and duration of the insult and the metabolic demands of the tissues at the time of the insult.

Some physical and chemical agents are well known for causing cell death. We are all aware of the devastating effects of dropping an atomic bomb and the mass destruction caused by chemical warfare. Radiation and chemicals produce cell death by the production of oxygen free radicals, which interfere with DNA structure and replication, resulting in mutations. The effects of these changes may be immediate, or can be subtle, manifesting many years

Table 2.1 Classification of extrinsic and intrinsic factors in disease

Category	Agent	Disease example
Extrinsic factors		
Physical	Trauma	Bone fracture
	Radiation	Cancer
	Temperature extremes	Frostbite/electric burn
	Environmental hazards	Drowning
Chemical	Toxic substances	Tobacco lung damage
	Inflammatory substances	Asthma
Biological	Bacteria	Various infections
	Virus	AIDS
	Fungi and parasites	Athlete's foot
	Prions	Creutzfeldt–Jakob disease
Nutritional	Various	Malnutrition and some cancers
Intrinsic factors		
Genetic		Sickle cell disease
		Cystic fibrosis
Metabolic		Diabetes
		Gluten-induced enteropathy
		Gallstones
Cellular		Autoimmune, e.g. rheumatoid arthritis
		Degenerative and ageing, e.g. Alzheimer's disease
Structural		Congenital, e.g. spina bifida
		Acquired, e.g. atheroma, biliary tract obstruction, osteoarthritis

after the initiating event. Temperature is another important factor. Heat applied to the skin in low doses may induce a coagulative type of necrosis, but with intense heat the tissue may simply vaporize! Those interested in Arctic exploration will be aware of the gangrene induced by extreme cold which is due to a combination of thrombosis in small vessels and ice crystal formation in tissues (frostbite). Water, that substance on which all life depends, can be lethal. Drowning is easily understood, but what is less well appreciated is that problems with water excretion in a patient with malfunctioning kidneys can be life threatening.

CLINICAL CASE – FROSTBITE

A 29-year-old skier lost his way after drinking a few beers in a mountain restaurant. He was discovered, unconscious, 20 hours later in an exposed location on the mountain face. He had obvious frostbite to his nose and fingertips, manifest as hard white areas. A weak, thready, but regular pulse was present and he was breathing shallowly. He was wrapped in a space blanket and rushed by helicopter to hospital. His rectal (core) temperature was found to be 30°C. He was warmed with blankets and hot water bottles. He suffered a cardiac arrest but was immediately resuscitated. His mild metabolic acidosis was corrected. As he regained consciousness he began to shiver violently and his limbs became reddened and swollen. He tried to raise himself up but promptly fainted. Over the next couple of days his fingertips and nose turned black and the skin began to slough off. At one point it appeared that he would lose the tips of most of his fingers, but after the skin had fallen off only two fingertips were lost and his nose was saved.

What has happened here?

Our patient was hypothermic, i.e. his core temperature was less than 35°C (normal temperature 37°C). The onset of hypothermia is dependent on many factors, including body build, ambient temperature, whether the individual is dry or wet, the presence of protective clothing, whether or not alcohol has been ingested (even small amounts can greatly increase the risk of hypothermia). Alcohol plus exercise is probably the worst combination, since not only is blood glucose depleted by exercise but the alcohol interferes with the generation of new glucose from body stores by reducing the amount of pyruvate available. Hypothermia is characterized by listlessness and confusion. Unconsciousness supervenes at temperatures from 26 to 33°C.

How does the body respond to cold?

Initially the heat gain centre in the hypothalamus directs the body to shiver violently and shut down peripheral blood vessels by vasoconstriction, but if this fails to restore core temperature the cooling of the heart interferes with cardiac output. Below 26°C the cardiac output is too low to sustain life. Oxygen combines more strongly with haemoglobin at low temperatures, further depleting tissues of oxygen. Anoxic effects on the heart include arrhythmias. A patient whose body temperature is below 30°C is at risk of cardiac arrest and should be monitored by ECG. Respiration is diminished, usually in proportion with tissue requirements but slight CO_2 retention may cause a respiratory acidosis, compounded by the metabolic acidosis which occurs when lactic acid accumulates as a result of shivering.

Why did the patient faint as he began to recover?

In the hypothermic patient blood volume falls due to a combination of a 'cold diuresis', which occurs in response to a drop in core temperature, and damage to renal tubular epithelium due to cold, preventing sodium reabsorption; this causes a drop in plasma osmolality and water moves out of the vascular compartment into the tissues to balance this (see page 92 and Fig. 4.8). When the patient is warmed and vasodilation occurs the blood volume is insufficient for demand and there is hypotension.

What is frostbite?

Frostbite is the result of freezing of tissues, which occurs at temperatures below −0.54°C. Before

freezing, cooling to less than 12°C causes paralysis of muscles and nerves by interference with the membrane sodium pump. A lack of sodium ions renders nerves and muscles inexcitable. Damage is reversible after a few hours, but not if left longer. If the tissue freezes, the tissue proteins become denatured and the cell dies. Vascular endothelial cells are particularly susceptible. When they thaw, plasma leaks out of the small vessels through the damaged endothelium and the retained red blood cells sludge, obstructing the lumen and causing local infarction of tissue. Although it is dangerous to warm the body of a hypothermic person too quickly, if a patient is suffering only from frostbite it is best to warm the affected area as quickly as possible, so that sludging and infarction is reduced to a minimum due to quick restoration of blood flow. Although damage may seem extensive, the actual area of necrosis may be less than it first appears and it is worth waiting for a few days before amputation of an affected area. The process is painful and requires analgesic support, plus elevation of the affected area to reduce tissue swelling.

Let us discuss in more detail three groups of causes: one extrinsic, one intrinsic and one that is a combination of the two. We shall consider biological agents as an extrinsic cause, genetic causes as intrinsic, and hypersensitivity reactions as an abnormal intrinsic cellular reaction to an external agent.

BIOLOGICAL AGENTS AS CAUSES OF DISEASES

This is an enormous topic and could fill many books. Although we would only like to cover some common mechanisms, some short lists of microbes and their relevant diseases are included. Two common mechanisms are toxin production (endotoxin and exotoxins) and direct cell damage.

Toxin production by bacteria

Refer to Table 2.2 and Fig. 2.1.

Bacterial endotoxin

Endotoxin is a cell wall component that is shed when a bacterium dies. It is not secreted by living bacteria. The component that causes the toxicity,

Table 2.2 Simple summary of the ways of classifying bacteria

	Gram-positive	Gram-negative	Acid fast
Examples of aerobic and anaerobic bacteria			
Obligate aerobes	*Bacillus cereus*	*Neisseria*	Mycobacteria
Facultative anaerobes	*Bacillus anthracis*	*E. coli*	
	Staphylococcus	*Salmonella*	
Microaerophilic bacteria	*Streptococcus*	Spirochaetes	
Obligate anaerobes	*Clostridia*	Bacteroides	

	Gram-positive	Gram-negative
Examples of morphologically distinct Gram-positive and Gram-negative bacteria		
Cocci (spherical)	Streptococci (in chains)	*Neisseria*
	Staphylococci (in clusters)	
Bacilli (rod-shaped)	*Corynebacteria*	*Haemophilus*
	Clostridia	*Bordetella*
	Bacillus	*Klebsiella, Proteus, Shigella,*
		E. coli,
	Listeria	*Vibrio, Salmonella*
Spiral		*Treponema, Borrelia,*
		Leptospira (spirochaetes).
		Helicobacter, Campylobacter
Pleomorphic		*Chlamydia, Rickettsia*
		(intracellular obligates)
Branching	*Actinomyces, Nocardia*	

lipid A, is part of the lipopolysaccharide (LPS) in the outer cell wall of Gram-negative bacteria. It causes fever and macrophage and B cell activation by inducing host cytokines. Only Gram-negative bacteria have this endotoxin, with the one exception of the Gram-positive *Listeria monocytogenes*.

Endotoxin is a potent stimulator of a wide range of immune responses. To the immune system, the recognition of LPS spells danger and warrants an immediate and dramatic response, which is often detrimental to the host itself. Clinically, this manifests as fever and vascular collapse or shock. Macrophages are stimulated by LPS to produce tumour necrosis factor (TNF) and interleukin 1 (IL-1), which have many effects including direct activity on the hypothalamus to produce fever (page 103 and Fig. 4.19). LPS also stimulates, directly or indirectly, the complement and clotting pathways and platelets to produce DIC (disseminated intravascular coagulation), thrombosis and shock (pages 163 and 186). Shock results from increased vascular permeability produced by mediators from mast cells and platelets, combined with TNF and LPS affecting

endothelial cells. LPS also stimulates the liver to produce acute phase proteins (page 104) and hypoglycaemia. In Gram-positive organisms, lipotechoic acid within the bacterial wall causes problems similar to LPS in Gram-negative bacteria.

Bacterial exotoxins

Exotoxins are proteins released by living bacteria and there are a wide variety with different actions. Neurotoxins act on nerves or end plates to produce paralysis, cytotoxins damage a variety of cells, tissue-invasive toxins are often enzymes capable of digesting host tissues and pyrogenic toxins stimulate cytokine release and cause rashes, fever and toxic shock syndrome. A very important group are the enterotoxins that act on the gastrointestinal tract to produce diarrhoea by inhibiting salt absorption, stimulating salt excretion or killing intestinal cells. There are two broad categories: infectious diarrhoea and food poisoning with preformed toxin. In infectious diarrhoea, the bacteria proliferate in

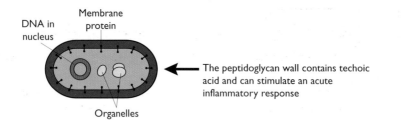

DNA in nucleus

Membrane protein

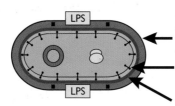

Organelles

The peptidoglycan wall contains techoic acid and can stimulate an acute inflammatory response

Gram-positive bacteria stain blue with cresyl violet, which lodges in their thick outer wall. Inside they have a double-layered phospholipid membrane, with membrane proteins, surrounding cytoplasm with organelles and a circular nucleus composed of double-stranded DNA

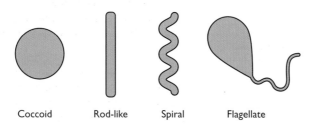

LPS

LPS

Outer coat contains lipopolysaccharide (LPS), a component of which causes endotoxic shock, fever and diarrhoea. Porin protein ■ allows nutrient transfer

Periplasmic space contains enzymes and proteins in a gel

Thin peptidoglycan coat

Gram-negative bacteria have an extra, double-layered coat that traps cresyl violet before it can reach the peptidoglycan coat (which is thinner than in G+ bacteria). The violet crystals are washed out by alcohol as part of the Gram staining process and the bacterium is visualized using a red counter-stain

Bacterial shapes

Coccoid   Rod-like   Spiral   Flagellate

Figure 2.1 Gram-positive and Gram-negative bacteria

the gut, continuously releasing enterotoxin. The symptoms do not occur immediately after ingestion but require a day or two for the bugs to become established in sufficient numbers. In food poisoning, the bacteria grow in the food, releasing their exotoxin. This acts very quickly after ingestion to produce diarrhoea, abdominal pain and vomiting, but the symptoms only last for 24 hours because no new toxin is created.

Bacterial exotoxins may be classified according to their site of action:

- Those that act at extracellular sites, e.g. epidermolytic toxin *Staphylococcus aureus*, which causes scalded skin syndrome.

- Those that have activity at cell membrane level (not transported into cell, but causes changes in intracellular cGMP), e.g. *E. coli* heat-stable enterotoxin (ST) responsible for travellers' diarrhoea and *Staphylococcus aureus* TSST 1 toxin which causes toxic shock syndrome.

- Those that act on the cell membrane, causing pore formation or disruption of lipid by enzymic activity, e.g. phospholipase C activity toxin of *Clostridium perfringens* and pore-forming toxins (thiol-activating haemolysins), such as streptolysin (*Streptococcus pyogenes*), pneumolysin (*Streptococcus pneumoniae*), listeriolysin (*Listeria monocytogenes*), perfringolysin (*Clostridium perfringens*; gas

Table 2.3 Main sources and effects of bacterial toxins

Toxin	Bacteria	Effect
Endotoxin	Gram-negative lipopolysaccharide	Fever and inflammatory cell stimulation
Exotoxins		
Neurotoxins	*Clostridium tetani*	Disordered neuromuscular transmission
	Clostridium botulinum	(tetanus & botulism)
Enterotoxins (infectious diarrhoea)	*Vibrio cholera, Escherichia coli, Bacillus cereus*	Diarrhoea
Enterotoxins (food poisoning)	*Staphylococcus aureus* *Bacillus cereus*	Diarrhoea and vomiting
Tissue-invasive toxins	*Staphylococcus aureus* *Streptococcus pyogenes* *Clostridium perfringens*	Tissue destruction by enzymes
Pyrogenic toxins	*Staphylococcus aureus* *Streptococcus pyogenes*	Toxic shock syndrome Scarlet fever
Verotoxins	*Escherichia coli* (O157:H7)	Haemolytic uraemic syndrome
Miscellaneous	*Bordetella pertussis* *Corynebacteria diphtheria* *Clostridium difficile*	Whooping cough Diphtheria (heart & nerve damage) Pseudomembranous colitis

gangrene) and cerolysin (*Bacillus cereus*; food poisoning).

- Type III toxins that act intracellularly by translocating an enzymic component across the membrane (A subunit of domain) that modifies an acceptor molecule in the cytoplasm. These can be grouped by the type of enzymic activity:
  - ADP-ribosylation (cholera, diphtheria, pertussis)
  - N-glycosidases (shiga toxin)
  - glucosyl transferases (*C. difficile* toxin A and B)
  - Zn^{2+}-requiring endopeptidases (tetanus and botulism toxins).

GTP-binding proteins are often the target for ADP-ribosylation by type III bacterial exotoxins. These proteins are involved in signal transduction and regulation of cellular function either by cAMP levels or kinase cascades leading to transcription modification: For example:

- G proteins (stimulatory or inhibitory of adenyl cyclase) – targeted by cholera, pertussis, *E. coli* LT toxin
- elongation factor 2 (translational control) – affected by diphtheria toxin

- Rho proteins (small G proteins that regulate actin cytoskeleton) – inactivated by *C. difficile* A and B toxins and can also be activated by deamination by pertussis-necrotizing toxin.

In structure, these toxins consist either of A:B5, i.e. one A (enzyme active) subunit and five B (binding) subunits, or A:B type with A and B domains on a single polypeptide chain. A:B5 types are seen in cholera and pertussis (whooping cough), *E. coli* LT1 and LT2. A:B types are encountered in diphtheria, botulism and tetanus.

It is fascinating to compare the contrasting actions between two structurally similar neurotoxins produced by members of the same bacterial family: *Clostridium tetani* and *C. botulinum*, which cause tetanus and botulism respectively. These diseases are caused purely by toxin-mediated action following infection and are quite different in pathology, yet the molecular action of the two toxins is identical. They are both endopeptidases specific for synaptobrevin, a protein found in the cytoplasm of synaptic vesicles. However, the binding (B) domains of the toxins show different specificities for cell receptors. Tetanus toxin binds to the gangliosides of the neuronal membrane, is internalized and moves by retroaxonal transport

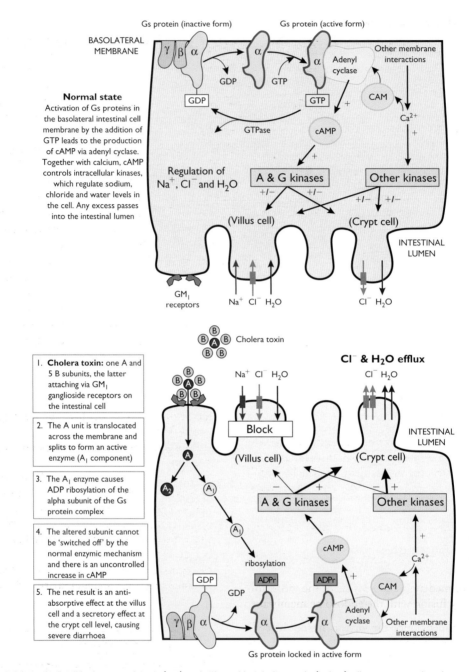

Figure 2.2 Intestinal cell in the normal state (top) and affected by cholera toxin (below); diagrams are mirror images with intestinal lumen in the middle. Na⁺ and Cl⁻ absorption by the villus cells is blocked by cholera toxin, but the main effect is on the crypt cells, where Cl⁻ secretion is stimulated. Water passively follows the active ion transport. Although the main Na⁺ absorption path (Na⁺/H⁺ exchange) is blocked by cholera toxin, Na⁺ can be co-transported with glucose or amino acids, which is why oral rehydration solutions using glucose are effective in cholera

from peripheral nerves to the CNS, where it is released from the postsynaptic dendrites and localizes in presynaptic nerve terminals. This blocks the release of the inhibitory neurotransmitter γ-aminobutyric acid, resulting in unopposed, continuous excitatory synaptic activity, and leading to spastic paralysis. Botulism toxin, on the other hand, binds ganglioside receptors of cholinergic synapses and prevents release of acetylcholine at the neuromuscular junctions, causing flaccid paralysis.

Table 2.4 Outline classification of viruses

Nucleic acid	Symmetry	Envelope	Strand	Family	Example
RNA	Icosahedral	No	SS+	Picorna	Polio, coxsackie
			DS	Reo	Rotavirus
		Yes	SS+	Toga	Rubella (rubivirus)
				Flavi	Yellow fever
	Helical	Yes	SS+	Corona	Colds
			SS−	Orthomyxo	Influenza A, B and C
				Paramyxo	Mumps, measles
				Rhabdo	Rabies
	Complex	Complex	SS+	Retro	HIV, HTLV
DNA	Icosahedral	No	SS linear	Parvo	Aplastic anaemia
			DS circular	Papova	Papillomavirus
			DS linear	Adeno	Colds
		Yes	DS linear	Herpes	Herpes simplex
					Varicella zoster
					Cytomegalovirus
					Epstein–Barr virus
			DS circular	Hepadna	Hepatitis B
	Complex	Complex	DS linear	Pox	Smallpox

SS = single strand; DS = double strand.

Direct cell damage by viruses

Microorganisms can also damage cells directly and this is particularly true of viruses. Viruses are obligate intracellular organisms requiring the host cell's machinery for replication. They use three main methods for entering cells:

- translocation of the entire virus through the cell membrane
- fusion of the viral envelope with the cell membrane
- receptor-mediated endocytosis of the virus, followed by fusion with the endosome membrane.

What happens once the virus is inside the cell? First the particle must uncoat and separate its genome from its structural components. It then uses specific enzymes of its own or present in the host cell to synthesize viral genome, enzyme and capsid proteins. These must be assembled and released, either directly (unencapsulated viruses) or by budding through the host cell's membrane (encapsulated viruses) (Fig. 2.4).

Viruses can damage the host cell directly in a variety of ways:

- through interference with host cell synthesis of DNA, RNA or proteins (e.g. polio virus modifies ribosomes so that they no longer recognize host mRNA)
- via lysis of host cells (e.g. poliovirus lyses neurons)
- by inserting proteins into host cell membrane so provoking an immune attack by host cytotoxic lymphocytes (e.g. hepatitis B and liver cells)
- by inserting proteins into host cell membrane to cause direct damage or promote cell fusion (e.g. herpes, measles, HIV)
- by transforming host cells into malignant tumours (e.g. EBV, papillomavirus, HTLV-1).

Dictionary box

Viral infection can be:

- **Persistent: Virions synthesized continuously, e.g. hepatitis B**

- **Latent: Virions temporarily inactive, e.g. herpes zoster in dorsal root ganglia**

- **Abortive: Incomplete viral replication**

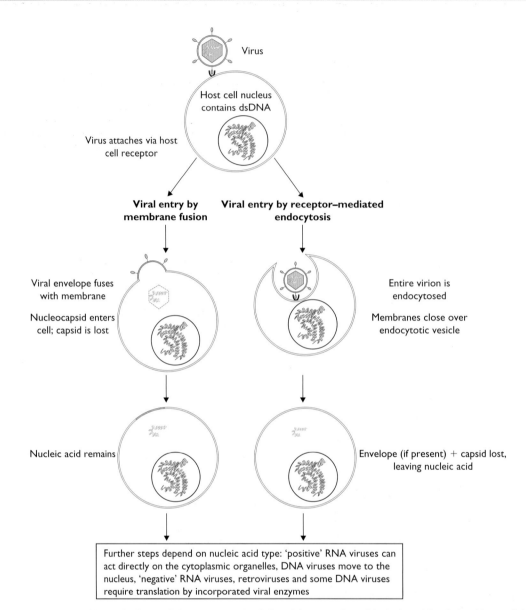

Figure 2.3 After attaching to the host cell via a receptor, the viral particle enters the cell by fusion of the viral and host cell membranes or by receptor-mediated endocytosis. It then uncoats and releases its nucleic acid. Replication occurs either in the cytoplasm alone, as with most RNA viruses and rare DNA viruses (the pox viruses), or involves both cytoplasmic and nuclear steps. DNA viruses can integrate directly with the host DNA but the only RNA viruses that can achieve nuclear integration are the retroviruses

Alternatively, the host cell may suffer secondary damage due to viral infection. This may be due to:

- increased susceptibility to infection due to damaged host defences (e.g. influenza viral damage to respiratory epithelium facilitates bacterial pneumonia with *Staphylococcus aureus*, HIV depletes CD4$^+$ T cells, allowing opportunistic infections such as *Pneuomocystis carinii* pneumonia)

- death or atrophy of cells dependent on the viral-damaged cell (e.g. muscle cell atrophy after motor neuron damage by polio virus).

Although the majority of infectious diseases are caused by bacteria and viruses, there are other organisms that are just as important, and many of these have evolved their own mechanisms for bypassing host defences and causing disease. Briefly,

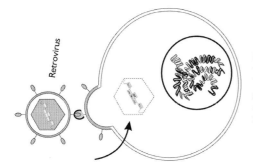

Retrovirus binds to a human surface receptor (e.g. HIV-1 virus binds using its gp120 antigen to human CD4 on T lymphocytes). The viral RNA contains the following genes: *pol* (encodes reverse transcriptase and integrase), *gag* (encodes viral structural proteins), *env* (encodes envelope proteins, including gp120), *reg* (encodes regulatory genes, e.g. *tat*, *rev*)

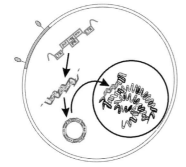

The viral and host cell membranes fuse, the viral capsid disintegrates and viral RNA enters the human cell. Viral reverse transcriptase catalyses the production of double-stranded DNA, which enters the host cell nucleus and integrates into host DNA under the influence of integrase

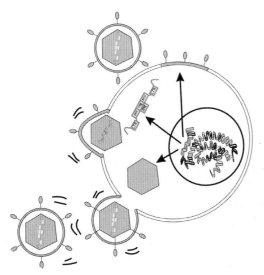

The host cell is induced to manufacture and assemble new virions by long terminal repeat sequences and genes *tat* and *rev*. The new virions peel off an envelope of host cell membrane as they exit

Figure 2.4 Retroviruses, like DNA viruses, can insert their genes into the host cell DNA, but require an additional step. Their RNA is translated into DNA by reverse transcriptase, supplied by the virus

these are the protozoa, helminths, fungi, parasites and prion proteins.

Protozoa

Protozoa are free-living, single-celled eucaryotes with nuclei, endoplasmic reticula, mitochondria and organelles. They ingest nutrients through a cytosome and can reproduce sexually and asexually. Most are able to form cysts when in hostile environments.

Helminths

Helminths or worms can usually be seen by the naked eye. They may be round (nematodes) or flat (platyhelminths).

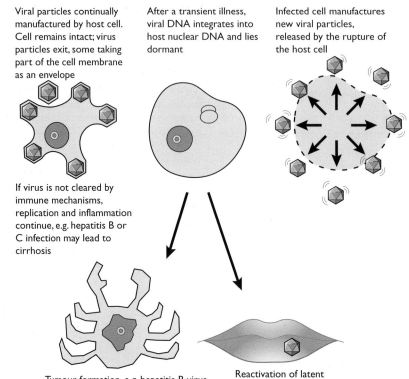

Viral particles continually manufactured by host cell. Cell remains intact; virus particles exit, some taking part of the cell membrane as an envelope

After a transient illness, viral DNA integrates into host nuclear DNA and lies dormant

Infected cell manufactures new viral particles, released by the rupture of the host cell

If virus is not cleared by immune mechanisms, replication and inflammation continue, e.g. hepatitis B or C infection may lead to cirrhosis

Tumour formation, e.g. hepatitis B virus (hepatocellular carcinoma), Epstein–Barr virus (Burkett's lymphoma, nasopharyngeal carcinoma, Hodgkin's lymphoma)

Reactivation of latent infection in a debilitated or immunosuppressed patient, e.g. herpes simplex (cold sore, genital ulcer), varicella zoster (shingles)

Figure 2.5 Possible outcomes in human cells infected by virus

Table 2.5 Examples of protozoa that cause human disease

Organism	Disease
Toxoplasma gondii*†	Cerebral, ocular, lymphoid and lung damage
Plasmodium (*falciparum, vivax, ovale* and *malariae*)	Malaria
Leishmania (various)	Cutaneous and visceral leishmaniasis
Trypanosoma (various)	Sleeping sickness and Chagas' disease
Pneumocystis carinii*†	Interstitial pneumonia
Entamoeba histolytica	Diarrhoea
Giardia lamblia	
Cryptosporidia*	
Isospora*	
Acanthamoeba*	Amoebic meningitis
Naegleri fowleri	
Trichomonas	Vaginal discharge

*People with defective immune systems are more liable to have significant problems with these organisms.
†Problems often relate to reactivation because the immune defences are reduced rather than there being a primary infection.

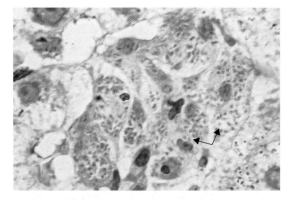

Figure 2.6 Leishmania, a parasitic flagellate protozoan (arrows)

Fungi

Fungi are eucaryotic cells requiring an aerobic environment. Athlete's foot is a common, but seldom

Table 2.6 Examples of helminths that cause human disease

Helminth	Disease
Platyhelminths	
Schistosoma (various)	Schistosomiasis (liver, lung, gut and bladder damage)
Echinococcus	Hydatid disease
Taenia solium, Taenia saginata and Diphyllobothrium latum	Tapeworm infestation from pig, cow and fish
Nematodes	
Necator, Trichuris	Hookworm, whipworm (gut infestation)
Wucheria, Onchocerca	Elephantiasis, river blindness, filariasis

Table 2.7 Examples of fungi that cause human disease

Fungus	Disease
Microsporum, Trichophyton (dermatophytes)	Ring worm, athlete's foot, etc.
Histoplasma capsulatum	Pneumonia or disseminated disease
Aspergillus (various)	Pneumonia or disseminated disease
Candida Cryptococcus Coccidioides	Disseminated disease in immuno-suppressed individuals

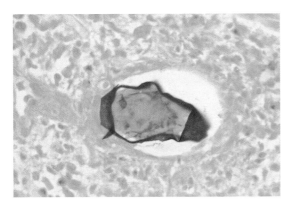

Figure 2.7 Schistosome, one of the platyhelminths

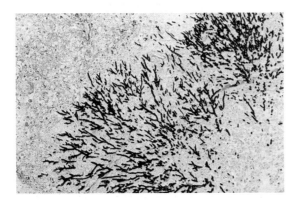

Figure 2.8 Aspergillus

life-threatening, fungal infection. Most fungal infection is relatively rare unless a person is immunosuppressed.

Subcellular infectious agents

This is a short section, but we should flag up our ignorance concerning certain diseases and some 'infectious' particles. There is great interest at present in transmissible spongiform encephalopathies, which can produce progressive and fatal brain damage in humans (kuru), sheep (scrapie) and cows (bovine spongiform encephalopathy (BSE) or 'mad cow' disease). These diseases are experimentally and naturally transmissible, but no viruses or bacteria are detectable. Prion proteins have been proposed as the cause. These are naturally occurring proteins in most mammals that may be induced to change shape, either spontaneously (as in sporadic Creutzfeldt–Jakob disease (CJD)) or if a mutant or foreign prion protein enters the cell (e.g. new variant CJD, thought to be the human equivalent of BSE, and caught from infected cattle). It is still speculation, but the suggestion is that 'infected' animals have abnormally folded proteins in nerve cell membranes. These lead to cell death and the release of prions, which then enter adjacent cells. It appears that strains can vary in virulence. This all sounds similar to viruses but the particle is protein without any evidence of nucleic acid.

HYPERSENSITIVITY AND AUTOIMMUNE DISEASES

The phenomenon of damage caused by the immune system while trying to combat an insult is referred to as hypersensitivity. As a cause, it is partially 'intrinsic' and partially 'extrinsic'. The precipitating factor may be an external agent but, instead of the immune system coping and restoring the body's homeostasis, the immune response is altered and becomes the 'internal' cause of the disease.

Four main types of hypersensitivity reaction have been described by Gell and Coombs, although several types may operate together:

- Type I (anaphylactic) hypersensitivity – release of allergic mediators
- Type II (antibody-dependent cytotoxic) hypersensitivity – binding of self-reactive antibodies to cells
- Type III (immune complex-mediated) hypersensitivity – damage to blood vessel walls and tissues by circulating immune complexes
- Type IV (cell-mediated) hypersensitivity – delayed tissue damage due to interactions between sensitized T lymphocytes and other inflammatory cells.

Type I: Anaphylactic hypersensitivity

This is the mechanism behind atopic allergies such as asthma, eczema, hay fever and reactions to certain food. After initial exposure to the allergen, such as grass pollen, house dust mite faeces or seafoods, the body produces IgE antibodies against it. These antibodies attach to mast cells via cell surface receptors. The next time the affected person is exposed to the allergen the reaction is immediate. The allergen binds to IgE on the surface of mast cells in the mucosa of the bronchial tree, nose, gut or conjunctivae, leading to release of chemical mediators. Some mediators, such as histamine, are already formed within mast cell granules and the cross-linking of IgE molecules attached to the mast cell surface stimulates the release of the granule contents into the tissues. This is why the effect of antigen exposure can be seen within 5 minutes – the granule contents elicit an inflammatory response which lasts up to an hour. In the meantime, the cross-linked IgE molecules stimulate the membrane of the mast cell to generate arachidonic acid and its metabolites within its

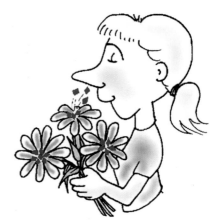

First exposure: nasal and bronchial mucosa exposed to pollen

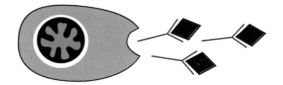

Soluble pollen antigen stimulates production of IgE antibodies

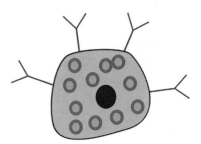

Fc component of IgE attaches to receptor on mucosal mast cell

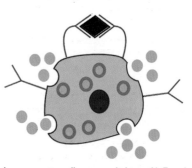

Second exposure to pollen: cross-linking of IgE molecules on mast cell stimulates release of primary and secondary inflammatory mediators

Figure 2.9 Type I hypersensitivity

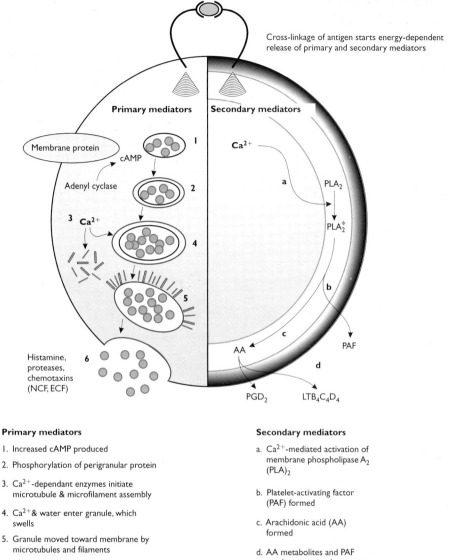

Primary mediators

1. Increased cAMP produced

2. Phosphorylation of perigranular protein

3. Ca^{2+}-dependant enzymes initiate microtubule & microfilament assembly

4. Ca^{2+} & water enter granule, which swells

5. Granule moved toward membrane by microtubules and filaments

6. Discharge of pre-formed mediators invokes inflammatory response in 5–30 min, lasting approximately 1 hour

Secondary mediators

a. Ca^{2+}-mediated activation of membrane phospholipase A_2 $(PLA)_2$

b. Platelet-activating factor (PAF) formed

c. Arachidonic acid (AA) formed

d. AA metabolites and PAF produce sustained response starting 8–12 hours after

Figure 2.10 Mast cell activation, stimulated by antibody cross-linkage. Note that mast cells can also be directly stimulated by some substances, e.g. mellitin from bee stings or C3a5a complement fragments, thus they do not always require cross-linkage of IgE

cell membrane; the release of leukotrienes, prostaglandins and platelet-activating factor by this mechanism sparks a response that starts 8–12 hours later and may last from 24 to 36 hours.

In general, the mediators released by these processes act locally, but they can also produce life-threatening systemic effects. Effects include constriction of smooth muscle in bronchi and bronchioles, causing wheezing; dilatation and increased permeability of capillaries, resulting in localized tissue oedema; increased nasal and bronchial secretions; red watery eyes; skin rashes; and diarrhoea. If laryngeal oedema or bronchospasm is severe, death may result from respiratory obstruction.

What can be done about this hypersensitivity? Antihistamines antagonize the action of histamine and can relieve many of the symptoms. Steroids, which inhibit the leukotriene pathway, can prevent

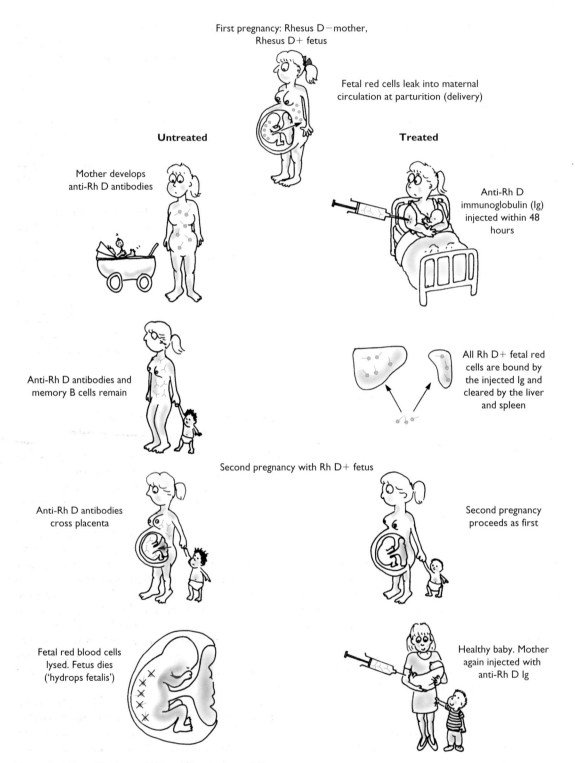

First pregnancy: Rhesus D−mother, Rhesus D+ fetus

Fetal red cells leak into maternal circulation at parturition (delivery)

Untreated

Treated

Mother develops anti-Rh D antibodies

Anti-Rh D immunoglobulin (Ig) injected within 48 hours

Anti-Rh D antibodies and memory B cells remain

All Rh D+ fetal red cells are bound by the injected Ig and cleared by the liver and spleen

Second pregnancy with Rh D+ fetus

Anti-Rh D antibodies cross placenta

Second pregnancy proceeds as first

Fetal red blood cells lysed. Fetus dies ('hydrops fetalis')

Healthy baby. Mother again injected with anti-Rh D Ig

Figure 2.11 Type II hypersensitivity – rhesus incompatibility

or alleviate the longer term symptoms. If an atopic patient knows they are likely to encounter an antigen on a particular occasion (e.g. pollen in a hay fever sufferer) they may be able to take drugs that stabilize the mast cell membrane, reducing or preventing its activation. A course of injections of a very dilute solution of the offending allergen can eventually lead to IgG instead of IgE being generated – since IgG does not stick to mast cells, the problem is avoided. But care must be taken with this approach not to generate anaphylactic shock – a life-threatening complication. In this condition, the patient must be injected immediately, subcutaneously, with adrenaline, which reverses the actions of the mediators causing bronchospasm and oedema. Patients known to be susceptible to this type of response (often to bee stings or peanut protein) carry an 'Epipen' with them, which can deliver a single dose of adrenaline (epinephrine). The action of adrenaline lasts only a finite time, and patients should also be given antihistamine or steroids as back-up.

Type II: Antibody-dependent cytotoxic hypersensitivity

In this type of hypersensitivity, antibodies react with antigens fixed to the surfaces of various types of cell and cause damage. The effects can be categorized as complement fixing, in which the antibodies cause the destruction of the target cell (cytolysis) (e.g. rhesus incompatibility, in which rhesus antibodies from a Rh-negative mother cross the placenta to damage the red cells of a Rh-positive baby) or damage the surrounding structures (e.g. Goodpasture's syndrome, in which antibodies to basement membrane in renal glomeruli damage the ability of the kidney to act as a filter); or functional, in which antibodies interfere with cell function (often by interfering with hormone receptors, but also with cell growth and differentiation or cell motility). Included in this group are antibodies that block cell function (as in some forms of Addison's disease, in which autoantibodies develop to several adrenocortical proteins) or which stimulate receptor function (as in Grave's disease, causing thyrotoxicosis). Some people split off the last group into a separate hypersensitivity type (type V, stimulatory hypersensitivity).

It is worth remembering that the body is not only on the lookout for foreign organisms, but is also generally pretty xenophobic when it comes to cells from another human. Consider, for example, blood transfusion. It is essential that any blood which is transfused into a patient is first crossmatched to ensure that the recipient does not possess antibodies to antigens on the donor red blood cells. This is because the donor red cells will become coated with antibody and/or complement which may promote phagocytosis due to opsonization, via Fc or C3b, or fix complement to produce cell membrane damage through the C8 and C9 membrane attack complex.

Type II reactions are also involved in some drug reactions (e.g. chlorpromazine-induced haemolytic anaemia and quinidine-induced agranulocytosis). The binding of a drug may alter a normal self antigen and thus produce something that can no longer be tolerated.

Natural killer (NK) cells, which are not restricted by HLA type, can kill through antibody dependent cell-mediated cytotoxicity (ADCC), which may be important for killing large parasites or tumour cells.

Type III: Immune complex-mediated hypersensitivity

Like type II, this is an antibody-driven process, but the difference is that the antibodies react with free antigen and, under the right circumstances, they form soluble immune complexes that circulate in the blood, giving rise to 'serum sickness'. Immune complexes are only soluble when the ratio of antibody to antigen is roughly equal. The complexes can be insoluble and these are usually precipitated at the site where antigen first encounters antibody. This is known as the Arthus reaction, after an experimental model of the disease which involved injecting pre-sensitized animals with an allergen. The animals developed tissue reactions at the site of injection. Don't confuse this antibody-mediated reaction with type IV (see next section).

Both the soluble and the insoluble types of complex can activate macrophages, aggregate platelets and initiate the complement cascade. Circulating immune complexes can lodge in the small vessels of many organs to cause a vasculitis (inflammation of the blood vessel wall), principally affecting the kidney (glomerulonephritis), skin and joints. An Arthus-type reaction is encountered clinically in the lung after an exogenous antigen is inhaled and precipitates locally within the alveolar walls. The inhaled antigens are usually animal or plant proteins and are often associated with specific occupations.

The resulting damage to lung alveoli, with repeated episodes of inflammation and scarring, leads to a restrictive form of lung disease called extrinsic allergic alveolitis.

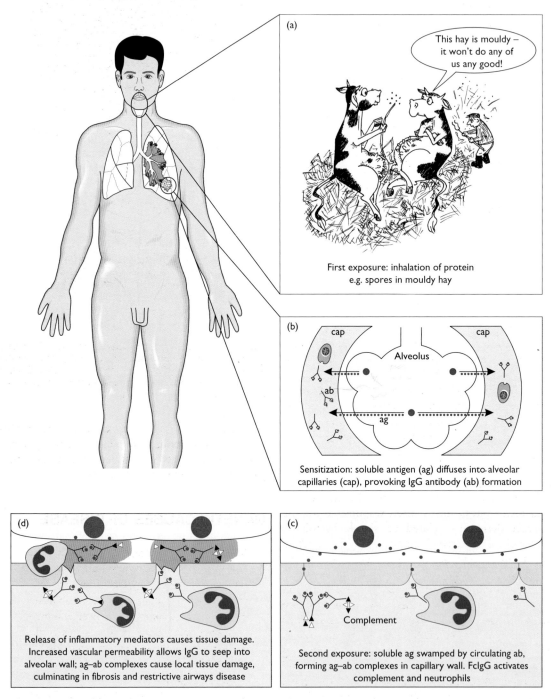

Figure 2.12 Type III hypersensitivity, e.g. farmer's lung (an example of extrinsic allergic alveolitis)

Type IV: Cell-mediated (delayed type) hypersensitivity

Unlike the other three forms of hypersensitivity, all of which involve antibody, type IV involves T lymphocytes which, over several hours and days, recruit and activate other T cells and macrophages and produce local tissue damage and granuloma formation. The antigen stimulates T cells to release IL-2, interferon γ and other cytokines, and recruitment of other cells follows the usual pathways (Fig. 2.13).

This type of hypersensitivity reaction can occur in response to many infective and non-infective causes, such as viruses, fungi, bacteria and insect bites, and is often responsible for the contact dermatitis related to simple chemicals. Clinically, it is extremely important in the rejection of transplanted tissue and graft-versus-host reactions.

Hypersensitivity can be useful! The Mantoux test (tuberculin test) takes advantage of this reaction to see whether a person has some T cell immunity to tuberculosis. This involves injecting a small amount of a (non-infectious) purified protein derivative of *Mycobacterium tuberculosis* into the skin and observing whether a localized red induration occurs over the next 48 hours; T cells and macrophages

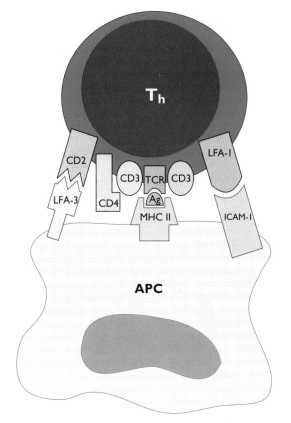

Figure 2.13 Surface receptor interactions between T$_h$ (helper T cells) and antigen-presenting cells (APCs). Many of the molecules involved (MHC II, T cell receptor (TCR), CD2, 3 and 4, and adhesion molecule ICAM) are members of the immunoglobulin gene superfamily

mount a type IV reaction in a sensitized person. This test is not 100 per cent certain, since some patients with overwhelming tuberculous infection are anergic and show no reaction (Fig. 2.14).

GENETIC CAUSES OF DISEASE

In considering the Origin of Species, it is quite conceivable that a naturalist, reflecting on the mutual affinities of organic beings, on their embryological relations, their geographical distribution, geological succession, and other such facts, might come to the conclusion that each species had not been independently created, but had descended, like varieties from other species.

Charles Darwin (1809–1882)

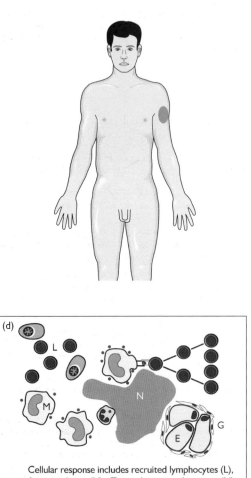

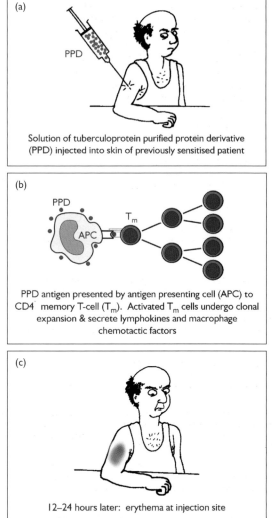

(a)

PPD

Solution of tuberculoprotein purified protein derivative (PPD) injected into skin of previously sensitised patient

(b)

PPD

T_m

APC

PPD antigen presented by antigen presenting cell (APC) to CD4 memory T-cell (T_m). Activated T_m cells undergo clonal expansion & secrete lymphokines and macrophage chemotactic factors

(c)

12–24 hours later: erythema at injection site

(d)

L

M

N

E

G

Cellular response includes recruited lymphocytes (L), & macrophages (M). Tissue damage and necrosis (N) occurs due to release of inflammatory mediators. Macrophages may become epithelioid cells (E) which aggregate to form granulomata (G)

Figure 2.14 Type IV hypersensitivity – Mantoux test reaction

Coeliac disease is an example of a predisposition to disease, in which inherited characteristics, dictated by the HLA antigens on the surfaces of the cells, render a person at increased risk of developing a disease. Susceptible individuals must encounter another agent, such as wheat protein, which mimics these HLA antigens and stimulates an immune response that cross-reacts with their own cells, before they develop the disease. After the case presentation below we will consider diseases that are predestined to occur due to inherited alterations within the genome itself.

Since genetic disorders are fundamental to so many diseases, we will illustrate the section on intrinsic causes of disease by using examples of disease mediated via the genes. As with the section on infective agents, this is a massive topic and one that is expanding rapidly.

It is a common misconception among medical students that pathology is an exact science. It is sometimes difficult to see why the examination of tissues at post mortem, both grossly and microscopically, cannot give a precise answer. Yet a short time in a laboratory will reveal that the terms 'possibility' and 'probability' are well known to the pathologist.

Clinicopathological case study – coeliac disease

Clinical

A slightly built, 25-year-old woman consulted her family doctor. She complained of tiredness and breathlessness on exertion, worse over the last six months. On examination, she was of medium height (1 m 65 cm), low weight (50 kg) (see BMI chart, Fig. 2.15) and had pale mucous membranes. Her doctor pointed out some bruising over her shins – she did not recall the injury but commented that she had bruised easily over recent months.

Investigations:
Hb: 9.6 g/dL (N 11–13.5)
MCV: 86 fL (N 78–95)
WCC: 3.8×10^9/L (N 3–5.5)
Platelets: 330×10^{12}/L (N 150–400)
Red cell folate: 152 mg/L (N 150–750)
Vitamin B12: 68 ng/L (N 150–1000)
Iron: 13 mmol/L (N 14–30)
INR: 2.5 (N 0.8–1.1)

Provisional clinical diagnosis: malabsorption, probably due to coeliac disease (gluten-induced enteropathy)

Management and progress:
She was referred for investigation at the gastroenterology clinic in her local hospital. The results of the investigations were as follows:

- upper GI endoscopy and duodenal biopsy: macroscopically normal, but biopsy showed subtotal villous atrophy and increased intraepithelial lymphocytes
- serology for antigliadin and other coeliac disease-related antibodies was positive
- bone density scan showed early osteoporosis.

The suspected diagnosis of coeliac disease (gluten-induced enteropathy) was confirmed and she was advised to exclude wheat from her diet (a gluten-free diet). She felt symptomatically improved after one month.

After six months she returns to clinic. She is bored with the gluten-free diet. She feels well and is putting on weight. She requests a return to a normal diet.

Repeat duodenal biopsy after six months showed greatly improved microscopical appearances, which were almost normal.

She is warned to remain on a strict gluten free diet, to prevent long-term sequelae.

Other members of her family are screened for occult coeliac disease.

Pathological

Pallor and symptoms suggest anaemia. Iron deficiency anaemia is the most common in a young woman and is likely to be due to menorrhagia, but bruising would be unusual.

Macrocytic anaemia indicates folic acid and/or vitamin B12 deficiency. Note that this patient also has a low serum iron.

Prolonged prothrombin time (measured as the INR – internal normalized ratio) is likely to be due to decreased vitamin K causing a deficiency of clotting factors (see Table 2.8).

The incidence of coeliac disease in the UK is approximately 1:300 people; Ireland has the highest rate at 1:100 people. Many patients have subclinical disease.

Subtotal villous atrophy with increased intraepithelial lymphocytes is the typical picture in coeliac disease, due to increased destruction of enterocytes by a T cell-mediated reaction (Fig. 2.16).

IgA anti-endomysial antibody is positive in 95 per cent of untreated coeliacs, IgA antigliadin in the majority of untreated coeliac children and 70 per cent of untreated coeliac adults. IgG antigliadin antibody is less specific for coeliac disease.

Bone density scan result: mild osteoporosis was due to vitamin D malabsorption, with resultant poor calcium absorption.

A gluten-free diet is difficult to sustain in Western countries: wheat is present in bread, cakes, biscuits, sauces. Any trace is sufficient to spark a recrudescence of disease. Social occasions are fraught with embarrassment and difficulty.

Short-term problems due to coeliac disease include vitamin deficiencies, growth retardation (in children), steatorrhoea, malnutrition and anaemia and osteoporosis. These are relatively quickly improved on a gluten-free diet.

The duodenal biopsy may take up to a year to return to normal (but just days to show subtotal villous atrophy again after a gluten challenge!).

Long-term problems include an increased incidence of malignant gut tumours, e.g. coeliac patients are at 50–100 times the normal risk of developing malignant lymphoma and there is a moderately increased risk of small and large bowel adenocarcinoma and squamous carcinoma of the oesophagus. It appears that the increased risk can be averted by adherence to a gluten-free diet.

The prevalence of coeliac disease in relatives is as follows:

First-degree relatives 10–15 per cent
HLA identical siblings 30 per cent
Dizygotic twins 25 per cent
Monozygotic twins 70–100 per cent

There are strong associations between HLA DQ2 and DQ8 and coeliac disease. Most coeliac patients inherit a particular HLA type, which renders them more likely to develop the disease, probably as a result of molecular mimicry between wheat protein antigen and epitopes on small intestinal mucosal cells, which are likely to be determined by the HLA type.

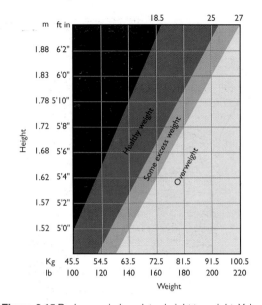

Figure 2.15 Body mass index relates height to weight. Values from 18.5 to 25 are healthy

Table 2.8 Clinical consequences of fat- and water-soluble vitamin deficiency

Vitamin	Clinical feature
A (retinol)	Xerophthalmia, night blindness, keratomalacia, follicular keratosis
D (cholecalciferol)	Rickets, osteomalacia
E (α-tocopherol)	Ataxia
K	Bleeding disorders
B1 (thiamine)	Beriberi
B2 (riboflavin)	Angular stomatitis
Niacin	Pellagra
B6 (pyridoxine)	Peripheral neuropathy
Pantothenic acid	
Biotin	Dermatitis
B12 (cobalamin)	Megaloblastic anaemia, neurological disorders
Folic acid	Megaloblastic anaemia
C (ascorbic acid)	Scurvy

From Lydyard *et al.* 2000: *Pathology integrated: An A–Z of Disease and its Pathogenesis*. London: Arnold.

Normal duodenum

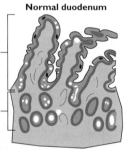

Normal slender villi with few intra-epithelial lymphocytes

Crypt to villus ratio 1:3

People with type II MHC antigens DQ2 or DQ8 are at risk of developing coeliac disease if wheat protein enters the lamina propria, possibly following an infection.

Some enteroviruses are thought to mimic wheat antigens.

An anti-inflammatory enzyme, tissue transglutaminase (tTG) deamidates gliadin, changing its three dimensional shape. The altered wheat protein 'fits' a groove in the DQ2 or DQ8 MHC antigens.

Intestinal epithelial cells present the wheat antigen associated with MCH II antigens to T cells. The T cells delete the epithelial cells bearing the foreign antigen, causing villous atrophy.

Removal of wheat from the diet restores normality in 3–6 months. Relapse occurs within days if wheat is eaten again.

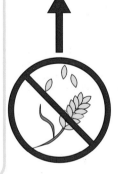

Gluten induced enteropathy (coeliac disease)

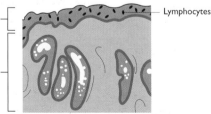

Near total villous atrophy

Lymphocytes

Crypt elongation inflammation in lamina propria (LP) and increased lymphocytes in the surface epithelium (arrow)

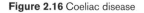

Figure 2.16 Coeliac disease

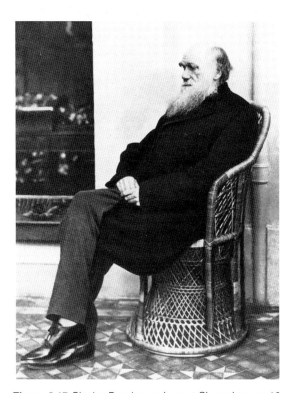

Figure 2.17 Charles Darwin was born at Shrewsbury on 12 February 1809. In 1825 he was sent to Edinburgh to study medicine. However, this was his father's choice, and Darwin later chose to study classics at Cambridge. He joined the *HMS Beagle*, which surveyed the coast of South America for 5 years. On this trip, Darwin pondered on the amazing diversity in nature. He was very religious and believed in the literal truth of the Bible. Thus he was reluctant to publish his heretical theory on evolution, preferring to direct his wife to publish it after his death. However, Alfred Russel Wallace had reached similar conclusions, which he sent to Darwin in 1858. This resulted in both Darwin's and Wallace's ideas being presented to the Linnean Society in London that year, followed in the next year by the publication of the *On the origin of species by means of natural selection*, or the *Preservation of favoured races in the struggle for life*. He died on 19 April 1882 and was buried in Westminster Abbey. © Bettmann/CORBIS

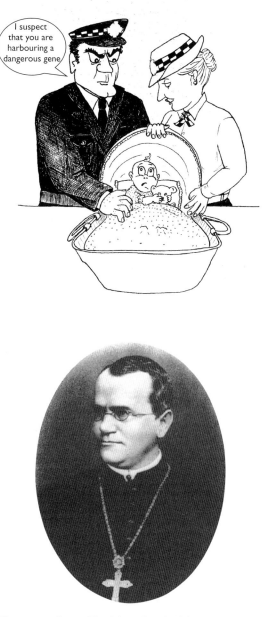

Figure 2.18 Gregor Mendel was born in Heizendorff, Moravia, on 22 July 1822. He joined the Augustine order in 1843 and, 10 years later, after studies at the University of Vienna, he went to the monastery at Brunn. His famous work with the peas began in 1856, but it was not until 1865 that he communicated the results to the Brunn Society of Natural Science. They remained in the archives until they were discovered in 1900, 35 years after publication, by three botanists pursuing a similar path. Mendel died in 1884 (Courtesy of Wellcome Institute for the History of Medicine)

If you encounter a patient with metastatic tumour in the liver, it is *possible* that the primary tumour may have arisen in the nose, but it is much more *probable* that it arose in the colon! The study of genetics involves appreciating how the inheritance of genes produces diseases so that the probability of a particular individual developing a disease can be calculated.

Most of us take our existence for granted, but life really is a source of constant wonder and it has occurred against probability. Let us begin when there was no life on earth. At some stage, molecules must have come into existence that were capable of self-replication and these molecules multiplied. If you have two molecules, one that manages to replicate and make copies without any mistakes while the other makes a lot of mistakes each time it is copied, then the correctly copied molecule is more likely to increase in number. Ironically, the molecule that copies perfectly will never change and it will still be the same molecule after 1 year, after 50 years and after a billion years. If a random mistake happens in the copying then there is the opportunity for change; possibly for the better, probably for worse. This is the basis for evolution recognized by Darwin in 1838. The other important factor is that there should be a 'struggle for survival', an evolutionary pressure that gives an advantage to the molecules or animals best adapted to the prevailing conditions.

Mendel and his peas

The probability of inheriting characteristics from parents was studied by Gregor Mendel. Mendel took garden peas with contrasting characteristics, seven to be exact, and bred from the plants which differed in only one characteristic. For the sake of discussion, let us consider violet and white flowers. He crossed plants with violet flowers with those bearing white flowers to produce the next generation, called the F1 generation. He found that the F1 generation plants all had the same colour flowers. Let us say that they were all violet. The F1 plants were then self-pollinated (inbred) to produce the next generation, called F2. Interestingly, there were three plants with violet flowers for every one plant with white flowers. He took this one step further and self-pollinated the white-flowered plants which gave rise to an F3 generation of plants that all had white flowers. Self-pollination of the violet-flowered plants produced an intriguing result: some plants produced only violet-flowered plants while others produced a mixture, some plants with white flowers and some with violet, in the ratio of 1 to 3 (Fig. 2.19).

As Mendel correctly deduced, although the violet-flowered plants in the F2 generation all looked the same, they had different inheritance factors. He postulated that each plant must possess two factors that determine a given characteristic, such as colour of the flower. If two plants are crossed, each will contribute one factor to the next generation and it is purely random as to which factor is passed on. This is the law of segregation, also known as Mendel's first law. We now know that these 'factors' are genes on paired chromosomes and that the two genes on the two chromosomes are alleles of each other.

In Mendel's experiment, violet is the dominant allele and white is the recessive allele. The F1 generation has one white plant, which is homozygous for the white allele, one violet plant that is homozygous for the violet allele and two violet plants that are heterozygous, i.e. they have one white and one violet allele but the violet one dominates. In simple examples like this, one allele dominates (i.e. if the plant has at least one violet allele then all the flowers will be violet). Sometimes the situation is more complicated and there is variable penetrance (i.e. the 'dominant' allele only dominates in a percentage of cases).

It was later appreciated by Thomas Hunt Morgan in 1934 that cell differentiation might depend on variation in the action of genes in different cell types. Towards the end of the nineteenth century, DNA, RNA and histones were discovered, and it was originally believed that the histone proteins were genes. However, in 1944, Oswald Avery, Colin MacLeod and Maclyn McCarty recognized that DNA was the structural component of the gene. In 1953, James Watson and Francis Crick elucidated the double-helical structure of DNA that provides the basis for its ability to replicate.

Obstetrics forms a major part of the medical curriculum, and during your training, you will meet pregnant women who are naturally concerned about their unborn baby. Let us briefly consider a clinical scenario to illustrate a possible problem you might encounter.

Clinical case: Turner's syndrome

A 34-year-old woman was seen in the antenatal clinic complaining of abdominal pain and 'spotting' of blood. This was her first pregnancy and examination revealed a uterus of approximately 20 weeks size. The gestation should have been 22 weeks according to her estimated date of delivery. The doctor failed to hear a fetal heart sound and arranged an ultrasound scan of her abdomen. This revealed an intrauterine death and evacuation of the fetus was carried out.

Let us consider some of the questions you may be faced with in clinical practice.

- What are the commonest genetic diseases?
- How can you diagnose them?
- Who should have their genes examined?

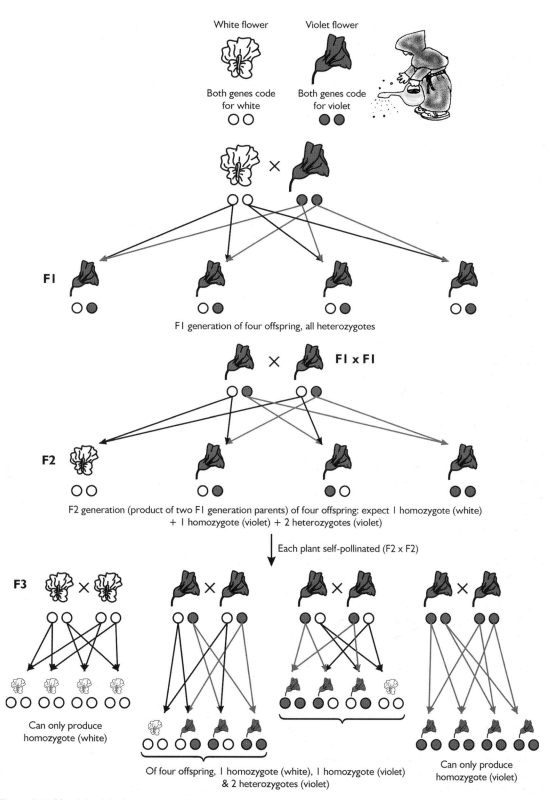

Figure 2.19 Mendelian inheritance

Pathological examination

Name: Fetus of A. Smith
Consultant: Mr I.M. Obs
Date of operation: 12.5.97
Gestation: 20 weeks

Post mortem examination of the aborted fetus was carried out to elucidate the cause and the report is illustrated below:

External examination:
The body was that of a female fetus and external measurements were consistent with a gestation of 18 weeks. There was generalized subcutaneous oedema and a cystic hygroma (benign cystic tumour of lymphatic vessels) was noted in the posterior aspect of the neck. The placenta was pale and bulky.

Internal examination:
The organ weights were consistent with a gestation of 18 weeks. The main abnormality was in the cardiovascular system. The left ventricle was small and the aorta proximal to the ductus arteriosus was narrowed – a severe infantile coarctation.

Special investigations:
Placental tissue was sent for cytogenetic analysis. Chromosomal analysis revealed the karyotype 45,X confirming a monosomy X (i.e. Turner's syndrome).

What are the commonest genetic diseases?

Table 2.9 lists the incidence per 1000 live births of the commonest genetic disorders. It is helpful to subdivide them into abnormalities of chromosomal structure or number. The single-gene disorders are caused by abnormalities of structure, and will be inherited in a Mendelian fashion. Abnormalities of chromosomal number are not normally inherited.

There are several points to highlight. The first is that the incidence relates to live births, which means that genetic abnormalities causing intrauterine death will be under-reported. This principally influences the figures for the chromosomal abnormalities, as their incidence in spontaneous abortions and stillbirths is 50 per cent while the incidence in live births is 6.5 per 1000. In spontaneous abortions with chromosomal abnormalities, around 50 per cent will have a trisomy, 18 per cent will be Turner's syndrome (XO) and 17 per cent will be triploid.

The commonest condition is X-linked red–green colour blindness, which, fortunately, is only a very minor handicap (and is not an excuse for avoiding histology sessions!). Klinefelter's syndrome is due to an extra X chromosome in males (47,XXY). Affected individuals are generally of normal intelligence and are tall, with hypogonadism and infertility. XYY syndrome also produces tall males. They may have behavioural problems, especially impulsive behaviour.

In familial hypercholesterolaemia patients have increased plasma low-density lipoprotein (LDL) levels and a predisposition for developing atheroma at an early age which gives them an eight-fold increased risk of ischaemic heart disease. The primary defect is a deficiency of cellular LDL receptors so that the liver uptake is reduced and plasma levels are two to three

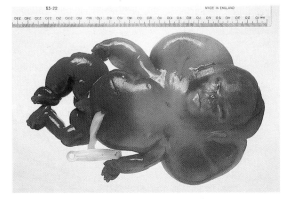

Figure 2.20 Hydropic fetus at 18 weeks – Turner's syndrome (Courtesy of R. Scott, UCLMS)

times normal. Around 30 different mutations of the LDL receptor gene have been identified. About 1 in 500 people are affected and they are heterozygotes that have half the normal number of LDL receptors. One in a million people are homozygotes and they usually die from cardiovascular disease in childhood.

Adult polycystic kidney disease occurs as a result of a defect on the short arm of chromosome 16 that is inherited in an autosomal dominant fashion. Both kidneys are enlarged, with numerous fluid-filled cysts, and may weigh a kilogram or more (normal = 150 g). The patients develop symptoms of renal damage and hypertension in their third or fourth decade.

Triple X syndrome produces tall girls who may have below average intelligence and, although gonadal function is usually normal, there may be premature ovarian failure. Fragile X syndrome was first described in 1969 and is now recognized as the second commonest cause of severe mental retardation after Down syndrome. Affected males have a reduced IQ, macro-orchidism and a prominent

Table 2.9 Common genetic disorders

Condition	Estimated freq/ 1000 live births	Abnormality
Red-green colour blindness	80*	X
Total autosomal dominant disease	10	AD
Dominant otosclerosis	3	AD
Klinefelter's (XXY)	2*	N
Familial hypercholesterolaemia	2	AD
Total autosomal recessive disease	2	AR
Trisomy 21 (Down's)	1.5	N
XYY	1.5*	N
Adult polycystic kidney disease	1	AD
Triple X syndrome	0.6#	N
Cystic fibrosis	0.5	AR
Fragile X-linked mental retardation	0.5*	X
Non-specific X-linked mental retardation	0.5*	X
Recessive mental retardation	0.5	AR
Neurofibromatosis	0.4	AR
Turner syndrome (XO)	0.4#	N
Duchenne muscular dystrophy	0.3*	X
Haemophilia A	0.2*	X
Trisomy 18 (Edward's)	0.12	N
Polyposis coli	0.1	AD
Trisomy 13 (Patau's)	0.07	N

AD = autosomal dominant; AR = autosomal recessive; X = sex-linked disorder; N = disorder of chromosomal number.
*per1000 male births; #per 1000 female births.

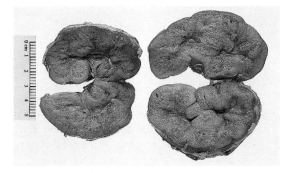

Figure 2.21 Abnormal recessive polycystic kidney disease. Smaller normal kidneys are included for comparison – 37 weeks' gestation (Courtesy of R. Scott, UCLMS)

cent of affected pregnancies will abort. Those surviving to delivery will be less severely affected and generally show short stature, webbing of the neck, normal intelligence, infertility, aortic coarctation and altered carrying angle of the arm (cubitus valgus).

Although we have listed the common genetic disorders and their karyotypes, this does not answer the question: 'How are they caused?' This is really two questions:

- How does the genetic abnormality produce disease?
- How does the genetic abnormality arise?

How does the genetic abnormality produce disease?

From our list so far, we have only explained the pathophysiology of familial hypercholesterolaemia. Now we shall discuss the recent discoveries that have increased our understanding of cystic fibrosis.

forehead and jaw. Heterozygote females can show mild retardation but counselling is difficult because not all female carriers show the chromosomal abnormality on testing. Turner's syndrome (monosomy X, i.e. 45,X) is a common cause of fetal hydrops and spontaneous abortion. About 95 per

Patients with cystic fibrosis present in infancy with pancreatic insufficiency, malabsorption and lung damage. This is an autosomal recessive disease and occurs in about 1:2000 live births. Approximately 1:25 people are heterozygotes. The pathological manifestations result from thickened secretions that lead to obstruction, inflammation and scarring. The tenacious secretions are an indicator of a fundamental problem in water and electrolyte handling. This has been recognized for a long time and used as a diagnostic test called the sweat test, which looks for elevated levels of sodium in the sweat.

The reason for the increased electrolytes in sweat is that there is defective cyclic-AMP-mediated regulation of chloride channels. The gene has now been identified on the long arm of chromosome 7 (7q31) and called the cystic fibrosis transmembrane conductance regulator (CFTR). The CFTR gene codes for a protein of 1480 amino acids, the structure of which is similar to that of the family of ATP-binding proteins. It is not yet clear whether the CFTR protein transports chloride directly or regulates chloride indirectly via another protein, but it is clear that a change in CFTR protein would affect electrolyte transport.

In about 70 per cent of cases of cystic fibrosis, there is a mutation referred to as the Delta F508 mutation. This is a deletion in the codon at position 508 that leads to loss of a phenylalanine molecule in a highly conserved region of the CFTR protein. This

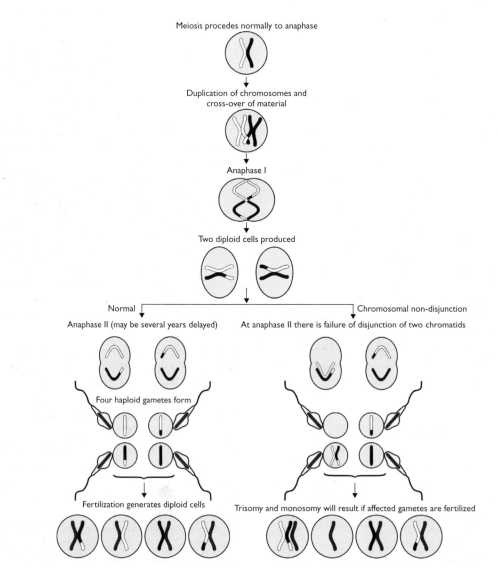

Figure 2.22 Abnormal chromosome numbers may arise because of non-disjunction during anaphase II

is thought to alter the folding of the protein. The abnormal protein that is produced is unable to respond to cyclic-AMP. In the pancreas and lungs, this leads to reduced chloride and water secretion so the mucus is thick. In the sweat test, the sweat glands secrete water and chloride normally but the secretory coil does not respond to β-adrenergic stimulation and does not reabsorb the chloride ions, hence allowing increased chloride and sodium in the sweat.

How does the genetic abnormality arise?

We need to consider abnormalities of chromosome number separately from abnormalities in chromosome structure or single gene disorders, as different mechanisms operate.

ABNORMAL CHROMOSOME NUMBER

This occurs because of problems at the anaphase stage of meiosis, leading to unequal sharing of the chromosomes so that one daughter cell will have an extra chromosome (trisomy) while the other is missing a chromosome (monosomy). A pair of chromosomes or sister chromatids may fail to separate, so-called non-disjunction, or there may be delayed movement (anaphase lag) of chromosomes so that one is left on the wrong side of the dividing wall. The cause is unknown but the incidence increases with maternal age as in Down syndrome. It may also be associated with irradiation, viral infection or familial tendencies.

Polyploidy means that the cell contains at least one complete extra set of chromosomes. Most commonly, this is one extra set (i.e. 69 chromosomes or triploidy). Affected fetuses usually die *in utero* or abort in early pregnancy. Polyploidy can result from fertilization by two sperm (dispermy) or from fertilization in which either the sperm or ovum is diploid because of an abnormality in their maturation divisions.

ABNORMAL CHROMOSOME STRUCTURE

Abnormalities in chromosome structure occur when chromosomes are inaccurately repaired after breaks have occurred. Chromosomal breakage can happen randomly at any gene locus but there are some areas that are particularly liable to breakage. The rate of breakage is markedly increased by ionizing radiation, certain chemicals and some rare inherited conditions. Structural abnormalities, such as translocations, deletions, duplications and inversions (Fig. 2.23), occur when two break points allow transfer, loss or rearrangement of chromosomal material.

Single-gene disorders

Single-gene disorders can also result from structural abnormalities involving minute areas of the chromosome. These are produced by the same mechanism, i.e. breakage resulting in deletions, etc. Alternatively, single-gene disorders result from a point mutation at the gene site. Point mutations are usually spontaneous and of unknown cause, but are probably mostly due to copying errors. Substitution of one base within a codon may lead to a different amino acid being inserted into the protein and major pathological effects (e.g. sickle cell disease). However, this is not inevitable because although there are only 20 amino acids, there are 64 possible codons ($4 \times 4 \times 4$), which is the basis of the 'degeneracy of the genetic code'. For example, an mRNA sequence of either GAA or GAG will code for alanine, thus some point mutations can alter the codon but have no effect on the amino acid sequence. Approximately 25 per cent of point mutations have no effect.

As well as coding for amino acids, codons also act as start and stop instructions. Messenger RNA employs UAA, UAG or UGA as stop codons. If a point mutation produces a stop codon, the amino acid chain will terminate too early and this is the effect of about 5 per cent of point mutations. The ultimate problem is a frameshift mutation, in which gain or loss of one or two bases produces a nonsense message because it alters every codon.

By way of illustration, take a look at the following sentences.

SHE HAD ONE MAD CAT AND ONE SAD RAT
SHE HAD ONE BAD CAT AND ONE SAD RAT
THE MAD BAD CAT ATE THE ONE SAD RAT
THE MAD **SHE** CAT ATE THE ONE SAD RAT
THE MAD HEC ATA TET HEO NES ADR AT

- The first sentence is the normal code.
- The second has a point mutation without a frameshift so there is a 25 per cent probability that it will not have any effect.
- The third sentence has a length mutation, possibly a translocation.
- The fourth sentence is a mutation of the third where SHE represents a premature stop codon.
- The fifth sentence changes the sex of the cat and makes nonsense.

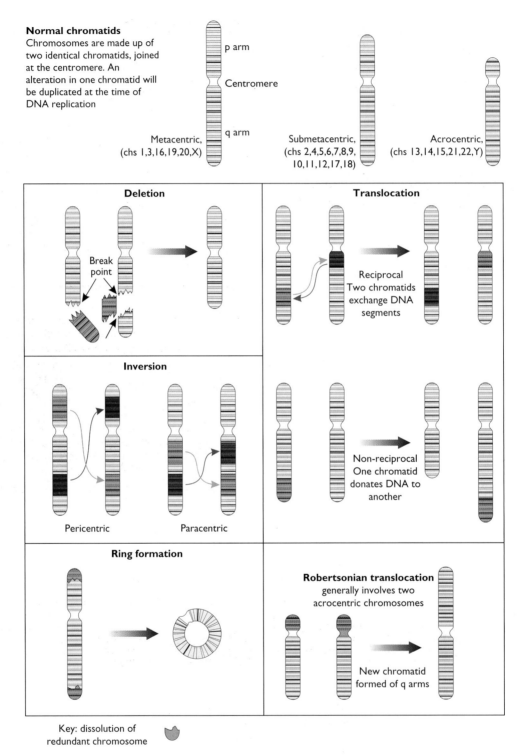

Normal chromatids
Chromosomes are made up of two identical chromatids, joined at the centromere. An alteration in one chromatid will be duplicated at the time of DNA replication

p arm

Centromere

q arm

Metacentric, (chs 1,3,16,19,20,X)

Submetacentric, (chs 2,4,5,6,7,8,9, 10,11,12,17,18)

Acrocentric, (chs 13,14,15,21,22,Y)

Deletion

Break point

Translocation

Reciprocal Two chromatids exchange DNA segments

Inversion

Pericentric

Paracentric

Non-reciprocal One chromatid donates DNA to another

Ring formation

Robertsonian translocation
generally involves two acrocentric chromosomes

New chromatid formed of q arms

Key: dissolution of redundant chromosome

Figure 2.23 Structural chromosomal abnormalities

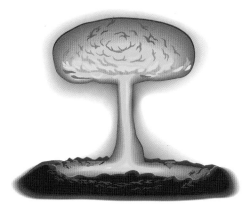

Immediate effects

Death from blast/burn injuries
Acute radiation syndromes:
• Bone marrow depression
• Gastrointestinal tract effects
• Cerebral effects

Delayed malignancies depend on age at time of exposure:

Childhood exposure
• Leukaemias*
• Thyroid cancer
• Breast cancer

Adult exposure
• Leukaemias*
• Lung/breast/salivary gland cancer
• All other cancers increased to some extent

* All leukaemias except chronic lymphocytic leukaemia are increased

Figure 2.24 Effects of irradiation, e.g. following a nuclear explosion, can be immediate or delayed

Multifactorial disorders

All new patients are asked about their 'family history', the idea being that if their parents and siblings suffer from a particular disease then they are at increased risk. Unfortunately, for most diseases it is not known how great that increased risk may be because the inheritance does not follow simple Mendelian principles but is multifactorial. It is likely that there will be a variety of genes involved which interact with a number of environmental factors.

Research into multifactorial disorders adopts a similar approach to single-gene problems. First, it is necessary to identify the diseases with a significant genetic component by comparing the incidence in family groups with the general population. This genetic contribution is termed heritability.

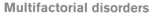

Small Print

Heritability = genetic contribution to the aetiology of the disorder

Disease	Estimate of heritability (per cent)
Schizophrenia	85
Asthma	80
Cleft lip and palate	76
Coronary artery disease	65
Hypertension	62
Neural tube defect	60
Peptic ulcer	35

MUTATION

New sequence in viable cell

Multiple breaks, and random joining of strands

DNA damaged by:
Irradiation
Drugs
UV light
Heat
(Spontaneous mutation)

Single strand break   Point mutation   Double strand break(s)   Cross-linkage

Changes
Loss of base
Alteration of base
Bulk lesion
Alkylation

Repair, using opposite strand as template

Irreparable damage, transcription impossible

RESTITUTION   **DELETION**

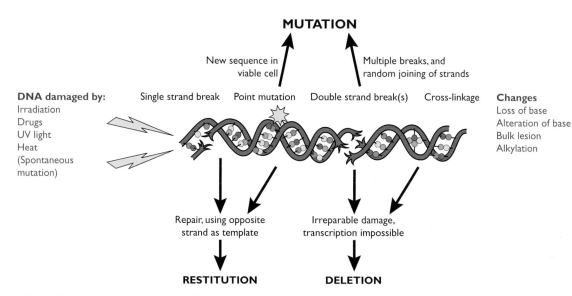

Figure 2.25 Causes of and types of DNA mutation and their consequences

The next step is to look for genetic, biochemical and immunological features that affected individuals have in common. It is well established that certain HLA types are associated with particular diseases and this may be helpful in counselling affected families. For example, in a family with ankylosing spondylitis, a first-degree relative has a 9 per cent risk of developing the disease if HLA-B27 positive but less than a 1 per cent risk if HLA-B27 negative.

The ultimate goal is to identify the gene or genes and the environmental factor(s), so that those at particularly high genetic risk can attempt to avoid the relevant environmental hazard. At a simple level, this would mean giving vitamin supplements to pregnant women at risk of producing babies with neural tube defects, or advising potential 'arteriopaths' to modify their diet and not smoke.

Diabetes is a disease in which a genetic predisposition is beginning to be better understood. The insulin-dependent (type 1) form was known to be associated with certain HLA types and thought to involve a viral infection in susceptible individuals. Although HLA association need not mean that the HLA genes are involved, in this case, study of the histocompatibility areas of chromosome 6 revealed that amino acid 57 in the DQ gene cluster was altered in susceptible individuals. Individuals with aspartate at position 57 had resistance to the disease, whereas mutations substituting alanine, valine or serine increased susceptibility.

HOW CAN GENETIC DISORDERS BE DIAGNOSED?

Non-invasive tests

Fortunately, the majority of pregnancies progress without any problems to produce a normal healthy baby after approximately 40 weeks' gestation. It would be unreasonable to subject all pregnant women to the stress and possible hazards of the many investigations that are available to detect fetal abnormalities. In recent years, the quality of ultrasound scanning has achieved a standard that makes it useful for detecting internal and external fetal malformations as well as giving accurate information on the rate of fetal growth through head circumference and body length measurements. In practice, early ultrasound (at 8–10 weeks) can be used to date the pregnancy and identify anencephaly. Spina bifida can be identified on ultrasound after 16 weeks' gestation and the scan is usually done between 17 and 20 weeks. The tests mentioned so far are non-invasive and no risks have been identified to either mother or baby.

Invasive procedures

One of the simplest tests is to measure the mother's serum α fetoprotein (AFP) concentration. Ultrasound is very good at picking up neural tube defects, so the AFP test is mainly useful for small defects that are missed. It is measured at about 16–18 weeks' gestation and will be raised in 90 per cent of mothers bearing children with open neural tube defects and 95 per cent of anencephalic cases. Obviously, this means that 5–10 per cent of cases will remain undetected, so it is essential to offer more sensitive techniques to mothers at particularly high risk. AFP levels are also raised in multiple pregnancies, threatened abortions and a variety of fetal malformations. The level is lowered in Down syndrome.

Screening for fetal well-being has developed rapidly over the last decade and many centres use a 'triple test' for Down syndrome. This includes AFP, human chorigonadotrophin (hCG) and oestriol. Such screening tests are particularly useful in detecting Down syndrome in younger women who do not have any particular risk factors for fetal abnormalities.

Amniocentesis can be performed between 15 and 16 weeks' gestation and involves removing about 20 mL of amniotic fluid, which contains small numbers of amniotic cells that can be cultured. The fluid can be tested for AFP and acetylcholinesterase activity to detect neural tube defects, or it can be used for more specialized tests to detect rare inborn errors of metabolism. The cells are cultured and used for karyotypic (chromosome) analysis.

Fetoscopy, which involves introducing a scope into the amniotic cavity, has also been used to perform fetal blood sampling and for therapeutic procedures such as intrauterine transfusion. It does carry a risk of inducing an abortion.

METHODS OF GENETIC ANALYSIS

Cytogenetic analysis

The human nucleus contains 23 pairs of chromosomes – 22 pairs of autosomes and one pair of sex chromosomes. It has been apparent for some time that certain diseases are associated with specific chromosomal abnormalities and it is logical to divide these into those affecting the autosomal chromosomes and those affecting the sex chromosomes. As discussed earlier, these groups can also be divided into abnormalities affecting numbers of chromosomes and those affecting the structure of chromosomes.

At metaphase, the two chromatids of each chromosome are joined by a centromere; the long arm is termed 'q' and the short arm is 'p'. There is a convention for reporting karyotypes so that the total number of chromosomes is given first, followed by the sex chromosomes. Examples are illustrated in Table 2.10.

The child with mosaicism has two genetically different cell types distributed in his or her tissues. These are not distributed evenly and some affected individuals may demonstrate only a normal phenotype in their peripheral blood lymphocytes. Therefore, it may be necessary to culture from other organs, such as skin, to confirm a suspected

Table 2.10 Examples of karyotypes

46XY	Normal male
46XX	Normal female
47XXY	Male with Klinefelter's syndrome

If there is a change in chromosomal number, then the affected chromosome is indicated with a + or −, e.g.

47XX + 21	Female with Down syndrome

If there is a structural rearrangement, the karyotype indicates the precise site affected and the nature of the abnormality, e.g.

46XXdel7 (p13-ptr)	Deletion of the short arm of chromosome 7 at band 13 to the end of the chromosome
46XYt(11;14) (p15.4;q22.3)	A translocation between chromosome 11 and 14 with the break points being band 15.4 on the short arm of chromosome 11 and band 22.3 on the long arm of chromosome 14

Mosaicism indicates that two different cell lines have derived from one fertilized egg and the karyotype specifies both cell lines:

46XX/47XX + 21	Down's mosaic
46XX/45X	Turner's mosaic

abnormality. Patients with mosaicism are generally less severely affected than those with the full disorder. This makes prenatal counselling difficult if mosaicism is detected in a fetus, as the clinical effects could be mild. There is also the complication that any mosaicism detected in chorionic villus samples may only indicate an abnormal genotype in some placental cells and the fetus need not be affected.

Chorionic villus sampling has some advantages over amniocentesis in that it can be performed between 8 and 12 weeks' gestation so that a diagnosis can often be made by 12–14 weeks' gestation, when termination is easier. It also provides material suitable for DNA analysis, which is necessary when the genetic changes are too small to be seen on light microscopic chromosomal preparations. It does, however, carry a greater risk of miscarriage.

Dictionary box

Mosaicism: The presence of two or more cell lines that are both karyotypically and genotypically distinct but are derived from the same zygote.

Fluorescence *in situ* hybridization

Recent advances in molecular biology have led to novel technologies for the assessment of chromosomes and genes. One such DNA-based technique is fluorescence *in situ* hybridization (FISH). This technique has been used extensively in research as well as in clinical diagnosis. The idea behind the technique is very simple. DNA probes labelled with fluorescence dyes are hybridized to the chromosomes to reveal their structure and number. An advantage of this method is that unlike classical karyotyping, it can also be used on interphase nuclei. This is particularly important for diagnosis in certain tumour types (e.g. leukaemias), where metaphase chromosomal spreads are difficult to obtain.

Comparative genomic hybridization (CGH) is an adaptation of the FISH technique that allows a global view of DNA copy number changes within a single hybridization. This has opened up avenues not only in tumour research but also in assessing genetic alterations in a clinical setting.

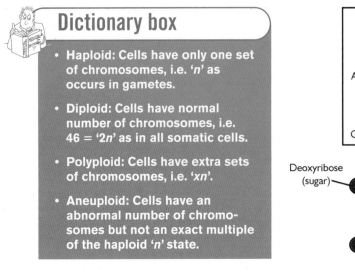

DNA analysis

First, let us remind ourselves of some basic facts about DNA (deoxyribonucleic acid). DNA consists of two antiparallel strands that have a backbone of deoxyribose sugars from which purine and pyrimidine bases project. The sequence of these bases determines the genetic code. It is estimated that there are approximately 6 billion bases in the human genome. The purine bases are adenine (A) and guanine (G) and the pyrimidine bases are cytosine (C) and thymine (T). The two strands form a right-handed double helix with about 10 nucleotide pairs per helical turn. They are linked through these purine and pyrimidine bases with G always pairing with C and A pairing with T. This point is fundamental to the use of probes for analysing DNA.

The binding of complementary purine and pyrimidine bases also allows DNA to act as a template for the production of messenger RNA (mRNA). This process is called transcription. The mRNA moves to the cytoplasm, attaches to a ribosome and is then used for protein production. This is termed translation and involves binding of transfer RNAs (tRNA) carrying a specific amino acid. The amino acids then combine to form a polypeptide chain and are released (Fig. 2.27). RNA differs from DNA in three respects: it is a single-stranded molecule, it contains ribose sugar instead of deoxyribose and the base thymine (T) is substituted by uracil (U).

There have been three major advances in recent years that have made DNA analysis possible: the

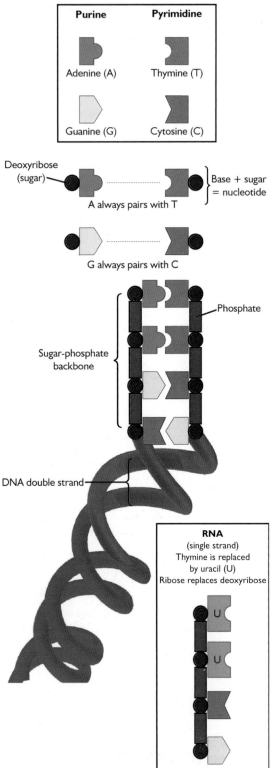

Figure 2.26 Structure of DNA, showing the bases

ability to cut DNA, the ability to sort the resulting fragments and the ability to amplify pieces of DNA. Certain bacteria can produce enzymes that are capable of cutting DNA at specific sites and only at those sites. These enzymes are called restriction endonucleases and the DNA fragments are known as restriction fragments. Different bacteria produce enzymes that cut DNA at different sites. How is this

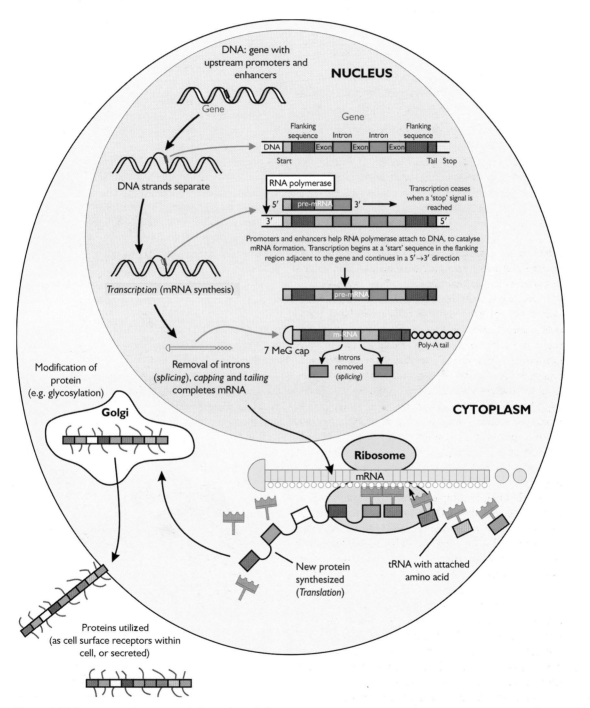

Figure 2.27 Gene expression – transcription and translation

useful in diagnosis? If you consider the sentence below, there are two identical sentences:

> The capacity to blunder slightly is the real
> marvel of DNA, without this special attribute,
> we would still **be**
> anaerobic bacteria and there would **be**
> no music.

> The capacity to blunder slightly **is**
> the real marvel of DNA, without this special
> attribute, we would still be anaerobic bacteria
> and there would be no music.

One has been cut whenever a 'be' appears and the other whenever 'is' appears. You can see that the fragments produced are of different lengths. In the first case, there are three fragments with the smallest composed of 'no music'. In the second case, there are two large fragments. The same principle applies to the endonucleases. Once fragments of different sizes are produced, they are run on an electrophoretic strip, which separates the fragments according to their size, and then 'stained' with a DNA probe.

The details of these electrophoretic methods are not important, suffice it to say that the method used for DNA fragments is called Southern blotting, after its inventor, and the corresponding technique for RNA is Northern blotting. The technique for analysis of proteins is called Western blotting. There is no Eastern blotting!

The binding of the probe to its complementary sequence is called hybridization. The DNA probe or oligonucleotide is a short length of DNA whose nucleotide sequence is known. These are labelled, for example with a radioactive element or fluorescence dye, so that their position on an electrophoretic strip can be identified. Their importance lies in their ability to bind only to a specific section of the patient's DNA, i.e. to a piece with an identical sequence of complementary bases.

This use of restriction endonucleases relies on the enzyme digesting at exactly the point that mutates to cause the disease. Often we do not know the precise mutation responsible for an inherited disease, but it may be possible to identify which section of DNA it is in by comparing the DNA of affected family members with healthy family members. Given that the human genome has approximately 6 billion bases, how do we start looking for differences?

First we can look for restriction fragment length polymorphisms (RFLPs). These are variations in DNA fragment lengths that can be produced by using a restriction endonuclease and probe appropriate for detecting a particular disease. For example, the DNA from family members with Huntington's disease was investigated with an enormous range of enzymes and probes. It was discovered that digestion with an enzyme called *Hin*dIII, combined with hybridization with a probe called G8, identified variations in the short arm of chromosome 4 that segregated with the disease. What is the principle behind this technique? It relies on variations in the genetic code that influence restriction endonuclease digestion but do not cause any clinical problems. We know that a change of just one base causes sickle cell disease, so why do other common mutations have no effect? It is because only about 10 per cent of DNA codes for proteins, while the rest has no clearly defined function. The coding regions (structural genes) are fairly constant from person to person and mutations in these regions generally cause disorders. The non-coding regions can vary from person to person and this diversity is useful for producing the 'DNA fingerprint'.

If a mutation has occurred in a non-coding region that is fairly close to the gene responsible for a disease, then it will be inherited with the disease gene. Obviously, the same mutation must not have occurred near to the normal gene or no difference will be detected. Provided that an enzyme exists which digests at the altered non-coding area, then the disease gene can be tracked. There is the inevitable problem of new mutations or crossover of chromosomal material that might 'unlink' the mutant non-coding region from the disease gene, but this technique is useful for counselling families for future pregnancies after an affected child is born.

So far, we have only mentioned the use of oligonucleotide probes as 'stains' for the altered fragment produced by restriction endonuclease digestion. They can also be used on DNA without digestion to demonstrate deletions that are too small to see on light microscopic chromosomal preparations. Haemophilia A, Duchenne muscular dystrophy, alpha-thalassaemia and some cases of beta-thalassaemia can be detected in this way.

Their most sophisticated use, however, is for 'staining' the gene that causes the disease. Provided that the same genetic change is always responsible for the disease, then this approach can be used without the need for family studies. In sickle cell disease, an oligonucleotide probe has been produced that detects the normal beta-globin gene sequence and another probe detects the mutant sickle gene. Each probe binds only to its specific complementary nucleotide sequence so the 'normal' probe binds to the normal gene, the 'sickle' probe binds to the mutant gene and, in heterozygous people, both probes will bind – one to each chromosome 11. How do the oligonucleotide probe sequences differ? Since we know that sickle cell disease involves a change from GAG to GTG, then the probes must be:

normal probe   xxxxxx CTC xxxxxx
sickle probe   xxxxxx CAC xxxxxx

Polymerase chain reaction

One of the problems of analysing DNA by the means so far described is that a relatively large amount of material is required. An ingenious technique that harnesses DNA's normal role, to act as a template for producing complementary DNA or RNA strands, has been developed. It is called the polymerase chain reaction (PCR) and is without doubt one of the most significant technological advances of the last century. The method involves amplifying a specific segment of DNA through successive rounds of replication (Fig. 2.28). This amplified segment, which must contain the area suspected of containing the mutant code, is then cut with the appropriate restriction enzyme and run on an electrophoretic agarose gel. It is not necessary to use a specific probe to stain the digested fragments because it is the relevant area that has been amplified. Instead, the DNA bands themselves can be viewed under ultraviolet light after staining with ethidium bromide. This is much faster than using autoradiography and can provide a result within 2 days of taking the sample. PCR is also used in forensic work to produce the well-known 'DNA

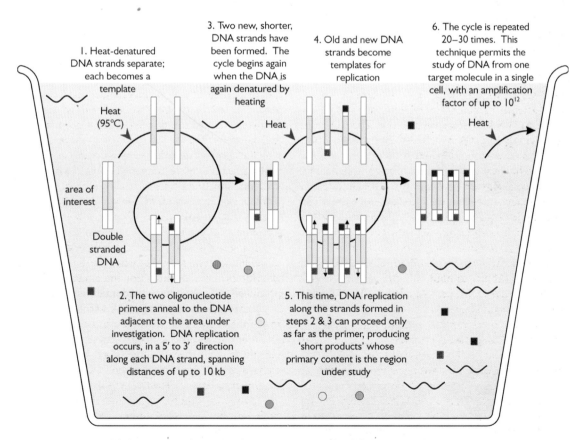

1. Heat-denatured DNA strands separate; each becomes a template

Heat (95°C)

area of interest

Double stranded DNA

2. The two oligonucleotide primers anneal to the DNA adjacent to the area under investigation. DNA replication occurs, in a 5′ to 3′ direction along each DNA strand, spanning distances of up to 10 kb

3. Two new, shorter, DNA strands have been formed. The cycle begins again when the DNA is again denatured by heating

Heat

4. Old and new DNA strands become templates for replication

5. This time, DNA replication along the strands formed in steps 2 & 3 can proceed only as far as the primer, producing 'short products' whose primary content is the region under study

6. The cycle is repeated 20–30 times. This technique permits the study of DNA from one target molecule in a single cell, with an amplification factor of up to 10^{12}

Heat

Medium contains oligonucleotide primers ■ ■ which will flank the area of interest by binding adjacent complementary sequences in the DNA molecule, thermostable DNA polymerase and the four deoxyribonucleoside triphosphates Ⓐ Ⓣ Ⓖ Ⓒ

Figure 2.28 Polymerase chain reaction

fingerprint' from small samples of blood, semen or hair left at the scene of a crime.

WHO SHOULD HAVE THEIR GENES EXAMINED?

It is not difficult to appreciate that a person with a strong family history of a disease may need to be tested. It is not quite that simple though, as one needs to be sure what is meant by a 'positive family history'. One also needs to decide which of the enormous range of diseases are due to a genetic abnormality that can be transmitted to the offspring. This requires careful observation of the incidence of a disease in the general population and within a family group. Many disorders, however, are multifactorial in nature, with both genetic predisposition and environmental agents influencing the outcome.

We will illustrate the importance of family history by considering the example of sickle cell disease.

Sickle cell disease

Patients with this recessive haemoglobin disorder may present clinically with abdominal pain, joint pains, cerebral symptoms, renal failure and cardiac failure, which result from thrombotic and ischaemic damage. This occurs because the red cells 'sickle', thus altering their shape and occluding capillaries. The red cells have an abnormal haemoglobin

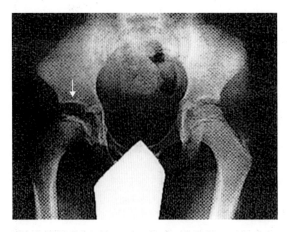

Figure 2.29 Pelvic X-ray showing avascular necrosis of the right femoral head in a patient with sickle cell disease

which, under hypoxic conditions, polymerizes and alters the cell's shape.

In 1949, Linus Pauling analysed the haemoglobin from patients with sickle cell anaemia and discovered that its mobility on electrophoresis differed from that of normal haemoglobin. He called it haemoglobin S (HbS). Later, family studies suggested that the gene for sickle cell haemoglobin was an allele of the normal gene on chromosome 11 for the beta-chain of the haemoglobin molecule, i.e. an alternative gene at the same locus on the chromosome. The difference between the normal haemoglobin gene and the sickle cell gene is a change in one base pair: GAG becomes GTG. This causes valine to replace glutamic acid at position 6 of the beta-chain. That's it – a point mutation changing just one nucleotide leads to the translation of one different amino acid, which entirely changes the property of the protein!

Fortunately, genes are paired and people who are heterozygous (i.e. one normal allele, one sickle cell allele) do not usually have any problems unless they become unusually hypoxic (e.g. at surgical operation). They have a mixture of the normal and abnormal haemoglobin.

For practical purposes, we can regard sickle cell disease as an autosomal recessive disorder. How should we counsel a healthy pregnant woman who has a family history of sickle cell disease? The problem lies in deciding which members of the family are carriers of the gene because two people with sickle cell trait (heterozygotes) are likely to produce one healthy child, one sick child and two carriers (Fig. 2.30).

Carriers of the sickle cell gene can be identified by adding a reducing agent to the blood *in vitro*, which induces the red cells to sickle. More recently, techniques have been developed to analyse the DNA itself. This is particularly useful in prenatal diagnosis for testing the fetus before it has switched on to full production of the beta-chains. It is not possible to detect the abnormal beta-chains in fetal red blood cells because the fetus is relying on

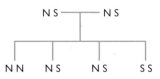

Figure 2.30 Possible outcomes for the offspring of two people with sickle cell trait. N = normal gene; S = sickle cell gene

haemoglobin produced from alpha- and gamma-chains, i.e. HbF. However, it is possible to remove a small piece of placenta (chorionic villus sampling) for DNA analysis, relying on the point mutation to alter the binding of specific oligonucleotide probes or interfere with restriction enzyme digestion as described earlier.

Other haemoglobinopathies

Sickle cell disease is not the only haemoglobinopathy, although it is one of the most common. Haemoglobinopathies can result from an abnormal chain being present or one type of chain not being produced. Haemoglobin is composed of two pairs of (i.e. four) polypeptide chains, each of which is linked to a haem group. The haem group is a protoporphorin molecule chelated with iron and able to carry

oxygen. For the moment, we shall concentrate on the polypeptide chains. The normal chains are called alpha (α), beta (β), gamma (γ) and delta (δ). All normal haemoglobin has one pair of alpha-chains combined with a pair of another type of chain. Hence there is haemoglobin A ($\alpha2\beta2$), haemoglobin A2 ($\alpha2\delta2$) and haemoglobin F ($\alpha2\gamma2$). HbF predominates in the fetus and HbA predominates in the adult.

Besides sickle cell disease, the other major group of haemoglobinopathies are the thalassaemias. In thalassaemias, the chains are normal in structure but not enough are produced. This condition is common in people originating from the Mediterranean, Africa and Asia and is due to a wide variety of underlying genetic changes. The severity of a person's symptoms depends on the chain involved and whether they are homozygous or heterozygous

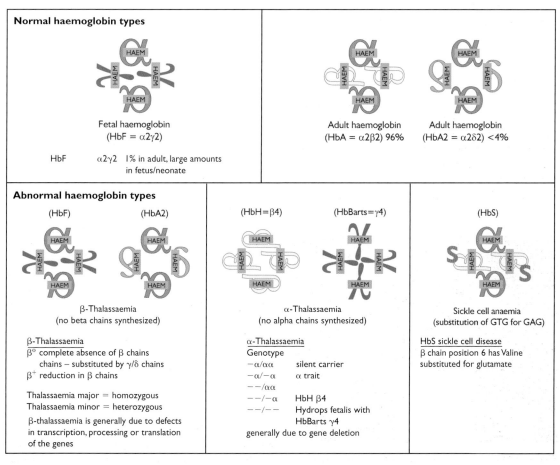

Normal haemoglobin types

Fetal haemoglobin
(HbF = $\alpha2\gamma2$)

HbF $\alpha2\gamma2$ 1% in adult, large amounts in fetus/neonate

Adult haemoglobin
(HbA = $\alpha2\beta2$) 96%

Adult haemoglobin
(HbA2 = $\alpha2\delta2$) <4%

Abnormal haemoglobin types

(HbF)   (HbA2)   (HbH = $\beta4$)   (HbBarts = $\gamma4$)   (HbS)

β-Thalassaemia
(no beta chains synthesized)

α-Thalassaemia
(no alpha chains synthesized)

Sickle cell anaemia
(substitution of GTG for GAG)

β-Thalassaemia
β^{0} complete absence of β chains
   chains – substituted by γ/δ chains
β^{+} reduction in β chains

Thalassaemia major = homozygous
Thalassaemia minor = heterozygous

β-thalassaemia is generally due to defects in transcription, processing or translation of the genes

α-Thalassaemia
Genotype
$-\alpha/\alpha\alpha$ silent carrier
$-\alpha/-\alpha$ α trait
$--/\alpha\alpha$
$--/-\alpha$ HbH $\beta4$
$--/--$ Hydrops fetalis with
   HbBarts $\gamma4$
generally due to gene deletion

HbS sickle cell disease
β chain position 6 has Valine substituted for glutamate

Figure 2.31 Normal and abnormal haemoglobin types

for the abnormality. All normal haemoglobin has alpha-chains so complete absence of alpha-chains is incompatible with life and an affected fetus will be oedematous (hydropic). In the absence of any alpha-chains, the other chains do their best to produce a haemoglobin molecule by combining together as HbBart's (γ4) and HbH (β4). This is the position with deletion of all four genes and, predictably, the severity decreases with the addition of each alpha-chain. This group of conditions is called alpha-thalassaemia.

Since around 95 per cent of adult haemoglobin is HbA, composed of alpha- and beta-chains, the other important disease is beta-thalassaemia, in which beta-chains are absent or reduced and the body attempts to compensate by producing HbA2 and HbF using gamma- and delta-chains respectively.

The main clinical problems in thalassaemia result from haemolysis of the red cells with the abnormal haemoglobin. These cells have a reduced lifespan and are removed in the reticuloendothelial system, particularly in the spleen and marrow. Here the red cell components are broken down for re-use or excretion. The iron is stored in the tissues as ferritin and haemosiderin and, if excessive, can cause tissue damage called haemochromatosis. The protoporphyrins are degraded to produce bile pigments and any excess gives the patient a yellow tinge to their skin and sclerae, i.e. jaundice.

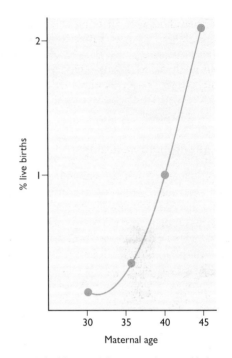

Figure 2.32 Incidence of Down syndrome with increasing maternal age

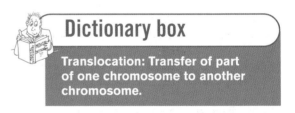

Dictionary box

Translocation: Transfer of part of one chromosome to another chromosome.

Maternal age

Separate from the desirability of testing the genes of people with a strong family history of a particular disease, is the need to consider the increased risk in pregnancies in older women. There is a dramatic increase in the number of chromosomally abnormal fetuses in women over the age of 35 years. This affects a wide variety of disorders with the commonest being trisomy 21 or Down syndrome.

People with Down syndrome are mentally retarded, may have congenital heart disease and an increased incidence of infections and leukaemia. In 1959, Jerome Lejeune and his colleagues showed that these patients have an extra chromosome 21. This most commonly arises because of non-disjunction of chromosome 21 during meiosis in one of the parents, so that either the egg or the sperm carries two copies of chromosome 21.

In about 5 per cent of cases, there is a translocation of chromosome 21 to 14 and occasionally translocations of chromosome 21 to chromosome 22, or 21 to 21.

For Down syndrome, the risk of producing a baby with the syndrome is 10 per cent when the mother is the carrier of the translocation and 2.5 per cent if the father is the carrier. Obviously, it is important to investigate the parents of children with such inherited disorders to look for balanced translocations, although non-disjunction is the commonest cause.

About half of all fetuses affected by Down syndrome do not survive to term. The incidence in live births is 1 in 650; however, that is an average figure for all ages. The risk at maternal age 30 is 1 in 900, which doubles by age 35, stands at 1 in 100 at age 40 and 1 in 40 at age 44. This age distribution makes it sensible to screen women over 35 years by examining chromosomes cultured from amniotic cells and measuring α fetoprotein levels which are *lowered* in Down syndrome. (N.B. they are *raised* in many other abnormalities, e.g. neural tube defects.)

Molecular family planning

With the advent of modern molecular biology techniques combined with *in vitro* fertilization, the potential to 'design' babies has become a reality in the last few years. Several companies have publicized that they can now perform sex selection by means of sperm sorting. Briefly, owing to differences in the nuclear morphology and genetic content of spermatozoids harbouring X or Y chromosomes, they can be sorted by DNA analysis with fluorescence *in situ* hybridization (FISH) and then separated by flow cytometry. Currently, this technique has been widely tested in animals and a specificity of up to 90 per cent has been claimed. Other methods are based on *in vitro* fertilization coupled with biopsy and genetic analysis of the polar body.

In most of the Western countries, sex selection is currently only allowed for medical reasons, such as the prevention of certain (X chromosome-linked) genetic disorders that are serious, untreatable and prematurely fatal (i.e. Duchenne muscular dystrophy or Lesch–Nyhan syndrome or some forms of inherited Alzheimer's disease).

However, since the early 1990s, shortly after the description of these and other techniques for sex preselection, several ethical issues have been raised, not least of which relates to eugenic practices. It is not difficult to envisage that, in the future, a couple could go to their molecular obstetrician and pick out several phenotypic characteristics for their babies, including hair and eye colours, personality and behaviour characteristics. This possibility is likely to cause much debate as technology evolves over the next decade.

As an amusing digression, it is interesting that several disputable methods for 'designing babies' have been publicized. Most of them have no scientific basis. Included in this category are special diets, complicated coital and postcoital practices, as well as the 'Selnas Method', which has received great popularity in Europe. This method requires knowledge of the mother's age, blood group and menstrual history and the proponents claim that using this information it is possible to 'conjure up the dates in the year when intercourse will result in a baby of the couple's choice'. So far, no papers describing the efficacy of these techniques have been reported in peer-reviewed journals.

Family history of cancer

This is covered in detail in Chapters 11 and 12. Where there is a strong family history of cancer, it may be necessary to screen for mutations in specific genes in order to counsel the patients regarding risk to themselves or their family members. Examples include the *BRCA1/2* mutations in breast and ovarian cancer.

The first staggering fact about medical education is that after two and a half years of being taught on the assumption that everyone is the same, the student has to find out for himself that everyone is different, which is really what his experience has taught him since infancy. And the second staggering fact about medical education is that having been taught for two and a half years not to trust any evidence except that based on the measurement of physical science, the student has to find out for himself that all important decisions are in reality made, almost at unconscious level, by that most perfect and complex of computers, the human brain, about which he has as yet learnt almost nothing, and will probably go on learning nothing to the end of his course – this computer which can take in and analyse an incredible number of data in an extremely short time. And the data are mostly not of the hard crude type with which that simple fellow the scientist has to deal, but are of a much more subtle, human and interesting character, each tinted in its own colours of personality and emotion. All this the student has to discover by himself while his teachers strangely pretend to believe that the secrets of medicine are revealed only to those whose biochemical background is beyond reproach.

Sir Robert Platt (1965)

Clinicopathological case study – alcoholic liver disease

Clinical
A 60-year-old man with long-standing history of alcohol abuse presented with a three-week history of general malaise, weight loss, loss of appetite and productive cough.

Examination:
He was noted to be short of breath with an increased respiratory rate and was jaundiced. He had a fever and tachycardia of 110 beats/min. He also had supraclavicular lymphadenopathy and a mildly enlarged and tender liver. Auscultation of his chest revealed coarse crackles over both his lung fields.

Investigations:
The liver function tests were abnormal with a raised bilirubin of 45 μmol/L and a raised γ-GT of 90 IU/L. His chest X-ray showed bilateral consolidation with a small right pleural effusion. A lymph node and liver biopsy were carried out.
   The lymph node showed numerous caseating granulomata with calcification. The Ziehl–Neelson stain showed abundant acid-fast mycobacteria. The liver biopsy showed an acute alcoholic hepatitis with marked fatty change and liver fibrosis, but without cirrhosis.

Management and progress:
He was started on antituberculous therapy and was counselled for his alcohol abuse.
While in hospital, he had a bout of abdominal pain and diarrhoea. Endoscopy showed gastritis but sigmoidoscopy was unremarkable. The rectal biopsy revealed the presence of amyloid in the mucosa. He was discharged on antituberculous therapy and sent for rehabilitation for his alcohol abuse but he defaulted from his appointments and was lost to follow-up.

Pathological
He had a long history of alcohol abuse and this predisposes to many illnesses. Alcoholics tend to be malnourished as they derive most of their calories from alcohol and are therefore deficient in many vitamins, especially the B group. They damage the liver by episodes of hepatitis which heals with scarring, producing fibrosis and eventually cirrhosis. They are also predisposed to infections because of depression of the immune system caused by the alcohol, and, in this man, clinical examination revealed signs of a chest infection. Tuberculosis is a particular problem in alcoholics.

The liver function tests were in keeping with alcoholic damage with raised bilirubin and liver cell enzymes. The chest X-ray confirmed a pneumonic process involving both lungs.

Caseous necrosis with granuloma formation is a classical picture of tuberculosis and special stains revealed the mycobacteria. Immune suppression due to the alcohol abuse is responsible for the reactivation or secondary tuberculosis. In areas of necrosis, calcification is common and this type is called dystrophic calcification. The serum calcium levels are normal as opposed to metastatic calcification in which serum calcium levels are raised.

His liver showed the classical fatty change common in alcohol abuse with some hepatitis, i.e. inflammation of the hepatocytes with liver cell necrosis. The result is healing by scarring with resultant fibrosis. He did not have cirrhosis which is irreversible, unlike fatty change which is.

Alcoholics are predisposed to gastritis, i.e. inflammation of the gastric mucosa. They may also have gastric ulcers. Other complications include oesophageal varices if portal hypertension has developed due to cirrhosis. Patients with long-standing chronic inflammatory diseases such as rheumatoid arthritis and tuberculosis are prone to reactive amyloidosis (AA). Rectal biopsy is a good way of diagnosing amyloid. The amyloid may have been responsible for the diarrhoea but infective causes should be excluded.

Lack of compliance is a common problem with alcoholics.

QUESTIONS

How would you classify the causes of disease?
- Divide into extrinsic and intrinsic and then subdivide as shown in Table 2.1 or use subdivisions that are relevant to your clinical area.

Cell death has two major mechanisms. What are they and how do they differ?
- Apoptosis (programmed cell death) and necrosis. Comparison summary is on page 25.

What are the key cellular events in reversible cell damage?
- Describe the molecular biological and biochemical events and the changes in appearance and function as on page 12, Fig. 1.3.

What is the range of microbiological agents causing disease? Which are the most significant?
- Describe under the categories defined in Tables 2.2, 2.4–2.7. The second part of the question is not answered in this book and will depend on the part of the world and the type of clinical

practice. It is worth looking into your local epidemiology and also remembering that 'significance' is influenced by the severity of any illness produced by the infection and whether it is easily treated.

Which are the most common genetic disorders and how are they transmitted?

♦ Describe about half a dozen disorders that are exemplars of autosomal, sex-linked and chromosomal number problems, such as familial hypercholesterolaemia and adult polycystic kidney disease (AD), cystic fibrosis (AR), red–green colour blindness and X-linked mental retardation (X), Down syndrome and Klinefelter's syndrome (extra chromosomes). Make the point that the commonest (red–green colour blindness) is of little clinical significance and, hence, no survival disadvantage. Also that penetrance varies and disease severity can depend on the number of abnormal gene copies (e.g. haemoglobinopathies) (pages 55–61 and page 65, Fig. 2.31).

FURTHER READING

Gibson, R.M. (2001) Does apoptosis have a role in neuro-degeneration? *British Medical Journal* **322**, 1539–40.

Harding, K.G., Morris, H.L. and Patel, G.K. (2002) Science, medicine, and the future – healing chronic wounds. *British Medical Journal* **324**, 160–3.

Haslett, C. and Savill, J. (2001) Why is apoptosis important to clinicians. *British Medical Journal* **322**, 1499.

Lin, J.-D. (2001) The role of apoptosis in autoimmune thyroid disorders and thyroid cancers. *British Medical Journal* **322**, 1525–7.

Parton, M., Dowsett, M. and Smith, I. (2001) Studies of apoptosis in breast cancer. *British Medical Journal* **322**, 1528–32.

Renehan, A.G., Booth, C. and Potten, C.S. (2001) What is apoptosis and why is it important? *British Medical Journal* **322**, 1536–8.

Scott-Peck, M. (1990) *The Road Less Travelled*. Arrow Books, London.

Sjostrom, J. and Bergh, J. (2001) How apoptosis is regulated, and what goes wrong in cancer. *British Medical Journal* **322**, 1538–9.

Smith, R. (2002) Clinical review – in search of 'non-disease'. *British Medical Journal* **324**, 883–5.

Underwood, J.C.E. (2000) *General and Systematic Pathology*, 3rd edition. Churchill Livingstone, London.

PART 2
Defence Against Disease

Introduction: The role of epidemiology in disease

Defence against disease is essentially the art of survival. It is not only a response to a dangerous microbe, but also about ensuring that the body is kept healthy with the right supply of nutrients and avoidance of toxic agents. Malnutrition is a disease that we defend against by eating a balanced diet. As we learn more about the factors influencing cardiovascular atheroma formation and some gastrointestinal tumours, we could include diet as one of the defences against cancer and heart attacks. Putting suntan lotion and a hat on will reduce the risk of sun-induced skin cancers. Having warm clothes and shelter will prevent hypothermia in cold climates.

You will appreciate that defence against disease goes beyond merely considering the tissue defences protecting us from microbes. However, much of the contribution of medicine to improving people's health over the last century has been due to advances in understanding and treating infections, so we will devote this section to that topic. Later sections discuss both the causes and defences involved in cardiovascular disease and cancer.

We have learned already about how disease can come about. Obviously the body has defence mechanisms tailored to deal with many of the insults we have discussed in Part 1. Before we even consider these though we should appreciate the great contribution made in the 1800s by Dr John Snow in identifying the role of water in spreading disease. His work led to one of the first environmental measures taken to prevent the spread of infection. Since then, epidemiological studies have identified the causative agents responsible for many diseases.

JOHN SNOW AND THE BROAD STREET PUMP

It would be quite possible to go through the entire medical curriculum without ever hearing the name of John Snow (1813–1858). He was a man of simple habits and seemed to lack the charisma that is vital in attracting attention on the world stage. Yet his contributions to medicine were certainly 'world class'. If you think that epidemiological studies might be dull, Snow's biography is well worth a read. It demonstrates eloquently how such studies can have a truly dramatic impact on public health. Snow is

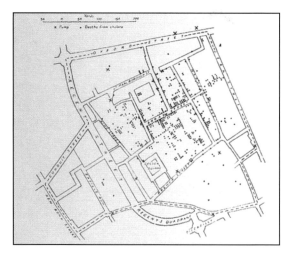

Figure 1 Deaths from cholera (*) in Broad Street, Golden Square, London, and the neighbourhood, 19 August to 30 September 1854. Water pumps are denoted by an x (Courtesy of the Wellcome Institute for the History of Medicine)

perhaps best remembered for having anaesthetized Queen Victoria in 1853 and 1857, giving credibility to the use of pain relief during childbirth! But it is his contribution to the understanding of cholera that is relevant here.

Snow's link with cholera evolved over a number of years. His first encounter with the disease was in Newcastle-upon-Tyne during the epidemic of 1831–1832, when he had just started his medical training. It was during the next cholera epidemic of 1848–1849 that he made his seminal contribution. By now Snow was in London and here he began to unravel the mode of transmission of the disease. Snow's work was a masterpiece in epidemiological investigation. He meticulously mapped the houses in which new cases of cholera were being diagnosed and observed a marked difference in the incidence and mortality of cholera in the south of London (8 deaths per 1000 inhabitants) compared with other areas (1–4 deaths per 100 inhabitants). This led him to hypothesize that cholera was spread by water. He identified the public pumps from which the families living in the affected and unaffected areas drew their water. He noticed that there were surprising sites of sparing within otherwise heavily affected areas. His suspicion that the infection was in the water supply grew when he found that those living in the spared areas worked at a local brewery and received free beer, which was made with water from a source away from that supplying their homes. Even before the identification of bacteria, he postulated that the transmission was the result of a living organism that had the ability to multiply and that social conditions and hygiene were of paramount importance in the spread of infection. Although there was no medical treatment for cholera, it became apparent that the way to stop an epidemic was through good sanitation and good hygiene. Snow urged that the handle be removed from the pump that supplied contaminated water in Broad Street in London during the epidemic of 1854. This led to a dramatic decrease in new cases in the area.

It follows from this that our first line of defence against infection is the prevention of the multiplication and spread of organisms. Open sewers, overcrowded living conditions, contaminated drinking water, poor food storage and preparation, inadequate personal hygiene and unprotected sexual contact are a recipe for disaster. This is not a text on public health medicine or politics, so we will not dwell on these points. But remember that each year in Asia, Africa and Latin America, between four and six million people die from diarrhoea and over a million die from malaria. One-third of the world's population is subclinically infected with tuberculosis and three million die from TB each year; 12 million people are infected with HIV world-wide. All these problems are more likely to be solved by engineers and politicians than by the latest advances in molecular biology!

CHAPTER 3

The body's response to disease

MAJOR ROUTES FOR THE TRANSMISSION OF INFECTION

Infections start from a reservoir of some kind, which acts as a source of pathogens. The commonest source of human infections is infected humans, although some diseases involve animal reservoirs or soil organisms.

It is not difficult to work out the main routes of spread from one infected human to another. Bugs in one person's respiratory tract are coughed out as aerosols, become air-borne and are inhaled by other people. A simple bus journey is laden with opportunities for bacteria and viruses to visit new human hosts. Direct mucosal contact is important in sexually transmitted diseases (HIV, herpes simplex, hepatitis B, papilloma virus, chlamydia, gonorrhoea and syphilis) and viruses infecting salivary glands (herpes and mumps).

Gut pathogens are excreted in the faeces and can re-enter the same or another gut via faecal contamination of water or food (faeco-oral route). Contamination of food generally results either from lack of human hand-washing or from failing to cover food to protect it from flies.

Then there is a much more sinister group of arthropods than the simple fly with dirty feet. These are insects that are themselves infected with an organism which they transfer by injection into humans (for example malaria and yellow fever). This is one means by which blood-borne spread can occur. An insect sucks up infected blood from a human or animal and transfers it to another human or animal when it next bites. In some instances (e.g. malaria) the insect is an essential component because part of the infective agent's life cycle takes place within its body. Humans traditionally fear rats, possibly because of their historical links with bubonic plague. But, like flies, they are relatively innocent,

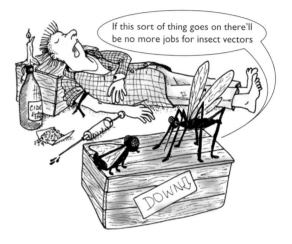

If this sort of thing goes on there'll be no more jobs for insect vectors

being mere vehicles for the ticks that live on their bodies and that carry the bug (*Yersinisa pestis*) to the human. Comparable methods of spread are via hypodermic needles shared by drug addicts (e.g. hepatitis B) or through use of contaminated blood products (e.g. HIV and hepatitis C in haemophiliacs).

Before we consider how the body can respond to disease we should consider its natural defences. For practical purposes, the defences of the body can be separated into three components: structural barriers, innate immunity and adaptive immunity. This is a rather artificial separation. As we will see, these three components are intimately linked and act together in many instances to protect the body. Let us start with the structural barriers.

WHAT ARE THE BODY'S NATURAL DEFENCES AGAINST INFECTION?

The body is covered by epithelium, inside and out. The skin, with its stratified squamous epithelium topped with a waterproof layer of keratin, covers the outside. However, it contains some large holes, leading to areas covered by more permeable epithelium. From the top down these are the eyes, nasal cavity, mouth, anus, urethra and vagina – and each one has its own defence system.

The eye drops its portcullis and floods the moat at the slightest provocation, determined to repel invaders before they can produce any tissue damage. Because the main parts of the eye must be transparent and able to transmit light without distortion, a scarred cornea can render the eye useless. Anything worse than a little inflammation of the conjunctiva can be devastating. Therefore the eye's defences include a nerve reflex to close the eyelids as danger approaches, and a lacrimal gland to secrete tears to wash away particles, chemicals and bugs in a matter of seconds. In addition, tears contain lysozyme, an enzyme capable of degrading bacterial cell walls. If you have ever had even the smallest scratch to the surface of your eye, you will know that the flow of tears and the desire to close the eyelids keeps going until the epithelial covering is re-established. Fortunately this generally takes less than 24 hours.

The nose can be considered with the respiratory tract, since both are covered predominantly by respiratory epithelium. This is characterized by the presence of mucus-secreting cells and cilia. Cilia are tiny hair-like structures that beat in a synchronous fashion to move particles up the respiratory tract. A layer of mucus lines the respiratory tract, providing a barrier against infectious agents and trapping inhaled particles. The mucous layer acts as a conveyor belt propelled by the underlying cilia. This is the mucociliary clearance mechanism and it is severely damaged by smoking. The airways also have a nervous mechanism of defence in coughs and sneezes, which forcefully expel unwanted material. This is good for the individual but potentially hazardous for those in the vicinity, as it is a super method of spread for airborne bugs. If microbes get past the mucociliary defence, there is a second line of defence involving the macrophages in the alveoli; often termed the sentries of the lung.

The mouth and anus form the ends of the gastrointestinal tract and both are protected by non-keratinizing stratified squamous epithelium and a layer of mucus from local glands. The mouth has teeth and an enzyme (amylase) both of which, it could be argued, have a defensive role but their main purpose is clearly related to digestion. There are similar dual-purpose roles for the hydrochloric acid and enzymes in the stomach or the secretions of the small intestine; their main role is digestive but they may also be harmful to many microorganisms. The gut, like the respiratory tract, has a layer of protective mucus. Immunoglobulins are specifically made for the lining of the gut and disable many bacteria and other organisms ingested with food. The gut, of course, is not sterile. It is colonized by a range of bugs that often live in peaceful coexistence unless something upsets the balance. This commonly occurs when a course of antibiotics destroys one type of bacterium, so allowing another to over-proliferate and cause problems, so-called antibiotic-associated or pseudomembranous colitis. *Clostridium difficile* is a bacterium that proliferates under these circumstances and secretes a toxin to produce bloody diarrhoea.

The urinary tract is normally protected by a one-way flow of urine from kidney to urethra, along tubes lined by a multilayered transitional epithelium. There is no mucus barrier here but it should not be needed, as the urine formed in the kidney is sterile. Its defences are the high volume of urine flushing the system, the physical barrier of the empty urethra and the natural variation of the pH of the urine. Women have a short urethra and are more prone than men to urinary tract infections, which often occur after sexual activity. This can cause perineal bacteria to be massaged up the urethra into the bladder ('honeymoon cystitis'). The urine may have an acidic or alkaline pH, favouring the growth of some bacterial strains over others. Hopefully, the natural variation in the urinary pH will prevent a particular bacterium from becoming established and proliferating. Diabetics can have particular problems if the urine contains glucose, which will nourish bacterial growth.

The genital tract of the female starts its defences with the vagina, which is lined by non-keratinizing stratified squamous epithelium and mucus and friendly colonies of Doderlein's bacillus, a lactobacillus that metabolizes glycogen to lactic acid to produce a pH of 5, which inhibits colonization by most other bacteria. Unfortunately, glycogen is only present when the vaginal epithelium is stimulated by oestrogens, between puberty and the menopause. At other ages, the vagina is alkaline and liable to infection with pathogenic staphylococci and streptococci. The main defence, however, is the mucus, lysozyme and ciliary action in the normal cervix. The uterus and tubes are specialized for their reproductive roles but it is possible that the monthly shedding of the endometrium may be a useful defence against

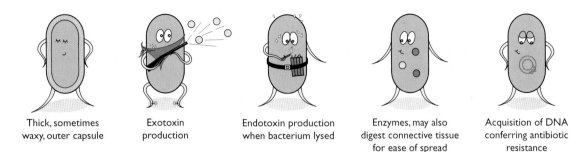

| Thick, sometimes waxy, outer capsule | Exotoxin production | Endotoxin production when bacterium lysed | Enzymes, may also digest connective tissue for ease of spread | Acquisition of DNA conferring antibiotic resistance |

Figure 3.1 Bacterial protection against attack

infection. The stereocilia in the Fallopian tubes, while wafting the ovum down, produce currents that may help to prevent bacteria from ascending.

Should the first line of defences fail, the body has a regular guard of armed and dangerous cells and molecules, whose brief is to resist attack (innate immunity). This army comes swiftly to the defence within seconds and minutes of damage occurring.

The innate immunity guard consists of neutrophil polymorphs and macrophages, which immobilize and engulf damaging agents, complement proteins, which attract inflammatory cells to the site of damage, molecules related to blood clotting and factors released from a variety of cells that assist in the inflammatory response. We will hear more of these when we come to discuss acute inflammation in Chapter 4.

Because bugs sometimes manage to break through the first and second line defences, we need another line of defence involving the inflammatory response and the immune system, so-called adaptive immunity. These are specific defences, which take time to develop, but because they are targeted specifically at the causative agent they generally cause less in the way of 'collateral damage' as they exert their effect than the innate defence mechanisms. T and B cells work to produce agents specifically against particular intruders. There are exceptions though (see tuberculosis later!).

HOW DO MICROORGANISMS EVADE OUR DEFENCES?

Entry through intact skin is most easily achieved if there is an animal vector designed for the purpose. Many microorganisms associate with biting insects that pierce human skin and so provide a route into the human body. The rabies virus relies on larger animals such as infected dogs or bats to bite humans and then on its acetylcholine-binding receptor to enter a neuronal cell. HIV, once in the blood (e.g. on a contaminated needle), binds helper T cells via the CD4 receptor, which binds to gp120 antigen on the viral surface. In these examples, the microorganism itself does not have special characteristics for skin penetration but some, such as the helminth larvae of hookworm or schistosoma, have lytic proteases to allow them to digest and burrow through intact skin.

Some viruses start out with a 'key to the door' in that they have receptors that bind specific molecules on the host cell surface, which allow them to gain entry. A good example of this is the rhinovirus, which binds ICAM-1 on mucosal cells.

Protective coverings, as in bacterial spores, protozoan cysts and thick-walled helminth eggs, can evade the digestive tract's acid and enzymes. Some parasites' eggs (e.g. *Giardia*) actually need stomach acid as a stimulus to cause them to hatch into the trophozoites that infect the intestine. Many of the non-enveloped viruses (hepatitis A, rotavirus, reovirus and Norwalk agents) are resistant to digestive juices and bacteria can 'hide' in food to avoid the acidity. *Helicobacter pylori* is the only pathogen that survives in the stomach acid. It does this by producing a urease that converts urea to ammonia and, thereby, changes the pH of its microenvironment.

The respiratory tract's mucociliary defence may be impaired by the host's own actions if they smoke or aspirate stomach acid. Neuraminidase-producing microorganisms may degrade the mucin layer and toxins produced by *Haemophilus* and *Bordetella* can paralyse mucosal cilia. Even if the mucociliary mechanisms are working well, some viruses can still avoid being expelled by having specific methods for adhesion to the epithelial surface, such as haemagglutinins on influenzavirus. Once the defences are damaged, for example by a bad cold or flu, bacterial pneumonias are common.

Many microorganisms avoid our second line of defences by not attempting to pass through the epithelial surface but being content to grow on the top. Skin fungi (dermatophytes, e.g. candida) and skin viruses (the papillomaviruses causing warts) live in the superficial layers. Gut pathogens, such as *Vibrio cholera*, multiply in the mucus layer releasing exotoxins that cause watery diarrhoea. Some bacteria cause us harm without even entering the body if they produce exotoxins that contaminate food (e.g. staphylococci) (see Fig. 3.1).

So the first line of defence has been breached, but the immune system and inflammatory mechanisms should still be able to defend us, shouldn't they? Thankfully, they normally do but the microbes have some clever tricks to avoid them.

First, the immune system must spot the invader, but the invaders change their surface antigens by shedding the antigens, changing the antigens during an infection or having numerous antigenic variants, so that infective episodes do not produce useful immune memory. The next phase is to kill the bugs by phagocytosis, complement-mediated lysis, antibody-mediated mechanisms or neutrophil activity. Yes, you've guessed. Somewhere there is a bug that will have evolved a way round each of these and a few examples are given in Table 3.1.

By now you will have realized that in any war a lot of innocent bystanders get hurt. The bugs need to survive, replicate and be shed to find new hosts. The normal flora or commensals manage this without causing damage but the pathogens are greedy, have more weapons and provoke a conflict with the inflammatory and immune cells. Damage to the host cells occurs because of competition for nutrients, release of inflammatory mediators and toxic substances by the host's inflammatory cells, production of substances by the microbes that damage the host's tissues and direct cellular damage by bugs.

Table 3.1 Mechanisms used by microbes to evade the immune system

Mechanism	Example
Shedding of antigens	Schistosoma mansoni
Changing antigens during infection	*Neisseria* altering pilins African trypanosomiasis
Many antigenic variants so no protective cross-immunity	Rhinovirus Influenza virus
Resistance to phagocytosis	Carbohydrate capsules of *Pneumococcus*, *Meningococcus* and *Haemophilus*
Interference with antibodies or complement	Protein A molecules of *Staphylococcus* blocking Fc portion of immunoglobulin Digestion by proteases of *Neisseria*, *Streptococcus* and *Haemophilus*
Resistance to complement-mediated lysis	K antigens on some *E. coli*
Resistance to macrophage killing	*Legionella*, *Mycobacterium* and *Toxoplasma* inhibit acidification
Inaccessible to immune system	Gut luminal proliferation of *Clostridium difficile* Papillomavirus or fungi in superficial layer of skin Direct viral transfer between adjacent cells
Specific damage to immune cells	*Pseudomonas* secretes a leucotoxin to kill neutrophils
Mimicry of host antigens	Group A streptococci and myocardium
Interference with MHC presentation of antigens	Herpes simplex inhibits peptide transporter CMV blocks MHC I presentation and expresses MHC I mimic
Bind to and inhibit cytokines	Vaccinia virus produces soluble interferon receptor
Immunosuppression	HIV, Epstein–Barr virus

ARE SOME PEOPLE MORE SUSCEPTIBLE TO INFECTION THAN OTHERS?

Let us consider a normal healthy individual; this person is not malnourished, not on immunosuppressive drugs nor just recovering from an operation. From a bug's point of view, what are the possible routes into the body? The surface of the body is covered by skin which, as we have discussed, has holes in it. Most of the holes lead down into sweat ducts, hair shafts and other skin appendage structures that still have an epithelial lining, albeit a more delicate one. Bugs can live down these holes without causing particular problems unless the environment is upset by something that disturbs the delicate balance between host and bug. This occurs, for example, in scarring acne when the composition of the sebaceous gland secretion is altered, leading to blockage of the neck of a hair follicle, proliferation of bacteria behind the blockage, and the destruction of the follicle's epithelial line of defence to provoke inflammation in the surrounding skin.

In fact, skin is built to take knocks and we are all liable to develop small cuts and grazes on a frequent basis. We know that when this defence is down we must be extra vigilant and keep the area clean and dry and do what mother says and resist picking at the delicate protective layer of scab that forms at the site of damage. This becomes even more important when the skin contains a large wound, as may follow a surgical operation. This is the time when

bacteria have a really good chance of successfully invading a human body, because they have a band of helpers. These are the doctors and medical students who move rapidly from one patient to the next in the post-op surgical wards, generously ensuring that all patients have the opportunity to acquire each other's skin flora.

> Since the antiseptic treatment has been brought into the full operation, and wounds and abscesses no longer poison the atmosphere with putrid exhalations, my wards, though in other respects under precisely the same circumstances as before, have completely changed their character: so that during the last nine months not a single instance of pyaemia, hospital gangrene or erysipelas has occurred in them. As there appears to be no doubt regarding the cause of this change, the importance of the fact can hardly be exaggerated
>
> *Joseph, Lord Lister (1827–1912)*
> *British surgeon*

The combination of overcrowding (i.e. many sick people living in a closed environment), difficulty with personal hygiene (just try having a bed bath!) and unprotected (non-sexual!) contact with a large number of strangers describes both a post-op surgical ward and a bacterium's idea of heaven. Add to this the likelihood of acquiring a bacterium which has been around in hospital for a while, and has learned a few tricks in terms of antibiotic resistance (see later) and an already weakened patient can have a big problem.

Diabetics are particularly prone to skin infections because, if their blood glucose levels are hard to control, all their body fluids can be high in glucose, and this provides an excellent culture medium for bacteria. Often diabetics have poor circulation due to vascular disease so bacteria can flourish relatively undisturbed by any immune response. The problem may be compounded by traumatic damage to the skin if they also have a loss of sensation due to diabetes-induced peripheral nerve damage, meaning that they might not feel, for example, the early stages of blisters or small abrasions.

Often the body's resistance mechanisms to bacterial infections must be assisted by the use of antibiotics. See Fig. 3.2 for the main mechanisms involved.

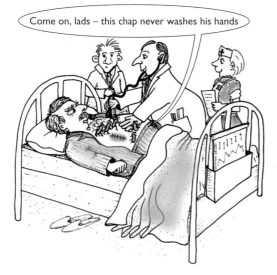

Come on, lads – this chap never washes his hands

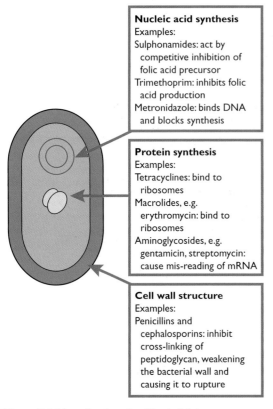

Nucleic acid synthesis
Examples:
Sulphonamides: act by
competitive inhibition of
folic acid precursor
Trimethoprim: inhibits folic
acid production
Metronidazole: binds DNA
and blocks synthesis

Protein synthesis
Examples:
Tetracyclines: bind to
ribosomes
Macrolides, e.g.
erythromycin: bind to
ribosomes
Aminoglycosides, e.g.
gentamicin, streptomycin:
cause mis-reading of mRNA

Cell wall structure
Examples:
Penicillins and
cephalosporins: inhibit
cross-linking of
peptidoglycan, weakening
the bacterial wall and
causing it to rupture

Figure 3.2 Sites of action of antibacterial drugs

ANTIBIOTIC RESISTANCE

Since the discovery of penicillin and sulphonamides in the first half of the twentieth century we have been able to treat many bacterial infections. However, superbugs have begun to emerge, resistant to many antibiotics. The first reports are now emerging of a strain of MRSA (methicillin-resistant *Staphylococcus aureus*), which is resistant to all known antibiotics. Drug-resistant tuberculosis is increasingly a problem. We know that the same genes encoding the various resistance factors can be found in several unrelated classes of bacteria. How do the bugs transmit resistance to each other?

It is now realized that spread of resistance involves the transfer of genes. This can be achieved in four main ways: transformation, transduction, conjugation and transposon insertion.

Transformation

Naked DNA fragments are released from a bacterium as it is lysed. These fragments then bind to

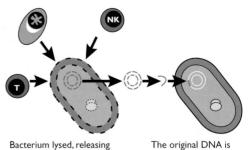

Bacterium lysed, releasing
DNA fragments, which bind
to a closely related bacterium

The original DNA is
endocytosed and incorporated
into the new bacterial DNA

Figure 3.3 Transformation

the cell wall of another bacterium, are taken in and become incorporated into the recipient's DNA. This sounds simple, but it generally only occurs between closely related bacteria with similar DNA (i.e. extensive homology) and suitable binding sites on the cell wall.

Transduction

Bacteria themselves can be infected by viruses, called bacteriophages. These viruses bind to specific receptors on the bacterial surface and then push a tube through the wall and inject the viral nucleic acid. The virus (bacteriophage) can take over the bacterial cell's replication mechanism in the same way as viruses replicate in human cells. New capsid proteins, nucleic acid and enzymes are produced and assembled so that, when the bacterial cell lyses, the phages are released. This is what happens with virulent phages, but there are also temperate phages that can insert their DNA into the host's DNA and lie dormant for long periods. Eventually these little time bombs go off; they can then replicate and lyse the host cell in similar fashion to virulent phages, but the fact that they have inserted into the bacteria's DNA is relevant to our discussion of transfer of resistance.

Generalized transduction involves virulent phages taking over the bacterial cell and accidentally packaging some bacterial DNA fragments instead of viral nucleic acid into one of the daughter phages. The mutant daughter phage will inject this bacterial DNA into the next cell it tries to infect and the bacterial DNA may incorporate into the host cell DNA (comparable to the changes in transformation). The host cell survives happily because no viral nucleic acid is

A **virulent phage** injects its DNA into a bacterium and utilizes the bacterial replication equipment to form further phage particles

The bacterial DNA becomes fragmented and a portion may be incorporated into newly formed phages, which are released as the bacterium lyses

A **temperate phage** injects its DNA into a bacterium; this becomes incorporated into the bacterial DNA and remains there until a stimulus to reproduce is received

Then the phage DNA is translated and often accidentally incorporates some of the adjacent bacterial DNA within the genome of the new phages, due to inaccurate splicing. The bacterium disintegrates as the phages are released

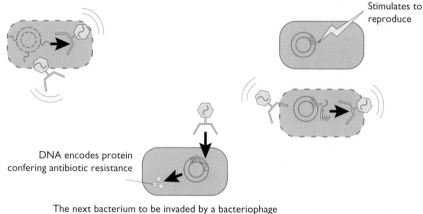

Stimulates to reproduce

DNA encodes protein confering antibiotic resistance

The next bacterium to be invaded by a bacteriophage receives DNA from another bacterium. If it is lucky, this will confer on it an advantage, such as antibiotic resistance

Figure 3.4 Transduction: bacterial DNA is transmitted via bacteriophages, of which there are two main types – virulent and temperate phages

injected and it may gain useful resistance or virulence factors, depending on the source of the fragment of bacterial DNA.

Specialized transduction utilizes temperate phages. When the phage DNA in the host genome (prophage) is reactivated, it is spliced out of the bacterial chromosome, replicated, translated and packaged into a capsid. The splicing may include taking some bacterial DNA immediately adjacent to the prophage and this will be incorporated into daughter phages. If the bacterial DNA confers resistance or virulence, this is a powerful method for sharing the information and it is called lysogenic conversion. The genes for exotoxin production by *Corynebacterium diphtheriae*, *Vibrio cholerae* and *Streptococcus pyogenes* (scarlet fever) can spread in this way.

Conjugation

Conjugation is the major mechanism for transfer of antibiotic resistance and involves the exchange of plasmids. Plasmids are pieces of circular, double-stranded DNA separate from the chromosome that carry a variety of genes, including some for drug resistance and some coding for the enzymes and proteins needed for conjugation. These are called self-transmissible or F plasmids and bacteria can be F^+ or F^-, depending on whether they contain the plasmid.

Bacterial sex involves a specialized sex pilus protruding from the surface of an F^+ bacterium. This binds to and penetrates the cell membrane of an F^- bacterium and a single strand of the F plasmid DNA passes from one cell to the other.

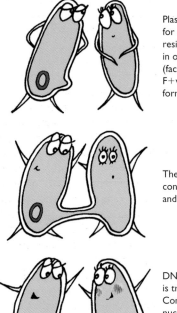

Plasmid determining, for example, penicillin resistance, is present in one bacterium (factor positive, F+ve). A sex pilus forms in the F+ve cell

The sex pilus connects the F+ve and F−ve bacteria

DNA from the plasmid is transferred. Complementary nucleotides are added, forming a complete plasmid in each bacterium

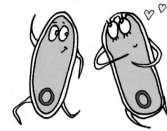

Both bacteria are now F+ve

Figure 3.5 Bacterial conjugation

The former F⁻ cell is now F⁺ and has the information for resistance and for conjugation with other cells. The plasmid DNA is not totally fixed but can acquire additional bacterial genes if it integrates into the bacterial chromosome in a similar fashion to a temperate bacteriophage, i.e. when it is spliced out of the host chromosome it includes some of the adjacent bacterial DNA and is called an **F prime** (F′) plasmid. An alternative is that the bacterial chromosome with the incorporated plasmid is all transferred to the F⁻ cell during conjugation.

Plasmids encode medically important enzymes, such as penicillinase, and virulence factors, such as exotoxin and fimbriae.

Transposons

Transposons are also DNA fragments that can carry genes for resistance and virulence, but differ in that they can insert into host DNA which is dissimilar (i.e. lacks homology) and so can spread resistance across bacterial genera. They can insert into phages, plasmids and bacterial DNA.

HOW CAN WE PREVENT OR OVERCOME BACTERIAL RESISTANCE?

Life is a struggle for survival, and the animal, plant or microorganism best adapted to a particular environment is most likely to flourish. Humans can have an enormous impact on the environment, and we must use this ability with care. In this context, we are concerned that we might alter the microbes' environment

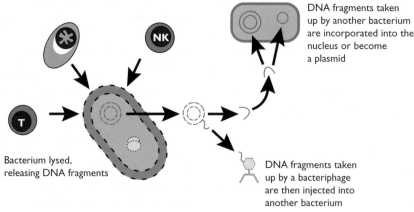

DNA fragments taken up by another bacterium are incorporated into the nucleus or become a plasmid

Bacterium lysed, releasing DNA fragments

DNA fragments taken up by a bacteriphage are then injected into another bacterium

Figure 3.6 Transposon insertion

in such a way as to give the resistant bacteria a survival advantage. If everyone was taking a particular antibiotic, only microbes resistant to that drug would survive and so that specific environmental niche would become populated with resistant bugs and the antibiotic would be useless. This is the fear with tuberculosis as the incidence of dormant multiple drug-resistant tuberculosis increases. Of course, we don't have everyone on the same antibiotic and we have to hope that the non-resistant bugs will predominate when the antibiotic is stopped.

Problems occur when antibiotics are widely used, particularly in a hospital setting, and the resistant bug gains a clear advantage. We shall consider methicillin-resistant *Staphylococcus aureus* (MRSA) as an important example of how man and microbe each develop strategies to defy the other. *Staphlococcus aureus* is a Gram-positive coccus that was originally sensitive to penicillin. By the 1950s, the bug had developed enzymes (β-lactamases) to destroy penicillin. Man then produced a penicillin analogue called methicillin, with a side chain that reduced lactamase binding to the enzyme. Further drug development led to the widely used flucloxacillin, so humans had the upper hand until the late 1970s and early 1980s, until *Staph. aureus* strains resistant to multiple antibiotics, including methicillin and gentamycin, emerged.

These bugs are an enormous problem in hospitals, particularly on surgical wards where wound infections are a major concern. The only effective drug against such staphlococci is vancomycin which is somewhat toxic and requires intravenous administration. The recent identification of vancomycin-resistant enterococci in a patient with MRSA sets the scene for a nightmare scenario in which resistance to vancomycin is transferred from the enterococci to the MRSA, both of which may be found in the gut or surgical wounds. The truly 'superbug' MRSA produced would then be unstoppable. It is just a matter of time before this happens, and nothing we have done with antibiotics suggests that we could contain such an event!

There are four main strategies for trying to avoid or overcome bacterial resistance:

- the control of antibiotic use
- the modification of existing antibiotics
- development of new antibiotics capable of bypassing the bacterium's method of resistance
- the use of combinations of antibiotics employing different mechanisms.

The best approach is preventative. If antibiotics are used less and are only used appropriately, then resistant strains are less likely to evolve. There should be great caution about the use of antibiotics as growth promoters in animal feeds; this could result in resistant bugs that may be transferred to humans. In humans, antibiotics should not be used unnecessarily and care should be taken to avoid incomplete treatment. Incomplete treatment is a particular problem in tuberculosis, where lengthy treatment with multiple drugs may be necessary to eradicate the organisms, but patient compliance may be poor. Incomplete treatment will allow the most resistant bug to survive, regrow and spread to other susceptible individuals. Multiple drug-resistant TB strains now represent more than 20 per cent of cases in some areas of New York, and are now being found in Europe and the UK.

Common sense also demands that, particularly in hospitals, transfer of bugs from one patient to another must be minimized. This requires special attention to the disinfection of endoscopes, bronchoscopes, etc. which cannot be autoclaved.

The second strategy involves the modification of existing drugs. The idea is that once the mechanism for bacterial resistance is understood, it should be possible to redesign the molecule to get around the problem. We have already mentioned the example of methicillin with its side chain to prevent it from binding to the enzyme β-lactamase. Another example involves the tetracyclines. These have little effect on certain bugs that have developed a highly efficient mechanism for excreting the drug from the bacterial cell through specific 'efflux proteins'. A new group of tetracyclines called glycylcyclines have an altered side chain that prevents their excretion via efflux proteins.

Thirdly, unusual sources of new antibiotics are being investigated. For example a peptide called crocodillin has been identified in crocodile blood that prevents the creatures from developing wound infections after fighting with other crocs.

The fourth approach to bacterial resistance is to use combinations of antibiotics. Sometimes the combinations have been developed empirically, but some have been specifically designed to overcome resistance. This is the case with clavulanic acid, which is only a weak antibiotic but binds irreversibly to many β-lactamases and can thus protect β-lactam antibiotics from destruction. This is used clinically as Augmentin, which is a combination of amoxycillin and clavulanic acid.

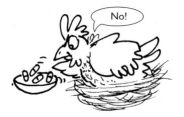

Caution should be exercised in the use of antibiotics in animal feeds

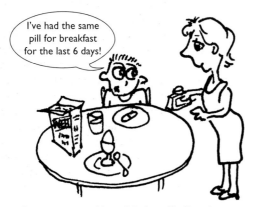

Incomplete treatment with antibiotics will allow the most resistant bugs to survive and spread

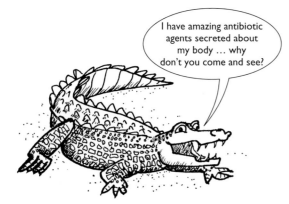

Seek new antibiotics in unusual places e.g. Crocodillins

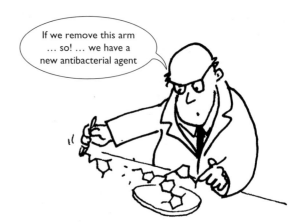

Bacterial resistance can be countered by the development of new drugs or the modification of existing ones

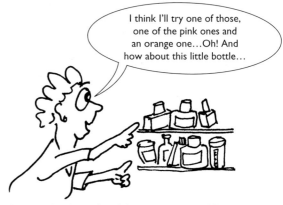

Use combinations of antibiotics employing different mechanisms of action

Figure 3.7 Mechanisms of overcoming or avoiding the development of antibiotic resistance

HOW DO VIRUSES DEVELOP RESISTANCE TO ANTIVIRAL AGENTS?

Viruses can also become resistant to antiviral agents through the selection of naturally occurring mutants, which have amino acid changes at the active site or binding site of the antiviral agent. This is only normally seen in immunocompromised hosts where the number of viral particles (viral load) is high, thus increasing the chances of a natural mutant occurring. Viruses have small genomes (HIV = 9 kb; herpes = 500 kb; bacteria = 3 Mb; human = 4000 Mb), so the chance of a mutant occurring is dependent on the number of virions and the size of the genome. HIV is a good example of this both in terms of drug resistance and immune evasion.

The first part of HIV replication is the conversion of its RNA genome into DNA prior to integration into the host cell chromosome as proviral DNA. This reaction is unique to retroviruses and is mediated by the virally encoded RNA-dependent DNA polymerase reverse transcriptase (RT). RT is the target for the antiviral AZT drug used in the treatment of AIDS. AZT is an analogue of thymidine with an azide group at the 3′ OH group of the ribose moeity. When incorporated into DNA by RT, AZT causes chain termination and stops DNA synthesis and halts the viral life cycle. Fortunately, AZT has higher affinity for RT than for cell-encoded DNA polymerases, hence its selective toxicity. AZT-resistant HIV mutants have amino acid substitutions in the active site, so AZT no longer binds. The RT of HIV does not possess any of the proofreading activity seen in cellular DNA polymerases, and has an error rate of 10^{-4} (i.e. it makes a mistake every 10 000 bases which is about once every time a genome is copied). Thus, if 10^8 virions were made, there would be a chance for each base to be changed in the viral progeny (genome size = 9000 bases).

During HIV infection, about 10^9 virions are made and destroyed by the immune system every day, so it is easy to see that a random mutation in the active site of RT is highly likely. Use of AZT selects out the resistant mutant, which continues to replicate and spread within the body; thus, AZT resistance can emerge readily in a few months or less. Combined anti-HIV chemotherapy is now used that includes several anti-RT compounds and a protease inhibitor, because it is much less likely that any one virus will acquire mutations in two or three separate sites to affect the binding and activity of all of the inhibitors.

HIV also uses this natural mutation rate to its advantage to change the amino acid sequences of its exterior glycoprotein (gp120), which binds the cell CD4 receptor. The V3 region of gp120 shows epitope changes in isolates from the same patient infected with HIV, and these have been shown to permit escape from a cytotoxic T cell immune response. Thus, RT error rate provides a mechanism for generating immune escape mutants and drug resistance.

It is hardly surprising that infection is still a challenge, and the next chapter is devoted to inflammation, which includes conditions of infective and immune aetiology.

CHAPTER 4

The inflammatory response

> No natural phenomenon can be adequately studied in itself alone, but to be understood must be considered as it stands connected with all nature.
>
> *Sir Francis Bacon (1561–1626)*

WHAT IS INFLAMMATION?

Inflammation is a mechanism by which the body deals with an injury or insult. It is stimulated by tissue injury caused by physical, chemical or biological agents. When living tissue is damaged, a series of local processes are initiated in order to contain the offensive agent, to neutralize its effect, to limit spread and hopefully to eradicate it. As part and parcel of this process, there is initiation of healing and repair of the injured tissue. Inflammation, healing and repair are like the black and white stripes of the zebra; in order truly to understand the zebra, one cannot study the stripes in isolation. In the same way, the processes of healing and repair have to be addressed in their relationship to the process of inflammation.

The circulatory system is of fundamental importance in the inflammatory response. In general terms, the offending agent, whatever it may be, causes a change in the microvasculature of the injured area leading to a massive outpouring of cells and fluid. This collection of cells and fluid is known as the inflammatory exudate, and within this exudate we find ingredients that are needed to combat the offending agent and to begin the process of healing and repair. However, this is only half the story. It is romantic to imagine an army being sent to deal with an invading force and to restore the peace and tranquillity of the area. But in reality life is not quite so simple; there is a price to be paid for war! The ugly side of it includes cosmetic problems, such as keloid scars, and life-threatening illnesses, such as autoimmune diseases.

John Hunter, surgeon to St George's Hospital from 1768 to 1793, was a pioneer in the study of inflammation and repair. He was a remarkable man, whose aim was the total understanding of mankind! Hunter was born in Scotland on 14 February 1728, the last of 10 children. He spent the first 20 years of his life there and his childhood has been described as 'wasted and idle'. This is because he 'wanted to know all about the clouds and the grasses, and why the leaves changed colour in the autumn'. Hunter's inquisitiveness and fascination with nature stood him in good stead when he began to unravel the mysteries of the human body. His book, *A Treatise on the Blood, Inflammation, and Gun-shot Wounds*, published posthumously in 1794, is a monument to his thoroughness and powers of observation in delineating the processes of disease. Hunter was one of the first to observe that

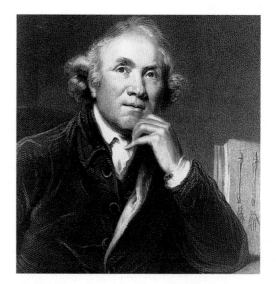

Figure 4.1 John Hunter (1728–93) © CORBIS

Table 4.1 Cells involved in inflammation

Cell category	Cell type	Origin	% white cells	Major function
Circulating cells				
Granulocytes (polymorphonuclear leukocytes)	Neutrophils	Bone marrow	75	Acute inflammatory cell involved in bacterial killing and phagocytosis. Granule contents for increasing vascular permeability, chemotaxis, killing organisms and digesting extracellular matrix
	Eosinophils	Bone marrow	1	Acute inflammatory cell particularly common in allergic and parasitic conditions. Granules include major basic protein
	Basophils	Bone marrow	<1	Circulating cells that give rise to **mast cells.** Granules include histamine
Lymphocytes	T cells	Lymphoid organs and thymus	20	Various subtypes involved in antigen recognition and presentation, cell killing and regulation of immune responses (e.g. helper, suppressor and natural killer cells)
	B cells	Lymphoid organs and bone marrow		On antigen stimulation, proliferate and give rise to specific **plasma cells,** which synthesize specific immunoglobulins
Macrophage system	Monocytes	Bone marrow	4	Migrate into tissues to be macrophages capable of phagocytosis, cytokine production and antigen processing and presentation
Non-circulating cells				
Kupffer cells (liver sinusoids) Macrophages (bone marrow, spleen and lymph nodes)				Fixed phagocytic cells lining sinusoids and filtering large molecules/particles from blood or lymph.
Megakaryocytes in bone marrow				Produce platelets which contain serotonin, platelet-derived growth factor, etc. Also important in haemostasis
Hepatocytes				Produce proteins important in: • clotting and fibrinolytic system • complement system • kinin system • acute phase proteins

inflammation was not a disease but a response to tissue injury whose attempts at repair were sometimes more harmful than the original disease.

Many of Hunter's experiments are absolutely fascinating as well as crazy and amusing, but more of that later, so keep reading!

Anyone who has had a boil or any other skin infection, will be familiar with the four cardinal signs of inflammation: rubor (redness), calor (heat), tumour (swelling) and dolor (pain). These were first described by a Roman physician, Cornelius Celsus, in the first century AD. A fifth sign was later added – laesio functae (loss of function), however, this is not a necessary accompaniment of the inflammatory process.

So what is the pathophysiology behind these clinical signs?

Microvasculature

The microvasculature plays a central role in inflammation. The redness is caused by vasodilatation, which is important for increasing the flow of blood to the affected area and delivering cells and plasma-derived substances needed to combat the infection.

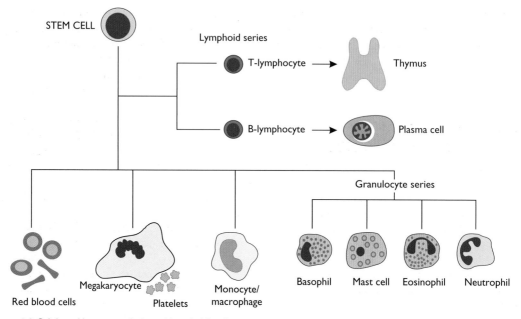

Figure 4.2 Origins of haematopoietic and lymphoid cells

Vasodilatation also produces the heat. The swelling results from increased permeability of vessel walls, leading to the outpouring of fluid and cells (the inflammatory exudate). In some circumstances, the swelling may cushion the affected part and lead to immobilization (loss of function). The sign that is the most difficult to explain is pain. This probably arises from the combination of stretching of tissue by exudate and the action of some of the chemical mediators involved in inflammation.

But what are the underlying mechanisms of this process? In broad terms, there are two aspects to consider: the cells of inflammation and the chemical mediators.

Cellular mediators

The principal cells of inflammation are the polymorphonuclear leukocytes or granulocytes (which include neutrophils, eosinophils and basophils) and the lymphocytes, plasma cells and macrophages. A Russian microbiologist, Elias Metchnikoff, working at the Pasteur Institute in Paris in 1884, demonstrated that leukocytes phagocytose bacteria and concluded that the purpose of the inflammatory response was to bring phagocytic cells to the area to kill the organisms. Inflammatory cells descend on a focus of tissue damage in 'waves'; the first cell type recruited is the neutrophil polymorph (an 'acute' inflammatory cell), which is followed by macrophages, lymphocytes and plasma cells ('chronic' inflammatory cells). Later, the tissue generates new blood vessels and fibrous scar tissue as reparative work begins.

Chemical mediators

In 1927, Sir Thomas Lewis identified histamine, present in tissue mast cells, as a mediator of acute inflammation. Since then a vast array of mediators have been identified, but not all have a proven role *in vivo*. They may be derived from the plasma, the participating inflammatory cells or from the damaged tissue itself.

The cell-derived products include:

- vasoactive amines
- cytokines and growth factors
- arachidonic acid derivatives (eiocosanoids)
- platelet-activating factor
- lysosomal enzymes
- oxygen-derived free radicals
- nitric oxide

The plasma-derived mediators include;

- the kinin system
- the coagulation and fibrinolytic system
- the complement system

Some of these are important in the amplification of the inflammatory response; others play their role in the elimination of the offending agent. The mediators and their roles in inflammation will be discussed in more detail later.

WHAT IS THE DIFFERENCE BETWEEN ACUTE AND CHRONIC INFLAMMATION?

Inflammation is divided into acute and chronic forms, based on the predominant inflammatory cell type. Acute inflammation, generally, is of short duration, lasting from a few minutes to a few days and the cellular exudate is rich in neutrophil polymorphonuclear leukocytes with some macrophages arriving after the initial insult. Chronic inflammation tends to be more variable, may last for months or years and the chief cells involved are lymphocytes, plasma cells

and macrophages. It is important to realize that in some instances chronic inflammatory diseases appear never go through an acute inflammatory phase, i.e. chronic inflammation may be the primary event and not a sequel to acute inflammation. This is the case in many viral illnesses. Equally, some predominantly chronic inflammatory states (as seen, for instance, in *Helicobacter pylori* colonization of the stomach) are preceded by an extremely brief acute inflammatory phase. In contrast, in some cases the opposite phenomenon may occur, and an acute inflammatory state becomes 'walled off' from the rest of the body and persists, as seen in abscesses and in osteomyelitis.

The inflammatory process, whether acute or chronic, may be modified by a whole host of factors such as the cause of the damage, the nutritional status of the patient, the competence of the patient's immune system and intervention with antibiotics, 'anti-inflammatory drugs' or surgery.

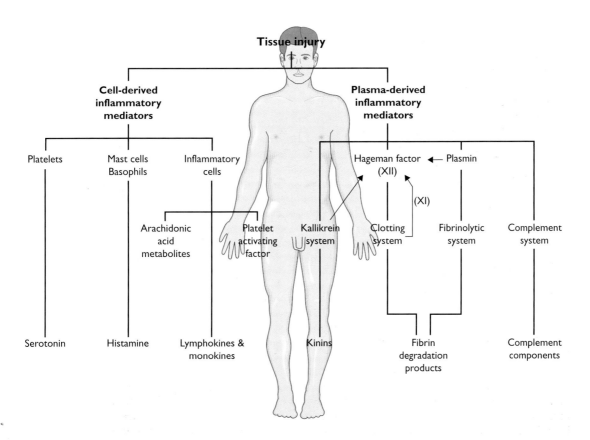

Figure 4.3 Origins of important mediators of inflammation

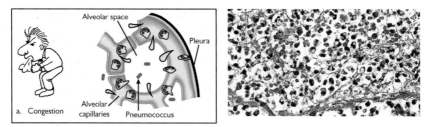

Acute congestion: Bacteria invade alveolar spaces of lung. Acute inflammatory response characterized first by increased vascular permeability, with the formation of a fibrin-rich exudate

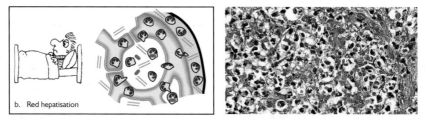

Red hepatization: Neutrophils are quickly attracted to the site, accompanied by red blood cells. The fluid spreads between alveolar spaces via pores of Kohn and soon the entire lung lobe is consolidated (solidified) due to a mixture of fibrin, red and white blood cells. Neutrophils phagocytose the bacteria. The texture and colour of the lobe resembles fresh liver

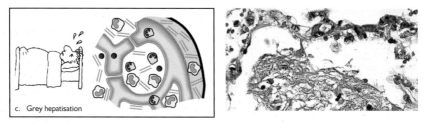

Grey hepatization: Macrophages are attracted to the site, also lymphocytes. Further phagocytosis occurs. Bacteria and dead red and white cells are removed and the fibrin mesh starts to be digested. The grey/white colour of the lobe is due to the high fibrin and white cell content; the texture resembles cooked liver (ugh!)

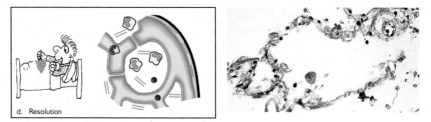

Resolution: The last few fibrin strands and white cells are removed, together with any remaining bacterial corpses and the lung returns to normal. This is possible because the basic skeleton of the lung (formed by reticulin, a type of collagen) is not damaged, unlike bronchopneumonia, in which the inflammatory process is centred on infected bronchioles and is characterized by destruction of the adjacent lung framework (this is usually followed by scarring of lung tissue)

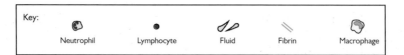

Figure 4.4 Lobar pneumonia

Lobar pneumonia

A disease exemplifying acute inflammation is lobar pneumonia, so named because the lung parenchyma is involved in continuity so that the process affects a whole lobe or contiguous lobes. The commonest cause of lobar pneumonia is *Streptococcus pneumoniae*, a Gram-positive diplococcus bacterium. This invades the lung, leading to changes in the microvasculature and a massive outpouring of fluid into the alveolar spaces, resulting in congestion (Fig. 4.4a). This fluid is rich in fibrin. Soon afterwards, neutrophils follow and the fibrin-rich fluid and cells spread from alveolus to alveolus via the pores of Kohn. The neutrophils attack the organisms and phagocytose them, leading to the death of both the organisms and many neutrophils. Not surprisingly, the alveoli are airless and the lung is now firm and red with the texture of liver, hence the term 'red hepatization' (Fig. 4.4b). As this process progresses, the macrophage is recruited not only to phagocytose dead neutrophils and bacteria but also to digest the fibrin mesh. The lung is still firm but the large inflammatory cell infiltrate and reduction in vasodilatation give it a grey colour. At this stage the term 'grey hepatization' is used (Fig. 4.4c).

The final outcome will depend on the competence of this system and whether the basic framework of the lung tissue is intact. Ideally, the alveoli will be cleared, re-aerated and resolution (Fig. 4.4d) will take place. If the alveolar framework has been destroyed or the exudate has not been cleared, organization will occur, leading to scar formation. The infection may persist, destroying lung tissue, but become localized so that an abscess is formed. This is a collection of pus walled off by fibrous tissue. Alternatively it may spread to the rest of the lung, involve the pleura, cause an empyema, or disseminate via the bloodstream to other areas of the body and can lead to death due to septicaemia or respiratory failure.

ACUTE INFLAMMATION

The patient with the boil on the bum will be less impressed than we are with the inflammatory processes taking place. He may regard the fact that the injury has caused microvascular changes via mediators, leading to cellular and humoral factors accumulating at the site of injury as of less importance than the burning question, 'What will happen next?'

There are several possibilities. The inflammatory and healing process may restore the tissue to its normal state, with nothing to suggest that anything has been amiss. Healing may take place but leave a scar. The injury and the inflammation may grumble on for a long time or the injury, particularly if infected, may completely overwhelm the body and lead to death. This last outcome is especially likely where inflammatory defences are deficient, such as in AIDS, cancer patients treated with cytotoxic drugs or patients receiving immunosuppressive drugs for autoimmune disease or following organ transplantation. The final outcome depends on the interactions between the various processes involved in inflammation. Just as the zebra is neither black with white

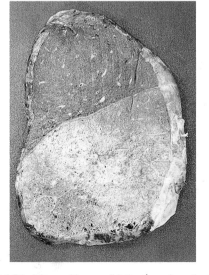

Figure 4.5 Left lung with consolidation (grey hepatization) of the lower lobe

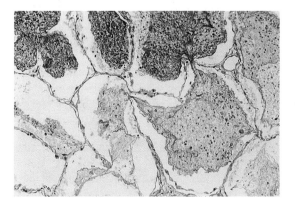

Figure 4.6 Photomicrograph of lung alveoli filled with inflammatory exudates and fibrin passing through the pores of Kohn

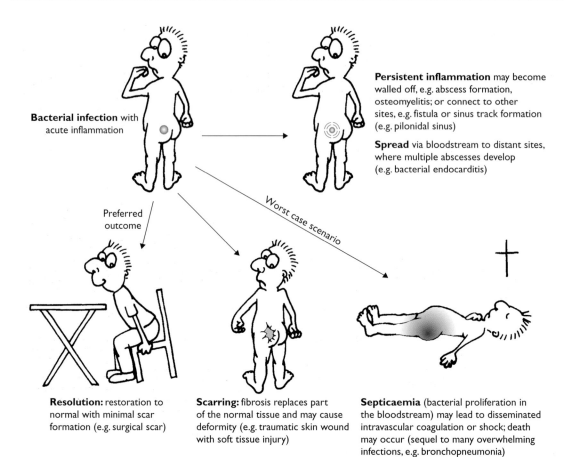

Bacterial infection with acute inflammation

Persistent inflammation may become walled off, e.g. abscess formation, osteomyelitis; or connect to other sites, e.g. fistula or sinus track formation (e.g. pilonidal sinus)

Spread via bloodstream to distant sites, where multiple abscesses develop (e.g. bacterial endocarditis)

Preferred outcome

Worst case scenario

Resolution: restoration to normal with minimal scar formation (e.g. surgical scar)

Scarring: fibrosis replaces part of the normal tissue and may cause deformity (e.g. traumatic skin wound with soft tissue injury)

Septicaemia (bacterial proliferation in the bloodstream) may lead to disseminated intravascular coagulation or shock; death may occur (sequel to many overwhelming infections, e.g. bronchopneumonia)

Figure 4.7 Possible outcomes of acute inflammation

stripes nor white with black stripes, so it is the combination of the various inflammatory components that determines the texture of the whole.

Now that we have the overall concept of inflammation and its clinical relevance, we must look more closely at the complex cellular and molecular events of this process. We shall first examine the changes in the microvasculature.

Vascular changes

We are indebted to the German pathologist Julius Conheim (1839–1884) for investigating the pathophysiology of inflammation. A pupil of and later assistant to the 'father' of cellular pathology, Rudolf Virchow, Conheim delineated the vascular changes of inflammation using living preparations of thin membranes, such as the mesentery, and demonstrated the vasodilatation and the subsequent exudation of fluid. His experiments with frog mesentery beautifully demonstrated that injury produced vasodilatation, resulting in more blood entering the tissue but sometimes a slower flow of blood in capillaries. This allows white cells (leukocytes) to attach to the vessel wall (margination) and then move across the wall to the extravascular compartment (diapedesis or emigration).

Before we consider the causes of altered vascular permeability, it is worth revising the normal physiological factors that control the movement of fluid across a small vessel wall (Fig. 4.8). Fluid flows away from areas of high hydrostatic pressure and towards areas of high osmotic pressure. Thus, fluid leaves from the arterial end of the capillary network and is reabsorbed at the venous end (Fig. 4.8a), with any excess being removed via lymphatics. A rise in hydrostatic pressure within the vessel without changes in permeability will increase leakage of fluid out of the vessel but it will have no

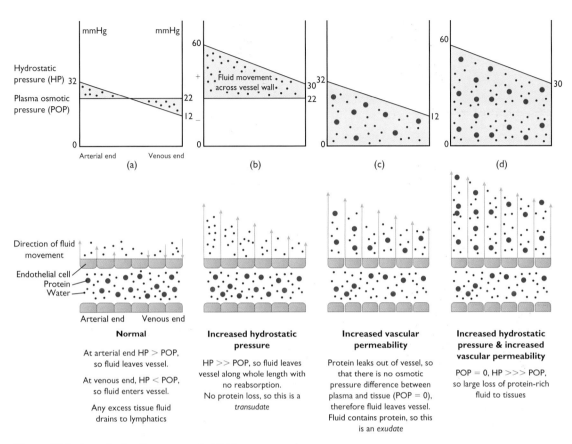

Figure 4.8 Factors affecting the movement of fluid across vessels

protein in it (Fig. 4.8b). However, if the permeability of the vessel wall increases, then fluid can move more readily and protein molecules may also leak across. Movement of protein molecules will alter the osmotic pressure gradient, such that less fluid is reabsorbed into the blood at the venous end of the capillaries and tissue fluid will increase (Fig. 4.8c). In areas of inflammation there is usually a rise in hydrostatic pressure and an increase in vascular permeability (Fig. 4.8d).

This is an appropriate time to introduce a number of new words. An exudate is the fluid within the extravascular spaces, which is rich in protein and hence has a specific gravity of greater than 1.020. On the other hand, a transudate has a low protein content and specific gravity of less than 1.020. Oedema simply refers to the presence of excess fluid within the extravascular space and body cavities and may be an exudate or transudate. Pus can be thought of as a special kind of exudate, a purulent exudate. Besides the protein-rich fluid, it contains dead or dying

bacteria and neutrophils. The consistency of the pus depends on the amount of digestion by neutrophil enzymes and the colour depends on the type of organism and the presence of neutrophil-derived myeloperoxidase, which imparts a yellow-green colour. Exudates generally contain fibrinogen, which is converted to fibrin through the action of tissue thromboplastin. The fibrin forms a mesh for cells to migrate on and later a scaffold for healing and repair.

If we examine the fluid that forms during an inflammatory reaction, we find that it is an exudate. This means that large protein molecules have leaked out of the microvasculature. What is the mechanism of the increased permeability? Most vessels are lined by endothelium that is termed 'continuous'. In endocrine organs, intestines and renal glomeruli, the endothelium is normally more permeable because it contains 'windows', hence the name fenestrated endothelium, while in the spleen, liver and bone marrow the endothelium is discontinuous. What happens following injury has been elegantly

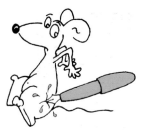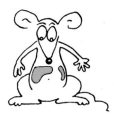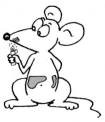

| Ink is injected intravenously | Ink escapes in organs with discontinuous endothelium | or if the endothelial cells are damaged |

Figure 4.9 Vascular endothelium is continuous everywhere except the liver and spleen – here the endothelium is fenestrated. Because of this, an intravenous injection of Indian ink will lead to the accumulation of ink particles in the liver and spleen. However, if endothelium elsewhere is damaged, e.g. by heat, gaps appear between the endothelial cells and ink particles can leak out of circulation at these sites

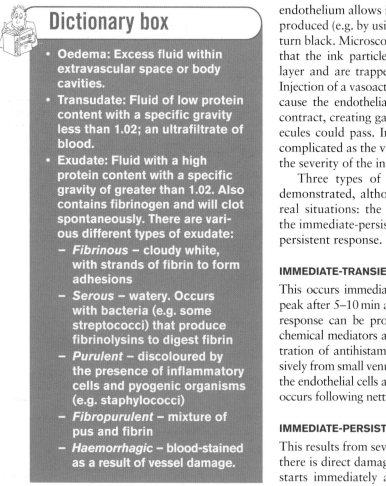

Dictionary box

- **Oedema: Excess fluid within extravascular space or body cavities.**
- **Transudate: Fluid of low protein content with a specific gravity less than 1.02; an ultrafiltrate of blood.**
- **Exudate: Fluid with a high protein content with a specific gravity of greater than 1.02. Also contains fibrinogen and will clot spontaneously. There are various different types of exudate:**
  - *Fibrinous* **– cloudy white, with strands of fibrin to form adhesions**
  - *Serous* **– watery. Occurs with bacteria (e.g. some streptococci) that produce fibrinolysins to digest fibrin**
  - *Purulent* **– discoloured by the presence of inflammatory cells and pyogenic organisms (e.g. staphylococci)**
  - *Fibropurulent* **– mixture of pus and fibrin**
  - *Haemorrhagic* **– blood-stained as a result of vessel damage.**

demonstrated using simple experiments involving the intravenous injection of Indian ink. The ink will remain within the vascular compartment, except in the liver and spleen, where the discontinuous endothelium allows ink to escape. If a mild injury is produced (e.g. by using heat), the damaged area will turn black. Microscopical examination would reveal that the ink particles have crossed the endothelial layer and are trapped at the basement membrane. Injection of a vasoactive substance, histamine, would cause the endothelial cells of the small venules to contract, creating gaps through which the ink molecules could pass. In reality, the situation is more complicated as the vascular changes will depend on the severity of the insult.

Three types of vascular response have been demonstrated, although they generally overlap in real situations: the immediate-transient response, the immediate-persistent response and the delayed-persistent response.

IMMEDIATE-TRANSIENT RESPONSE

This occurs immediately following injury, reaches a peak after 5–10 min and ceases after 15–30 min. This response can be produced by histamine and other chemical mediators and is blocked by prior administration of antihistamines. The leakage occurs exclusively from small venules which develop gaps between the endothelial cells as endothelial cells contract. This occurs following nettle stings or insect bites.

IMMEDIATE-PERSISTENT RESPONSE

This results from severe injury such as burns, where there is direct damage to endothelial cells. The leak starts immediately and reaches a peak within an hour. As the endothelial cells are damaged and may even slough off, the leak will continue until the vessel has been blocked with thrombus or the vessel is repaired. Unlike the previous example, it can affect any type of vessel.

DELAYED-PERSISTENT RESPONSE

This is a very interesting type of response, familiar to anyone who has overdone the sunbathing during a tropical holiday after a period under the clouds of England. There is an interval of up to 24 hours before the leak starts from both capillaries and venules. Small aggregates of platelets and endothelial cells are seen in some capillaries and it seems that the endothelial cells are damaged directly.

Cellular events

The principal cells of the acute inflammatory response are the neutrophils and macrophages. Following injury, the neutrophils migrate out of the vessels, the number recruited depending on the type of injury. For example, infections with bacteria attract more inflammatory cells than purely physical injuries. After the neutrophils, there is a second wave of cells, the macrophages. The movement of neutrophils out of the vessels and their role in combat can be divided into discrete steps. These are:

* margination
* adhesion
* emigration
* chemotaxis
* phagocytosis and degranulation.

MARGINATION AND ADHESION

When haemodynamic changes take place in the vasculature during inflammation, white cells fall out of the central axial flow and line themselves up along the wall (a little reminiscent of the school disco!). This is a result of rolling of leukocytes on the endothelial surface. It appears that there are specific complementary 'adhesion molecules' that stick leukocytes to endothelial cells, and the number of these molecules on the cell surfaces is increased by inflammatory mediators. One pair of such molecules is ICAM-1 (intercellular adhesion molecule 1) on endothelial cells and LFA-1 on leukocytes, which bind together like a 'lock and key', arresting the rolling leukocyte on the endothelial surface. Resting cells express very few adhesion molecules, but some inflammatory mediators increase expression of LFA-1 (e.g. complement fragments (C5a) and leukotrienes (LTB₄)), while other mediators enhance ICAM-1 expression (e.g. interleukin 1 and bacterial endotoxin). This adhesion is of great importance and people with a genetic deficiency in

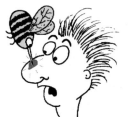

Immediate-transient response: Immediate onset, peaking in 5–10 minutes and lasting from 15 to 30 minutes. Small blood vessels are affected. The damage is caused by histamine, bradykinin, nitric oxide, complement (C5a), leukotrienes (e.g. LTB₄), platelet-activating factor (PAF). Causes include nettle sting, insect bite

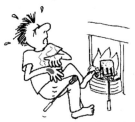

Immediate-persistent response: Caused by endothelial cell injury, arises immediately, peaking in about 1 hour and lasts until the vessel is plugged by thrombus or repaired. Any vessel type may be involved, the mechanism of injury being due to bradykinins, nitric oxide, complement, leukotrienes (e.g. LTB₄), platelet-activating factor (PAF), and potentiated by prostaglandins. Causes include severe direct injury, such as burns

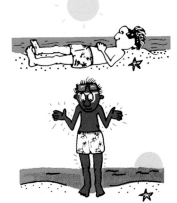

Delayed-persistent response: Caused by endothelial cell injury; arises in 18–24 hours and progresses for up to 36 hours (sometimes longer). Capillaries and venules are affected. Causes include sunburn, DXT (radiotherapy), bacterial toxins

Figure 4.10 Types of vascular response

these adhesion molecules suffer from repeated bacterial infections.

Our knowledge of adhesion molecules is expanding rapidly. Broadly, there are four families, three of which are involved in inflammation: the integrins, the immunoglobulin gene superfamily and

Table 4.2 Adhesion molecules

Family	Some family members	Principally expressed on	Main function
Integrins	β1 family, e.g. VLA-4 β2 family, e.g. LFA-1	Lymphocytes and monocytes	Mediates immune and inflammatory responses including binding immuno-globulin superfamily molecules on endothelial cells to provide firm adhesion to vessel wall prior to migration
Immunoglobulin superfamily	ICAM 1, 2 and 3 VCAM-1	Endothelial cells, lymphocytes and monocytes	As above by binding to integrins
Selectins	E-selectin L-selectin P-selectin	Endothelium Lymphocytes, polymorphs and monocytes Platelets and endothelial cells	Initial phase of leukocyte adhesion to vessel wall
Cadherins	B, E, M, N, P, R, T	Range of tissues	Homophilic calcium-dependent cell–cell adhesion, e.g. at sites of desmosomes and adherens junctions. Not specifically involved in inflammation

ICAM-1 = intercellular adhesion molecule 1; LFA-1 = leukocyte function-associated antigen 1; VCAM-1 = vascular cell adhesion molecule 1; VLA-4 = very late antigen 4.

the selectins. Some (but not all) of their family members are listed in Table 4.2. Their expression changes during inflammation so that different types of cells adhere at different stages. Some of these molecules have been termed addressins because they act as address labels to allow cells to leave the circulation in a specific tissue. This is particularly important in the recirculation and 'homing' of lymphocytes which is discussed on page 122.

EMIGRATION AND CHEMOTAXIS

Once the cells have firmly adhered to the endothelium they form foot-like processes termed pseudopodia that push their way between the endothelial cells. Eventually, the leukocyte lies between the endothelial cell and the basement membrane, where it releases a protease to digest the basement membrane so that it can reach the extravascular space. Neutrophils, basophils, eosinophils, macrophages and lymphocytes all use this route. Red blood cells may also pass through the gaps, but only as passive passengers.

The cells are able to move towards a chemical signal and this specific movement is termed chemotaxis. (Note that this is different to chemokinesis, which is an increased and accelerated *random* movement.) The Boyden Chamber is a popular system for demonstrating chemotaxis. It consists of two chambers separated by a micropore filter. The cells go into one chamber and the putative chemical mediator is placed in the other. If cells move from the first to the second chamber, then chemotaxis is demonstrated. The compounds that have been suggested as chemotactic agents include bacterial products, fragments of the complement system (e.g. C5a) and products of arachidonic acid metabolism (e.g. prostaglandins and leukotrienes).

How does this process work? Well, like so many cellular stimuli, the first stage depends on the chemotactic agents binding to specific receptors on the leukocyte cell membrane. This leads to an increase in ionized calcium within the cytoplasm which promotes construction of the contractile elements actin and myosin, responsible for movement.

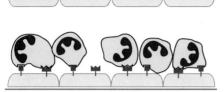

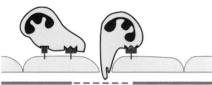

(a) Laminar flow: Polymorphs are carried in the central stream of normally flowing blood. The flow rate slows in acute inflammation and they 'fall out' of the axial stream towards the marginal stream. Acute inflammatory mediators, such as IL-1, TNF and endotoxins cause the upregulation of E-selectin on the lining endothelial cells. The polymorphs bind these loosely and roll along the endothelial surface.

(b) The endothelial cells express integrins (e.g. ICAM-1), which bind tightly to the Ig superfamily molecule, LFA-1, on the polymorph, tethering it to the wall. These are also induced by acute inflammatory mediators. Polymorphs and other inflammatory cells migrate into the extravascular space by extending a pseudopodium into the junction between endothelial cells. They dissolve the basement membrane with proteases.

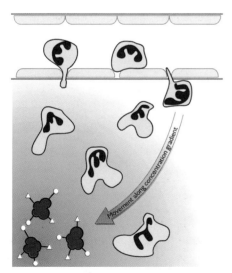

(c) The polymorph migrates between endothelial cells and the defect in the basement membrane seals behind them. Some red cells follow, but in acute inflammation there is generally little extravasation of red cells unless there has been vascular damage. The polymorph then moves along a chemotactic gradient set up by chemokines (which attach to matrix proteins in the soft tissues) to the inflammatory stimulus. Other inflammatory cells, particularly macrophages and eosinophils, use the same principles.

Figure 4.11 Polymorph movement across blood vessels in acute inflammation is mediated by adhesion molecules and then follows a chemotactic gradient to the source of the inflammatory response

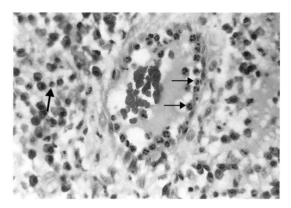

Figure 4.12 Photomicrograph illustrating margination (small arrows) and emigration (large arrow)

However, precisely how these interact to produce directional movement of the cell is not known.

PHAGOCYTOSIS

Once the neutrophils and macrophages have arrived at the site of injury, they ingest the debris and bacteria, a process termed phagocytosis. This requires a number of distinct steps; the material has to be recognized as foreign or dead, it has to be engulfed and ingested and, finally, it has to be killed or degraded.

Not all of the processes by which neutrophils and macrophages differentiate between normal tissue and foreign or dead tissue are known; however, it is clear that bacteria coated with certain substances are ingested more readily. The factors that coat bacteria are called opsonins and the process is termed opsonization. This is derived from the Greek word *opson* meaning 'to relish', i.e. to get ready for eating. There are two major opsonins:

- immunoglobulin (IgG)
- C3b component of complement.

In order for the neutrophils and macrophages to recognize these opsonins, there must be receptors on the cell surface. There are two such receptors, one for the Fc fragment of IgG (Fig. 5.4) and the other for C3b (page 103). After the opsonized fragment attaches to the receptor, the cell puts out a pseudopodium. This extension of cell cytoplasm encircles the particle so that it becomes wrapped in what was originally cell surface membrane. This new intracytoplasmic membrane-bound sac is termed a phagosome. Another such sac, normally present in the cell and packed with destructive enzymes, is the lysosome. When a lysosome fuses with a phagosome

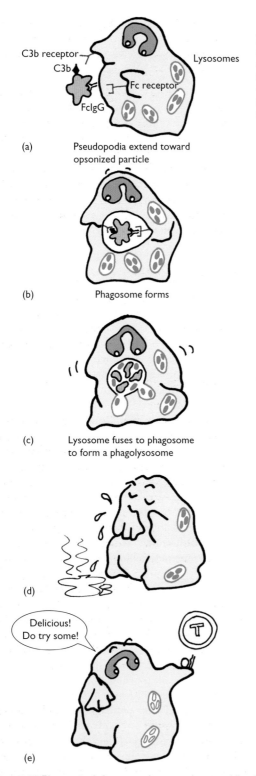

Macrophages and polymorphs must be activated (e.g. by cytokines, bacterial polysaccharides or endotoxin, C5a) before they can phagocytose particles. Opsonization is essential for polymorphs; this is achieved with complement C3b or the Fc component of antibody molecules. The phagocyte extends pseudopodia towards and attaches to the opsonized particle.

(a) Pseudopodia extend toward opsonized particle

By a process called endocytosis the phagocyte engulfs the bound particle to form a phagosome.

(b) Phagosome forms

Lysosomes packed with granules containing destructive enzymes, such as acid hydrolases, fuse with the phagosome to form a phagolysosome. Killing and digestion of the particle takes place. Polymorphs kill using O_2-dependent and -independent mechanisms.

(c) Lysosome fuses to phagosome to form a phagolysosome

'Regurgitation during feeding' may lead to the release of destructive enzymes into surrounding tissue, which is then damaged and may lead to the release of further inflammatory mediators.

(d)

The macrophage, unlike the polymorph, can release cytokines, such as TNF and IL-1 and present antigenic portions of the particle to lymphocytes in order to initiate a specific inflammatory response.

(e)

Figure 4.13 Phagocytosis by macrophages and neutrophil polymorphs

it produces a phagolysosome. This allows the enzymes to have access to the engulfed particle and it is within this vesicle that the killing takes place. If some proteolytic enzymes leak out of the phagolysosome, as may occur if the lysosome fuses with the phagosome while the phagosome is still open to the cell surface, they may damage adjacent tissue. This is a phenomenon described, rather poetically, as 'regurgitation during feeding'. Fusion of a lysosome with the cell membrane and, hence, local release of toxic metabolites is important for attacking large organisms, such as worms, that are too large to be ingested.

MECHANISMS FOR BACTERIAL KILLING

There are essentially two mechanisms for bacterial killing: oxygen-dependent and oxygen-independent.

The oxygen-dependent system involves toxic oxygen radicals that have an unpaired electron (indicated by a dot). These include superoxide (O_2^-·), singlet oxygen (O·) and the hydroxyl radical (OH^-·). These molecules are produced by the respiratory burst that occurs during the process of phagocytosis. Oxygen is reduced to superoxide ion which is then converted to hydrogen peroxide (H_2O_2). This is not, however, the most powerful bactericidal chemical. Neutrophils contain the enzyme myeloperoxidase, which converts H_2O_2 to HOCl (hypochlorous acid) in the presence of halide ions (e.g. chloride), and nitric oxide, produced by macrophages, reacts with superoxide anion to form the strong oxidant nitrogen dioxide. These are powerful oxidants active against bacteria, fungi, viruses, protozoa and helminths. This system is of clinical importance; its absence produces 'chronic granulomatous disease of childhood', an inherited disease in which the neutrophils are able to ingest bacteria but unable to kill them. This is because the child lacks the enzyme NADPH oxidase, which leads to a failure of production of superoxide anion, (O_2^-·) and hydrogen peroxide.

There are a number of oxygen-independent mechanisms that are useful in microbial killing. These include:

- lysozyme, an enzyme that attacks the cell wall of some bacteria (especially Gram-positive cocci),
- lactoferrin, an iron-binding protein that inhibits growth of bacteria,
- major basic protein (MBP), a cationic protein found in eosinophils and active principally against parasites,

- bactericidal permeability-increasing protein (BPI), which as the name implies, causes changes in the permeability of the membranes of the microorganisms.

Also the low pH found in the phagolysosomes, besides being bactericidal itself, enhances the conversion of hydrogen peroxide to superoxide. Unfortunately, the leukocytes are not successful in killing all organisms, and some bacteria, such as the mycobacterium that causes tuberculosis, can survive inside phagocytes, happily protected from antibacterial drugs and host-defence mechanisms.

We shall now go on to consider the chemical mediators involved in inflammation.

Chemical mediators

Since Sir Thomas Lewis first demonstrated the role of histamine, an enormous number of possible mediators have been put forward, some remaining putative rather than having an established role.

CELL-DERIVED MEDIATORS

Arachidonic acid derivatives

These are the prostaglandins and the leukotrienes. Just like the clotting and fibrinolytic system, they play a part in thrombosis as well as inflammation. They are best thought of as local hormones. They have a short range of action, are produced rapidly and degenerate spontaneously or are degraded by enzymes. Arachidonic acid, the parent molecule, is a 20-carbon polyunsaturated fatty acid that is derived either from the diet or from essential fatty acids. It is not found in a free state but is present esterified in the cell membrane phospholipid. The two pathways of arachidonic acid metabolism and its products are shown in Fig. 4.14, which also depicts some of the roles of the products in inflammation. Drugs such as corticosteroids, aspirin and indometacin act to reduce inflammation by inhibiting the production of prostaglandins.

Cytokines, lymphokines and monokines

A large array of these polypeptides are being identified. They act principally to regulate immune and haematopoietic cell proliferation and activity. In addition they have effects in the inflammatory response. They are produced by many different cells in the body; those produced by lymphocytes are called lymphokines and those from macrophages

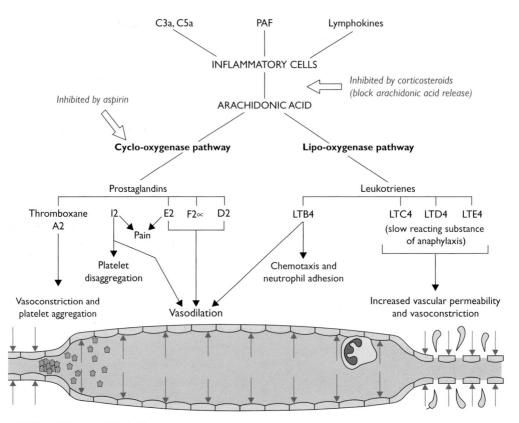

Figure 4.14 Arachidonic acid derivatives

are termed monokines. Two of the most important are interleukin 1 (IL-1) and tumour necrosis factor (TNF). They have a variety of important effects in inflammation as shown in Fig. 4.15.

Cytokines can be grouped broadly as:

- interleukins
- colony-stimulating factors
- interferons
- chemokines
- growth factors.

Growth factors have a role in chemotaxis as well as inducing healing and repair of tissues and playing a part in the development of malignant tumours. The principal growth factors are:

- epidermal growth factor (EGF)
- platelet-derived growth factor (PDGF)
- fibroblast growth factor (FGF)
- transforming growth factor (TGF).

Most of these can be produced by macrophages, which are numerous in areas of chronic inflammation.

Platelet-activating factor (PAF)

PAF is derived from antigen-stimulated IgE-sensitized basophils as well as neutrophils, macrophages and endothelial cells. In addition to activating platelets, it can cause vasodilatation, permeability changes, leukocyte adhesion and chemotaxis and can stimulate the production of other mediators, in particular the arachidonic acid metabolites.

Vasoactive amines

Histamine and serotonin (5-hydroxytryptamine) are stored in and released from mast cells, basophils and platelets. Their release causes vasodilatation and increases the permeability of venules. The action of histamine on vessels is mediated via H_1 receptors, while some of its other actions (e.g. bronchoconstriction) are effected via H_2 receptors.

Many factors can lead to release of these substances, including physical trauma, immunological reactions leading to formation of C3a and C5a, releasing factors produced by neutrophils, monocytes and platelets and interleukin 1. The role of

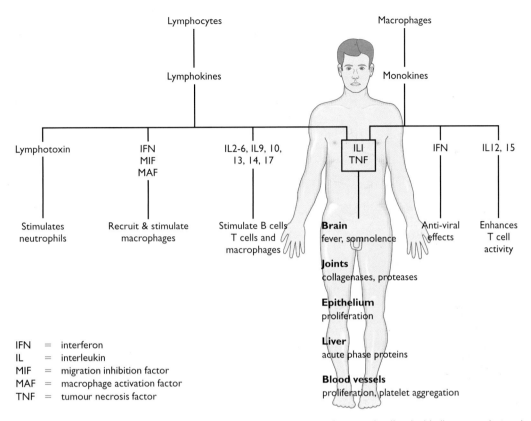

Figure 4.15 The effects of cytokines in inflammation. Chemokines achieve a chemotactic effect by binding to matrix proteins in the connective tissue, setting up a concentration gradient that directs polymorphs, eosinophils and macrophages to the site of tissue damage

these amines is thought to be in the early phase of inflammation as it has been shown that anti-histamines blocking H_1 receptors have no effect on the permeability that is present after 60 minutes.

Lysosomal contents

Lysosomal enzymes and accessory substances are present in neutrophils and monocytes, packaged in membrane-bound vesicles ('granules') to prevent them from damaging their own cell. There are two types of granules, the smaller specific and the larger azurophilic. These contain substances that increase vascular permeability and are chemotactic. The enzymes destroy many extracellular components, including collagen, fibrin, elastin, cartilage and basement membrane, as well as producing intracellular killing in the phagolysosome as already described. If these processes were unopposed there would be massive tissue destruction, so there are antiproteases within the serum and tissue fluids to neutralize these enzymes and therefore regulate the extent of tissue

damage. Does this seem a far fetched idea, distant from clinical practice? Well not so!

A deficiency of one such antiprotease, α_1-antitrypsin, leads to unopposed action of elastase and hence destruction of elastic tissue, especially in the lungs and liver. Clinically, a patient with α_1-antitrypsin deficiency may suffer from emphysema of the lungs and liver cirrhosis.

Nitric oxide (NO)

Nitric oxide is produced by endothelial cells, macrophages and specific neurons in the brain and has roles in smooth muscle relaxation and the reduction of platelet aggregation and adhesion. It also acts as a toxic radical to certain microbes and tumour cells. Macrophage nitric oxide production only occurs when induced by cytokines, such as gamma interferon, whereas endothelial and neural nitrous oxide is produced constitutively. Uncontrolled production by macrophages can lead to massive peripheral vasodilatation and shock (see page 186).

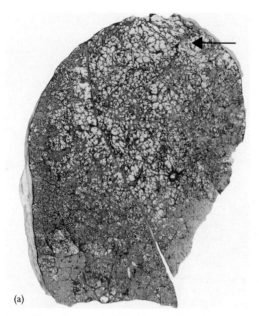

(a)

Lung with emphysema: the 'holes' (arrowed) are hugely distended, coalescent, alveolar spaces. If blood A1AT levels are less than 75% of normal, patients are at severe risk of developing emphysema. Any inflammatory stimulus exacerbates the risk – this patient was a coal miner.

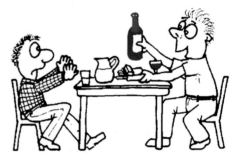

(b)

Mutations in the genes encoding A1AT lead to abnormally folded protein, which cannot be secreted into the blood by the liver. Instead, it accumulates within endoplasmic reticulum, shown here (arrows). These patients are at increased risk of cirrhosis. Drinking alcohol stimulates an acute inflammatory response in the liver and increases the risk of this complication.

Figure 4.16 Alpha-1-antitrypsin (A1AT) is a 394-amino-acid glycoprotein secreted by the liver that is produced during the acute inflammatory response. It inhibits serine proteases, especially neutrophil elastase, which can cleave a wide variety of extra-cellular matrix components, including elastin. Elastin confers elastic recoil to tissues such as lung. Inflammatory episodes are more severe and prolonged than normal, with more tissue damage leading to scarring. A1AT deficiency may occur due to defects at several molecular sites; thus some patients are more severely affected than others

Key facts

Lysosomal contents

Specific granules contain:

- Lactoferrin
- Lysozyme
- Alkaline phosphatase
- Collagenase
- Leukocyte adhesion molecule

Azurophilic granules contain:

- Myeloperoxidase
- Lysozyme
- Cationic proteins
- Acid hydrolases
- Neutral proteases (elastase)

PLASMA-DERIVED MEDIATORS

Kinin system

Bradykinin is the major active product of this system. This polypeptide is one of the most powerful vasodilators known to man. It increases vascular permeability and also induces pain when injected into the skin. The kinin cascade is activated by Hageman factor and its relationship to the coagulation system is shown in Fig. 6.3 (page 149). As with other cascades, this contains an amplification step because kallikrein itself acts to stimulate production of Hageman factor.

Clotting and fibrinolytic systems

This system is not only important in inflammation but also central to blood clotting, as discussed in Chapter 6. It is the end-product fibrinopeptides that act as chemical mediators in inflammation. These increase vascular permeability and are chemotactic for neutrophils. As in the kinin system, the cascade is

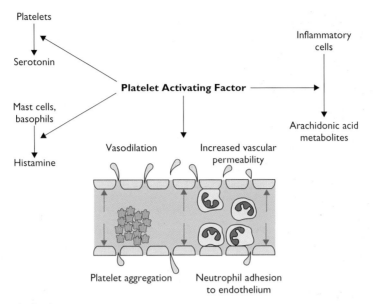

Figure 4.17 Platelet-activating factor

activated by Hageman factor and includes an amplification loop so that plasmin stimulates Hageman factor. Plasmin is a multifunctional protease that also lyses fibrin clots to produce fibrin-degradation products, which themselves induce permeability changes and also trigger the complement system by cleaving C3 (see Fig. 6.3).

The complement system

This system comprises a large number of proteins that are involved in increasing vascular permeability, chemotaxis, opsonization and direct lysis of organisms.

The most important components concerned with the inflammatory reaction are:

- C3a and C5a: increase vascular permeability and chemotaxis
- C3b and C3bi: opsonins
- C5b–9: membrane attack complex, involved in cell lysis.

Activation of this system occurs rapidly through the classical pathway initiated by antigen–antibody complexes, or more slowly through the alternative pathway (Fig. 4.18).

Systemic effects of inflammation

Having considered lobar pneumonia, we have an idea of the local effects of inflammation. We have alluded to the fact that, at the same time, there are many systemic effects that may take place, such as fever, rigors, tachycardia, drop in blood pressure, loss of appetite, vomiting, skeletal weakness and aching. These are known collectively as acute phase reactions.

Fever is a regular accompaniment of inflammatory responses and occurs due to the 'resetting' of the thermoregulatory centre in the anterior hypothalamus. The hypothalamus reacts to the new setting by causing a rise in the body's core temperature by constricting vessels in the skin, so reducing blood flow and limiting heat loss, and by promoting heat production in muscles by shivering. Biological substances that induce fever are called pyrogens. Many bacteria and viruses produce molecules that act as pyrogens and these are called exogenous pyrogens. Endogenous pyrogens are produced by the body. They include:

- tumour necrosis factor (TNF)
- interleukin 1 (IL-1)
- noradrenaline
- α-interferon
- prostaglandin E_1 (PGE_1)
- prostaglandin E_2 (PGE_2).

It is thought that exogenous pyrogens stimulate leukocytes to release the endogenous pyrogen IL-1, which acts on the hypothalamus by raising local PGE_2 levels. Aspirin is useful for lowering the temperature because it interferes with PGE_2 production.

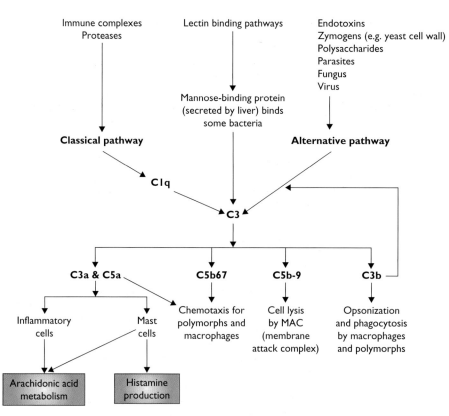

Figure 4.18 The complement system

Localized inflammatory responses lead to changes in plasma proteins due to alterations in liver metabolism. These proteins are called acute phase proteins and this change is thought to be mediated by IL-1, IL-6 and TNF. There is increased production of clotting factors and complement, which is of importance because they are consumed during the inflammatory process. Transport proteins, such as haptoglobins, may be important in regulating the amount of amines and oxygen free radicals. Many other acute phase proteins, such as mannose binding protein (MBP) and C-reactive protein (both opsonins) and serum amyloid A are produced.

The acute phase reaction varies depending on the cause of inflammation. Viral infection is a poor inducer of acute phase proteins, whereas bacterial infections produce a major response, probably by bacterial endotoxins acting indirectly through raised TNFα levels. When investigating a patient, C-reactive protein is the most useful acute phase reactant to measure. If symptoms are equivocal, it may help to establish that there is organic disease rather than psychosomatic disease. In those patients with chronic diseases, a rise

in the level may be an indication of an acute exacerbation or of intercurrent infection (Fig. 4.20).

The number of leukocytes in the peripheral blood increases in many forms of inflammation so that they are available to fight infection. It is assumed that cytokines act through colony-stimulating factors to increase the production and release of cells from the marrow. Again there are differences depending on the type of infection and this may be helpful in making a diagnosis. Bacterial infection provokes an increase in neutrophils, whereas viral infections cause a rise in lymphocyte numbers and allergic reactions or parasitic infections result in more eosinophils.

Trauma or stress of any kind also affects the hypothalamus-pituitary-adrenal axis, resulting in the production of growth hormone, prolactin, antidiuretic hormone (ADH), adrenocorticotrophic hormone (ACTH) and adrenaline. These hormones are responsible for the breakdown of glycogen, changes in fatty acid metabolism and sodium–potassium transport. It is these metabolic changes that are responsible for the malaise, weakness, loss of appetite and other varied systemic effects observed during injury.

Normal control of body temperature and the mechanism of fever:

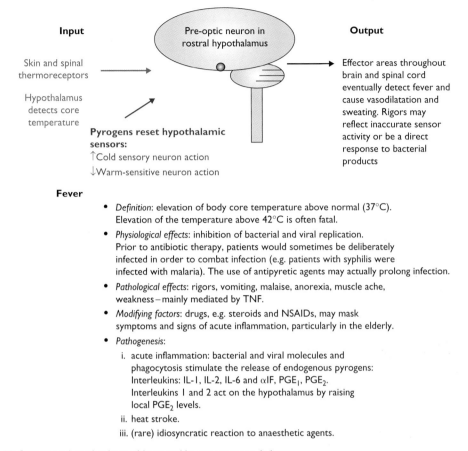

| Input | Pre-optic neuron in rostral hypothalamus | Output |

Skin and spinal thermoreceptors

Hypothalamus detects core temperature

Pyrogens reset hypothalamic sensors:
↑Cold sensory neuron action
↓Warm-sensitive neuron action

Effector areas throughout brain and spinal cord eventually detect fever and cause vasodilatation and sweating. Rigors may reflect inaccurate sensor activity or be a direct response to bacterial products

Fever

- *Definition*: elevation of body core temperature above normal (37°C). Elevation of the temperature above 42°C is often fatal.
- *Physiological effects*: inhibition of bacterial and viral replication. Prior to antibiotic therapy, patients would sometimes be deliberately infected in order to combat infection (e.g. patients with syphilis were infected with malaria). The use of antipyretic agents may actually prolong infection.
- *Pathological effects*: rigors, vomiting, malaise, anorexia, muscle ache, weakness – mainly mediated by TNF.
- *Modifying factors*: drugs, e.g. steroids and NSAIDs, may mask symptoms and signs of acute inflammation, particularly in the elderly.
- *Pathogenesis*:
    i. acute inflammation: bacterial and viral molecules and phagocytosis stimulate the release of endogenous pyrogens: Interleukins: IL-1, IL-2, IL-6 and αIF, PGE_1, PGE_2. Interleukins 1 and 2 act on the hypothalamus by raising local PGE_2 levels.
    ii. heat stroke.
    iii. (rare) idiosyncratic reaction to anaesthetic agents.

Figure 4.19 Causes and mechanisms of fever and its symptoms and signs

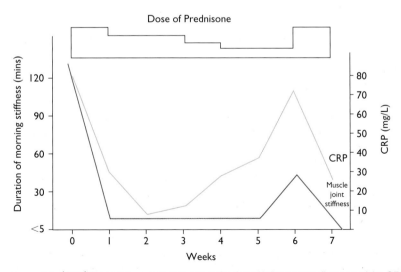

Figure 4.20 C-reactive protein (CRP) fluctuations are an accurate reflection of inflammatory disease activity. CRP levels rise within 4–6 hours and have a half-life of 12 hours. This graph, from a patient with polymyalgia rheumatica, shows the parallel between the patient's symptoms, CRP levels and requirement for prednisone (Acknowledgement: Jo Sheldon, St George's Hospital)

CHRONIC AND GRANULOMATOUS INFLAMMATION

Chronic inflammation differs from acute inflammation in a number of respects. The key features required for a diagnosis of chronic inflammation are:

- mononuclear cell infiltrate composed of macrophages, lymphocytes and plasma cells
- tissue destruction
- granulation tissue formation, i.e. proliferation of fibroblasts and small blood vessels (this is not the same as a granuloma)
- fibrosis.

The definition of chronic inflammation is not as clear-cut as one might like. You might expect that acute and chronic inflammation are the ends of a spectrum and that after a certain length of time has elapsed, an inflammatory process is considered to be chronic. There are instances in which this is the case, for example when acute inflammation fails to resolve, polymorphs may become walled off by fibrous tissue to form abscesses. Some of you will have experienced a dental abscess, in which bacteria enter the jaw through a cracked or carious tooth and thrive in the oxygen-poor environment of the dental root and surrounding bone. Microscopical examination of the abscess would show acute inflammation in the centre with many surrounding chronic inflammatory cells, as well as fibrous tissue. Osteomyelitis is another interesting example of 'chronic' acute inflammation, in which a nidus of infection within a bone becomes walled off (or 'sequestered') by new bone formation. A variety of bacteria may be responsible for osteomyelitis, particularly the Gram-positive coccus *Staphylococcus aureus*, and also the Gram-negative typhoid bacillus, *Salmonella typhi*. The infected bone suppurates and becomes greatly thickened, and the continuing inflammation can act as a source of infected material for dissemination via the blood to other sites in the body.

However, much of the time we find that chronic inflammatory diseases appear to have either a negligible or no acute component and that the disease is typified by a chronic inflammatory cell infiltrate from the start. Rheumatoid arthritis is a good example of a *de novo* chronic inflammatory condition, in which abundant plasma cells and lymphocytes expand the synovium of joints, which becomes greatly thickened and covered in a thick membrane, or 'pannus'

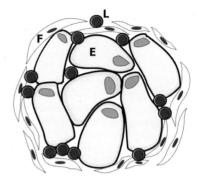

Group of epithelioid cells (E), with variable numbers of lymphocytes (L) and fibroblasts (F)

Figure 4.21 Non-caseating granuloma

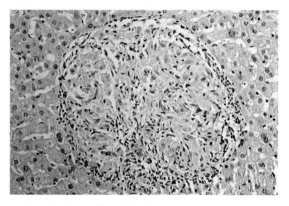

Figure 4.22 Non-caseating granuloma from a patient with sarcoidosis

of fibrin and chronic inflammatory cells. The inflammatory process destroys bone, leading to severe joint deformities, typically in the knee, wrists and the small bones of the hands.

Granulomatous inflammation is a special type of chronic inflammation, characterized by the presence of granulomata. A granuloma is a collection of macrophages frequently surrounded by a rim of lymphocytes. These macrophages are usually modified to become larger, with more abundant pink cytoplasm and are referred to as 'epithelioid' cells.

The factors influencing granuloma formation are largely unknown but a variety of cytokines appear to be involved. Animal experiments suggest that IL-1 is important in the initiation of granulomata and that TNF is responsible for their maintenance. IL-2 has been shown to increase their size and IL-5 can attract eosinophils to the site, as seen in parasitic disease. IL-6 is believed to have an important role in tuberculous granulomata.

Chronic inflammatory disorders are some of the most common, fascinating, devastating and mysterious diseases to affect humans. They include tuberculosis, sarcoidosis, syphilis, leprosy, Crohn's disease, rheumatoid arthritis, systemic lupus erythematosus and the pneumoconioses. Despite the availability of treatment and some information on prevention, tuberculosis remains a significant world-wide problem. For this reason, (and because it turns up in exams with frightening regularity!), we shall discuss tuberculosis (TB) as an example of a chronic granulomatous inflammatory disease.

Tuberculosis

The great German bacteriologist, Robert Koch, was the first to show that tuberculosis is an infective disease, a fact we now take for granted. Koch's original investigations in 1876 were performed with anthrax, which he demonstrated to be the cause of what was then known as 'splenic fever'. It was clear to Koch that in order to implicate a particular organism as the cause of a disease, he must:

- demonstrate the organism in the lesions in all cases of that disease
- be able to isolate the organism and cultivate it in pure culture outside the host
- produce the same disease by injecting the pure culture into a healthy subject.

These three criteria are known as Koch's postulates.

On 24 March 1882, Koch announced the discovery of the tubercle bacillus to the Berlin Physiological Society. His work proved that 'pulmonary consumption' was not a disorder of nutrition but an infective disease that ran a chronic course. Although Koch is best remembered for his contribution to tuberculosis, he did not confine his interests to that disease. He also discovered the cholera vibrio that had created havoc from India to Egypt, investigated bubonic plague in India, researched diseases caused by the tsetse fly in East Africa and studied malaria in Java.

Tuberculosis is caused by *Mycobacterium tuberculosis*, occasionally called the 'Koch Bacillus', and is a world-wide problem. Two strains – *M. tuberculosis hominis* and *M. tuberculosis bovis* – infect humans. Bovine tuberculosis is passed from cattle to humans in milk, entering through the gastrointestinal tract to produce abdominal tuberculosis. It is uncommon in developed countries now that dairy herds are generally free of mycobacteria and milk is pasteurized. Infection with *M. tuberculosis hominis* is the common form and it produces pulmonary tuberculosis.

The incidence of TB, having dipped in the early part of the twentieth century, is now rising: in 1998 the incidence was 10.9 per 100 000 in the UK. Tuberculosis is more common in the young and the very old and there are definite racial and ethnic differences in incidence. It is commoner in Asians (in the UK the incidence in this group is 121 per 100 000), black Africans (in the UK the incidence in this group is 210 per 100 000), American Indians, the Irish and Eskimos. By contrast TB is seen in only 5 per 100 000 in the UK white ethnic group. The incidence is generally due to reactivation of tuberculosis in migrants to the UK, born in countries with a high prevalence of tuberculosis. The disease also flourishes in socially deprived areas and poverty and malnutrition appear to be important predisposing factors. There is a higher incidence in males and in people suffering from alcoholism, chronic lung diseases and conditions causing immunosuppression, e.g. cancer and AIDS.

Patients with tuberculosis may present with a cough producing blood-stained sputum or, more subtly, with night sweats, weight loss and vague symptoms of ill-health.

Mycobacterium tuberculosis is a slender, rod-shaped organism, approximately 4 µm in length. It is not visible on haematoxylin and eosin-stained sections but can be stained using the Ziehl–Neelsen method. This reaction relies on the fact that, once stained, the organisms are resistant to decolorization with acid and alcohol (hence the term 'acid and alcohol-fast bacilli', AAFB). Mycobacteria grow very slowly in culture and may not be apparent for 6 weeks. Observing the bacilli in excised tissues will allow faster diagnosis and treatment, but they will not be seen in sections unless there are approximately one million bacteria per millilitre of tissue. Using the polymerase chain reaction (see page 63) to detect mycobacterial nucleic acid is both reasonably fast and more sensitive but technically more difficult and not generally available.

Mycobacterium tuberculosis does not possess any toxins with which to harm its host, however a number of cell membrane glycolipids and proteins, including bacterial stress proteins, act to provoke a hypersensitivity reaction. It is the hypersensitivity reaction that causes the tissue destruction so characteristic of this disease.

PRIMARY TUBERCULOSIS

Primary TB occurs in individuals who have never previously been infected with *Mycobacterium tuberculosis*.

Inhalation of the organism produces a small lesion (approximately 1 cm in diameter), usually in the subpleural region in the lower part of the upper lobe or the upper part of the lower lobe of lung. This is referred to as the Ghon focus. Lesions occur in these sites because the bacterium is a strict aerobe and prefers these well-oxygenated regions. When the tissue is first invaded by the mycobacteria, there is no hypersensitivity reaction, but an initial transient acute, non-specific, inflammatory response with neutrophils predominating. This is followed rapidly by an influx of macrophages, which ingest the bacilli and present their antigens to T lymphocytes, leading to the proliferation of a clone of T cells and the emergence of specific hypersensitivity. The lymphocytes release lymphokines, which attract more macrophages. These accumulate to form the characteristic granuloma, containing a mixture of macrophages, including epithelioid cells and Langhan-type giant cells. Tissue destruction leads to necrosis in the centre of the granuloma called caseous necrosis because, macroscopically, the necrotic area resembles cheesy material! Tubercle bacilli, either free or contained in macrophages, may drain to the regional lymph nodes and set up granulomatous inflammation, causing massive lymph node enlargement. The combination of the Ghon focus and the regional nodes is called the primary complex.

Thus, the development of hypersensitivity results in tissue destruction but also improves the body's resistance to the mycobacterium by promoting phagocytosis and reducing intracellular replication of bacilli. It is not known why the granulomatous response to mycobacteria produces caseation whereas most other granulomatous reactions do not. Another puzzle is why the attraction of macrophages in most inflammatory responses produces a dispersed infiltrate while in granulomatous reactions they form well-demarcated collections – granulomata.

In the majority of cases, the primary Ghon complex (Ghon focus plus enlarged hilar lymph nodes) will heal. There will be replacement of the caseous necrosis by a small fibrous scar and the lesion will be walled off. Calcification may also occur in these lesions. Despite this, the mycobacterial organisms may survive and lead to reactivation infection at a later date, especially if the host defences become

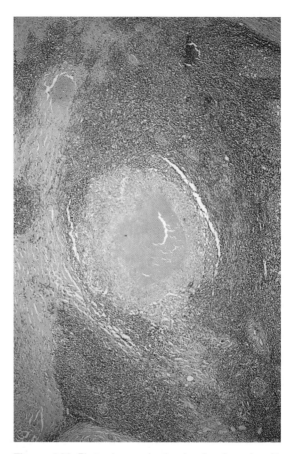

Figure 4.23 Photomicrograph showing lymph node with caseous necrosis

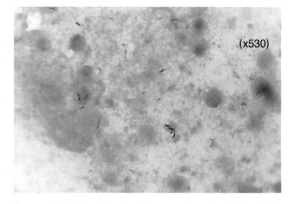

(x530)

Figure 4.24 ZN stain showing presence of acid-fast (red) bacilli (From Lydyard, P. *et al.* 2000: *Pathology Integrated: An A–Z of Disease and its Pathogenesis*. London: Arnold.)

lowered, as can occur with cancer or steroid treatment for diseases such as rheumatoid arthritis.

There are, however, alternative outcomes. If the hypersensitivity reaction is severe, it will lead to a florid inflammatory response and the patient may present with a systemic illness. If the caseous necrosis is extensive, the tissue destruction may erode major bronchi and allow air-borne spread of organisms to produce satellite lesions in either lung. Alternatively, tubercle bacilli may enter the bloodstream. If they enter a small pulmonary arteriole, then the bacilli will lodge in lung tissue. However, if they enter a pulmonary vein the bacilli may disseminate throughout the systemic circulation. If this occurs, numerous small granulomata may be encountered in almost any organ including meninges, kidneys and adrenals. This type of disease is called miliary tuberculosis, so-called because the lesions look like millet seeds! This is a disastrous complication, associated with a high risk of death. Fortunately, systemic spread is not a common event in primary disease.

SECONDARY TUBERCULOSIS

Secondary, or post-primary, tuberculosis refers to infection occurring in a patient previously sensitized to the mycobacteria. Most of these cases result from reactivation of latent mycobacteria following an asymptomatic primary infection. The latency period can vary tremendously and reactivation may not occur for many decades. (Occasionally there is reinfection from an exogenous source.)

Secondary infection tends to affect the subapical region of the upper lobe and although the reasons for this are far from clear, it is believed to be due to the higher oxygen concentration in this part. (If you remember, tubercle bacilli are obligate aerobes.) This focus of reactivation is called the Assman focus.

There are three possible outcomes of secondary tuberculous infection: healing, cavitation or spread.

Because there has been previous infection, the host will have some degree of immunity. If this is sufficient, the reactivated infection will heal, with scarring and subsequent calcification. Intervention with antituberculous drugs will also enhance and modify the healing process. If, on the other hand, the host's degree of hypersensitivity is high and/or the organisms are particularly virulent, there may be considerable lung tissue destruction and caseous necrosis, which can lead to the formation of a cavity.

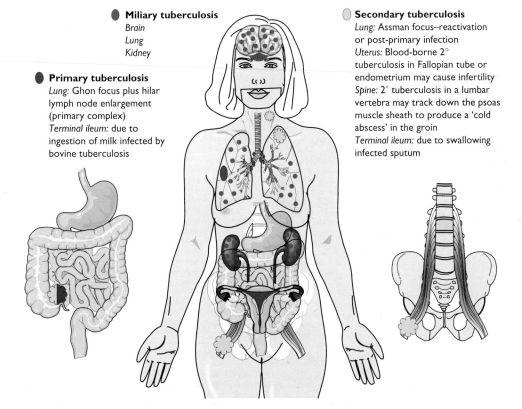

● **Miliary tuberculosis**
  Brain
  Lung
  Kidney

● **Primary tuberculosis**
  Lung: Ghon focus plus hilar lymph node enlargement (primary complex)
  Terminal ileum: due to ingestion of milk infected by bovine tuberculosis

○ **Secondary tuberculosis**
  Lung: Assman focus–reactivation or post-primary infection
  Uterus: Blood-borne 2° tuberculosis in Fallopian tube or endometrium may cause infertility
  Spine: 2° tuberculosis in a lumbar vertebra may track down the psoas muscle sheath to produce a 'cold abscess' in the groin
  Terminal ileum: due to swallowing infected sputum

Figure 4.25 Tuberculosis

The infected caseous material may spread through destroyed tissue or via bronchi to adjacent parts of the lung and extend the local disease. Patients with cavitation and bronchial erosion are usually highly

Key facts

Some causes of granulomatous inflammation

Bacterial
  Tuberculosis
  Leprosy
  Syphilis

Fungal
  Cryptococcus
  Coccidioides

Protozoal
  Toxoplasmosis
  Pneumocystis

Parasitic
  Schistosomiasis

Inorganic material
  Silicosis
  Berylliosis
  Foreign material

Autoimmune
  Rheumatoid arthritis
  Primary biliary cirrhosis

Unknown
  Sarcoidosis
  Crohn's disease

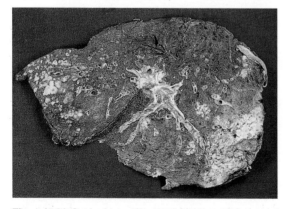

Figure 4.26 Cut surface of the lung showing white areas of caseation due to tuberculosis in the upper and lower lobes

infectious, since they can cough up large numbers of organisms. The pleura may become involved, with the production of an effusion, which can contain caseous and necrotic material – a tuberculous empyema. Infected sputum may be swallowed, spreading the disease to the gastrointestinal tract. Systemic spread to produce miliary tuberculosis is more common in post-primary tuberculosis because tissue destruction is greater and there is more likelihood of venous disruption and dissemination of organisms.

The natural history of the disease will depend on the host's immunity, hypersensitivity and factors such as nutritional status, associated disease and intervention with (preventative) BCG vaccination or treatment of active disease with antituberculous drugs. Tuberculosis is a treatable disease, yet despite this, it remains a major problem in developing countries and there is a worrying trend towards the development of antibiotic-resistant strains in developed countries. Inoculation with the BCG vaccine has greatly reduced the incidence of post-primary tuberculosis, but it has had less effect on reactivation tuberculosis.

Not all granulomas are caused by tuberculosis! Some other causes of granulomatous inflammation are listed below. Many are due to infections, some are of autoimmune aetiology and sometimes we do not know the cause, as in the case of sarcoid and Crohn's disease. A tissue biopsy is essential when trying to establish the cause of granulomatous disease.

Sarcoidosis

Sarcoidosis is a baffling systemic disease of unknown aetiology and is characterized by the presence of granulomata, which, unlike those in tuberculosis, do not exhibit caseous necrosis and so are termed 'non-caseating granulomas'.

Sarcoidosis is a systemic disorder of variable severity, and can present in numerous ways. Many patients are asymptomatic and diagnosis is only made at post mortem. Almost every organ in the body may be affected, the commonest being lung, liver, spleen, skin and salivary glands with the heart, kidneys and central nervous system slightly less commonly affected. Most patients present with respiratory symptoms (shortness of breath, haemoptysis and chest pain) but some have a more rapid course with fever, erythema nodosum and polyarthritis. Patients may also present with signs and symptoms of hypercalcaemia, and lytic bone lesions, especially in the phalanges, are strong supportive evidence for the disease.

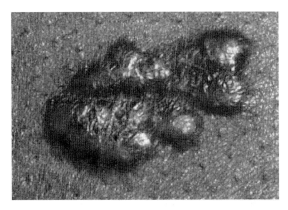

Figure 4.27 Raised skin lesion in sarcoidosis. Microscopy would show epitheloid granulomata

The only way to be certain of the cause of granulomatous disease is either to see it under the microscope, as for instance with fungal hyphae or acid and alcohol-fast bacilli, or to culture the organism. However, some macrophage variants are more common in specific conditions and the type seen may offer a clue as to the underlying cause. We will discuss the origin and activity of this remarkable cell in the following section, but for now will consider briefly the ways in which macrophages may adapt to fight particular diseases, becoming morphologically distinctive in the process.

Having learnt about acute inflammation, chronic inflammation and the immune system, you will appreciate the complex interplay between cells and mediators. It is a veritable orchestra but who is the conductor? As yet we do not know; perhaps there is not one, but a key player is undoubtedly the macrophage and it is useful to summarize inflammation and repair by reviewing macrophage function.

MACROPHAGES

Macrophages are involved in all inflammatory processes with their ability to phagocytose particles, process and present antigens and secrete an array of mediators. They are derived from stem cells in the bone marrow that also give rise to polymorphonuclear leukocyte precursors. The marrow cells produce monocytes that circulate in the blood for a day or two before migrating into the tissues where they are called macrophages or (a more old-fashioned term) histiocytes. As well as entering areas of inflammation and damage, there are also relatively fixed

macrophages, lining the endothelial aspects of vessels in the liver (Kupffer cells), spleen, bone marrow and lymph nodes; the so-called reticuloendothelial system. Other macrophages line parts of the central nervous system (microglial cells). Particularly in the spleen, sinusoidal macrophages remove from circulation those red blood cells that have either passed their sell-by date (the lifespan of a normal red cell is 120 days) or become battered and worn. This can happen in inherited diseases of the red cell membrane (e.g. hereditary spherocytosis, in which the red cells are round and incompressible, or sickle cell anaemia, in which a point mutation alters the shape of the red cell under conditions of poor oxygenation, and causes sludging of the sickled cells within blood vessels) or autoimmune diseases, in which antibodies are produced against the body's own red cells. The sinusoidal macrophages also phagocytose bacteria that have been opsonized with antibody.

A common misconception is that the spleen is redundant and can be removed with impunity: but splenectomy patients are particularly susceptible to severe infection by encapsulated bacteria, such as *Haemophilus influenzae* or *Streptococcus pneumoniae*. Splenectomized patients must receive lifelong antibiotic therapy if it has not been possible to vaccinate them prior to the removal of the spleen.

Just like neutrophils in acute inflammation, macrophages emigrate and activate under the influence of chemotactic factors, adhesion molecules and cytokines, etc. An activated macrophage increases its size and its lysosomal enzyme content and speeds up its metabolism and ability to phagocytose and kill microbes. A crucially important function is their ability to scavenge and phagocytose in areas of damage.

Macrophages possess scavenger receptor molecules, which are important in self/non-self discrimination and appear able to bind to a wide range of modified molecules. Most important of these is modified LDL (low-density lipoprotein), but modified albumin and probably other molecules can also be bound and phagocytosed. Unlike LDL receptors on other tissue cells, these surface receptors are not downregulated as the LDL content of the cytoplasm increases. This means that macrophages keep taking up lipid etc. and become foamy macrophages, seen in areas of tissue damage and atheromatous plaques (page 173).

Macrophages are also important because they synthesize and secrete factors that promote granulation tissue formation and enhance healing and repair. For example, macrophage-derived growth factor stimulates endothelial cells, resulting in new vessel formation, and fibroblasts for collagen and extracellular matrix production.

After an acute insult, macrophages will assist in healing and repair and then depart. However, in chronic inflammation, macrophages are potentially harmful because they produce a variety of substances that maintain the inflammatory process and attract and stimulate other inflammatory cells, contributing to local tissue injury and fibrosis. Their continued presence is due principally to continued emigration from the blood, a reduction in movement out of the tissues and some local proliferation.

Macrophages in specific diseases

Epithelioid cells occur in all types of granulomatous disease. They have some resemblance to epithelial cells, possessing abundant pink cytoplasm, packed with endoplasmic reticulum, Golgi apparatus and vesicles. Thus the cells are well adapted to synthesize

macrophage products, such as arachidonic acid metabolites, complement, coagulation factors and cytokines. However, they are less mobile and less proficient at phagocytosis than ordinary macrophages. Multinucleate giant macrophages principally form by fusion of epithelioid cells. Each may have 50 nuclei or more and it is the arrangement of these nuclei that distinguishes the types. The Langhan giant cell is typical of tuberculosis or sarcoid and has its nuclei arranged as a horseshoe at the periphery. The foreign body giant cell, predictably, often contains identifiable foreign material (for instance suture material or shards of glass) in its cytoplasm. Its nuclei are randomly arranged throughout the cell. Foreign

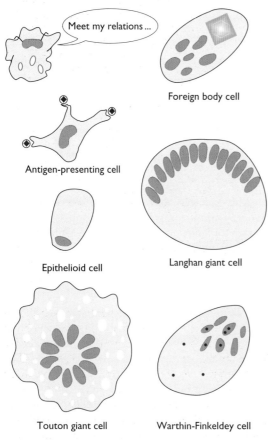

Figure 4.28 Types of macrophage

Meet my relations ...

Foreign body cell

Antigen-presenting cell

Epithelioid cell

Langhan giant cell

Touton giant cell

Warthin-Finkeldey cell

Key facts

The role of the macrophage in chronic inflammation

In chronic inflammation, macrophages:

- present antigen to T cells and B cells, leading to clonal expansion
- scavenge abnormal cells, particles, large molecules, immune complexes, etc.
- produce chemotactic factors for other leukocytes
- stimulate endothelium for adhesion molecule activation and granulation tissue formation
- fuse with other macrophages to form giant cells
- phagocytose and kill some organisms
- harbour some organisms
- exocytose attacking parasites or damaging tissues.

Macrophage products involved in tissue injury include:

- Toxic oxygen metabolites
- Nitric oxide
- Proteases
- Eicosanoids
- Coagulation factors
- Neutrophil chemotactic factors.

body giant cells are also seen often in parasitic infections, such as schistosomiasis ('bilharzia').

These are the most important macrophage variants but, for completeness, we will mention two others. These are the Warthin-Finkeldey cell, pathognomonic of measles and characterized by the presence of eosinophilic nuclear and cytoplasmic inclusions, and Touton giant cells, which have a central cluster of nuclei surrounded by foamy lipid-laden cytoplasm. Touton cells occur in xanthomas, which are benign tumorous collections of lipid-laden macrophages in the skin. (Antigen-presenting cells will be discussed in Chapter 5).

CLINICAL CASE – WOUND HEALING AND REPAIR

Edward, a 22-year-old student, is rushed to Accident and Emergency. He has been rescued from the wreck of a small car entangled with a juggernaut, the result of a miscalculated overtaking manoeuvre on a rainy night. He is unconscious on admission, but he almost immediately regains consciousness and appears lucid and in pain. He has obviously broken his left thigh, which is swollen and shows early bruising. A grating sensation is palpable when the thigh is gently pressed. He has a gaping wound on his right thigh, about 6 cm diameter and 1 cm deep, through which the underlying fatty tissue can be seen, along with much oozing and crusted blood. His blood pressure is low, at 95/40 mmHg, and his pulse rate is 120 beats per minute: these features indicate that he is probably bleeding internally. He may have lost a litre of blood or so into the tissues surrounding his broken femur. However the presence of tenderness and guarding over his upper left abdomen point at a ruptured spleen. Whilst his blood is being cross-matched for transfusion, fluids and plasma expanders are infused to maintain his circulation. An emergency scan indicates that he does indeed have a ruptured spleen. Edward undergoes an emergency splenectomy. His fractured femur is set at the same time, and the gaping wound in his right thigh is debrided (the injured tissue is scraped away) and the site is packed with gauze impregnated with iodine (a disinfectant). By the time his parents have been tracked down and retrieved from a party by the police, Edward is settled in intensive care, in traction, and is beginning to regain consciousness after the anaesthetic.

Once Edward's parents have recovered from the shock of the events they begin to ask questions of the

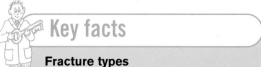

Key facts

Fracture types

- Simple fracture: no communication between bone and skin surface

- Compound fracture: bone fragments breach skin, thus has potential for infection

- Comminuted fracture: multiple bone fragments due to more than one breakage site

- Greenstick fracture (typical in young children): incomplete fracture, with part of a fractured long bone remaining intact

- Stress fracture: the result of abnormal stresses applied to bone (similar to metal fatigue)

- Pathological fracture: the bone is abnormal and fractures easily. There are four types: congenital disease, such as osteogenesis imperfecta; inflammatory disease, such as osteomyelitis; neoplastic disease, such as primary or metastatic tumour in bone; metabolic disease, such as osteoporosis.

Fracture management

- Reduction: to restore bony alignment

- Immobilization: to maintain the alignment until union has occurred – if this cannot be achieved by external fixation in a plaster cast, internal fixation with pins, screws or plates may be required

- Rehabilitation: to restore normal function if possible, or cope with residual disability.

consultant orthopaedic surgeon. Edward was unconscious on arrival – will he suffer any permanent brain damage? He is a keen rugby player with possible hopes for the national squad – when, if ever, will he be able to play again? And what about the loss of his spleen – isn't it important? How long will his operation scar take to heal? He supplements his student grant by stacking supermarket shelves late at night – a job that involves lifting heavy boxes and crates. When will he be able to return to work?

The surgeon tackles the questions when he can get a word in. It is too early to tell whether Edward has any lasting brain injury, but the speed of his return to consciousness bodes well. The spleen *is* an important organ, with a particular role in removing certain bacteria from the blood. Without going into too much detail, he tells them that Edward must be inoculated against pneumococci and will have to take lifelong antibiotic prophylaxis against other bacterial infection, but should otherwise manage very well. Edward will not be fit for shelf stacking for at least three months. His fracture is uncomplicated and should heal well – as long as all goes according to plan, he should be walking on crutches in 6 weeks and be ready for rugby after several months of rehabilitation.

Edward's parents are content with this, but let us examine the surgeon's statements about wound and bone fracture healing in a bit more detail. We know already that any tissue injury will initiate acute inflammation (see Chapter 4) and that neutrophil polymorphs will soon arrive at the scene of the damage, along with macrophages, to start phagocytosing the debris. If any microorganisms have penetrated the skin wounds, they will be immobilized and phagocytosed, opsonized by a combination of circulating antibody and complement. But what happens next?

Cell capacity for regeneration

What happens when injury causes loss of normal tissue and leaves a defect, for example a cut in the skin? In this situation the end result depends on the size of the defect and the capacity of the tissue to regenerate. Not all tissues of the body have the same capacity to regenerate and cells can be divided into three major types: labile, stable and permanent.

The labile cells include epithelial and blood cells; these divide and proliferate throughout life and the cells have a set lifespan. Stable cells normally divide extremely slowly but can proliferate rapidly if required. If you remove half the liver, the cells will regenerate and return it to its original size! Other examples of stable cells are fibroblasts, vascular endothelial cells, smooth muscle cells, osteoblasts and renal tubular epithelial cells. Permanent cells cannot divide but may be capable of some individual cell repair if the nucleus and synthetic apparatus are intact. Examples include neurons and cardiac muscle cells. If a permanent cell is damaged but not destroyed, as in injury to a nerve axon, there may

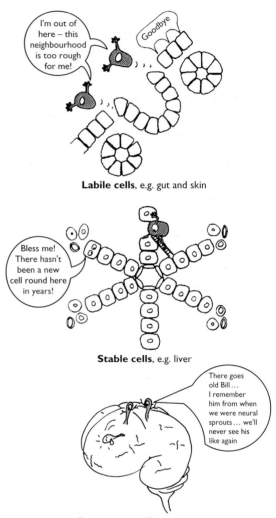

Figure 4.29 The capacity for cell regeneration after damage depends on the type of tissue involved

be regrowth of the damaged portion. However, if the whole cell is destroyed, it must be replaced by a small scar because its neighbouring cells are incapable of proliferating to replace it.

When injury takes place and the processes of inflammation are set in motion, the elements of repair and healing are also activated. Briefly, the processes that take place during and after the injury are:

- removal of dead and foreign material
- regeneration of injured tissue from cells of the same type
- replacement of damaged tissue by new connective tissue.

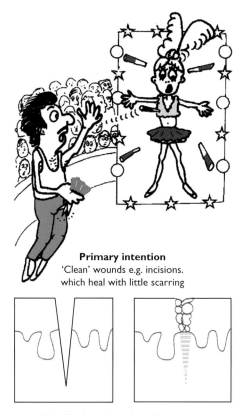

Primary intention
'Clean' wounds e.g. incisions.
which heal with little scarring

Figure 4.30 Healing by primary intention

Wound healing requires:

- haemostasis
- inflammation
- cell proliferation and repair
- adequate nutrition.

Ideally, adequate tissue repair will occur within 3 weeks. This process of restoring the tissue to pristine condition is called resolution. Resolution requires that the inflammatory process deals quickly with the insult, the tissue has not lost its basic scaffolding and any damaged specialized cells are capable of regeneration. The size of the defect is very important, as any destruction of the tissue scaffold will result in scarring.

Although the basic mechanisms involved in wound healing are the same, by convention, the healing of cleanly incised wounds, where the edges are in close apposition, is considered separately from those in which there is extensive loss of epithelium, a large subepithelial tissue defect which has to be filled in by scar tissue and where the edges cannot be

brought together with sutures. These two circumstances are described as 'healing by primary intention' or 'healing by secondary intention'. These terms first appeared in a surgical treatise published in 1543, although John Thomson (1813) in *Lectures on Inflammation*, gives the credit for introducing these terms to Galen.

Healing by primary intention

Let us return to Edward and consider his abdominal surgical incision, made at the time of splenectomy. This is about the cleanest type of wound you can get – in both senses. Not only is surgery performed using aseptic technique, but also a sharp knife makes the wound, with the minimum of tissue trauma. The healing in this type of instance, in which the two sides need merely to be pushed back together and held still (by sutures) in order to heal, is known as 'healing by primary intention'.

The skill of the surgeon has a role to play in the outcome of course, not least in the selection of an incision site that will not come under undue tension, which would tend to pull the wound sides apart as soon as the sutures have been removed.

Healing by secondary intention

What about the large gash on Edward's thigh? You will recall that this was not sutured, but left open, packed with gauze. How will this wound heal? And why not suture the sides together, so that the skin can form a barrier to infection from marauding bacteria?

This was a very large wound – almost the size of the palm of Edward's hand – it would have been impossible to appose the sides without generating unbearable tension on the tissues. Also, there was severely damaged tissue at the wound base, not the clean edges of a surgical excision. Dead tissue may form a nidus for infection, and it is quite possible that microorganisms had already entered the wound site by the time Edward arrived at the A&E department. The surgeon has cleared away the obviously dead tissue. By allowing this wound to granulate up, i.e. heal by what is called 'secondary intention', the patient will stand a good chance of an uncomplicated repair, though at the expense of an unsightly scar. Luckily Edward does not rely on the appearance of his thighs to make a living.

WHAT DOES WOUND HEALING LOOK LIKE AT THE TISSUE LEVEL?

Damage to the small blood vessels of the skin causes haemorrhage which helps to 'glue' the edges together and provides the protective dry surface scab (Fig. 4.31a). First, neutrophils migrate from the vessels to the damaged area and epidermal cells proliferate at the surface. Within a few hours of wounding, a single layer of epidermal cells starts to migrate from the wound edges to form a delicate covering over the raw area exposed by the loss of epidermis. Normal keratinocytes are non-motile but can alter their phenotype in order to re-epithelialize a surface defect. Epidermal cell movement can provide an initial covering for very small wounds, but in most instances new cells are derived from the stem cell compartment of the epidermis. From about 12 hours after wounding, there is a marked increase in mitotic activity in the basal cells lying close to the cut edges. The new epidermal cells grow under the surface fibrin/fibronectin clot and for a little distance down the

gap between the cut edges to form a small 'spur' of epithelium which afterwards regresses. If the wound has been sutured, a similar downgrowth of new epidermis occurs in relation to the suture tracks and, on occasion, these may form the basis of keratin-forming cysts within the dermis – so-called 'implantation dermoid cysts'. This ability of epidermal cells to grow along tracts created by sutures or other foreign material is of course the basis for piercing of tissues for earrings, nose rings, etc. Once re-epithelialization is complete, basement proteins will reappear and the epithelial cells revert to their normal non-migratory phenotype.

Meanwhile, there is an influx of macrophages, proliferation of fibroblasts and ingrowth of many fine capillaries (granulation tissue) (Fig. 4.31b). The macrophages are involved in the demolition and removal of any inflammatory exudate and tissue debris and in restoring the tensile strength of the subepithelial connective tissue. They accomplish this by secreting chemoattractants, which recruit

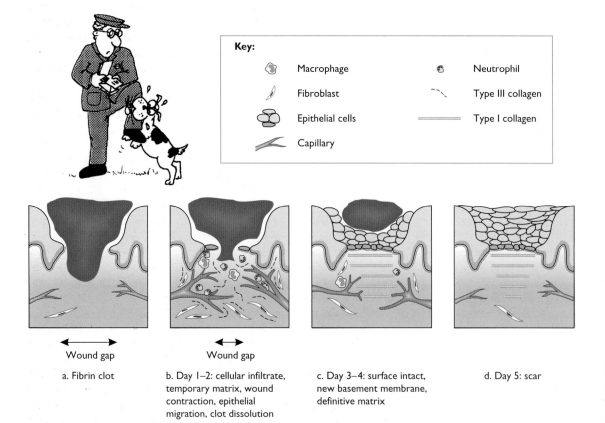

Key:

Macrophage		Neutrophil	
Fibroblast		Type III collagen	
Epithelial cells		Type I collagen	
Capillary			

Wound gap

Wound gap

a. Fibrin clot

b. Day 1–2: cellular infiltrate, temporary matrix, wound contraction, epithelial migration, clot dissolution

c. Day 3–4: surface intact, new basement membrane, definitive matrix

d. Day 5: scar

Figure 4.31 Healing by secondary intention

the cells that synthesize and secrete collagen and other connective tissue proteins (i.e. fibroblasts). The macrophages also expand the existing small fibroblast population by stimulating the cells to proliferate, and stimulate these new fibroblasts to secrete extracellular connective tissue proteins.

Fibroblast growth factors (FGFs) stimulate the endothelial cells of capillaries and postcapillary venules to secrete proteases that digest the surrounding basement membrane. The endothelial cells then proliferate to produce a bud of cells protruding through the gap in the wall towards the source of the stimulus. At first the bud of endothelial cells is solid but eventually it canalizes to allow the flow of blood, although quite how the circulatory loop is completed is not known.

The ingrowth of new small blood vessels (angiogenesis) into the area undergoing repair is thought to be a result of the secretion of factors such as vascular endothelial growth factor β, angiogenin, angiotropin and TNFα, hypoxia and the accumulation of lactate that occurs in anoxic tissues. Angiogenesis involves the budding of new endothelial cells from small intact blood vessels at the edges of the wound, and chemoattraction of these new endothelial cells into the fibrin/fibronectin gel within the wounded area. This combination of a richly vascularized gel in which both inflammatory cells and collagen-producing fibroblasts are present is known as granulation tissue. The term is derived from the observation that the raw surface of a wound shows a granular appearance, rather like that seen on the surface of a strawberry. Each of these 'granules' contains a loop of capillaries and hence bleeds easily if traumatized.

At this stage, there is a temporary matrix of type III collagen. Epithelial migration halts by contact inhibition and a definitive matrix (type I collagen) is laid down. The vessels and inflammatory cells reduce in number (Fig. 4.31c). By day 5, bundles of collagen have been laid down across the damaged tissue to form a scar and the epidermis has returned to normal thickness (Fig. 4.31d). The ultimate development of tensile strength in a wound depends on the production of adequate amounts of collagen and on the final orientation of that collagen. Within a few weeks, the amount of collagen in the wounded area is normal, though preoperative tensile strength is not regained for some months. Replacement and remodelling of the collagen formed early in wound healing is an important part of the healing process. Initially the scar is red, because of the increase in small vessels, but it will blanch over the next few weeks as the vessels regress and the collagen thickens.

If the cut is fine and there is good wound apposition, the scar tissue is limited and the cosmetic result good, but how strong is the repair? Immediately after surgery, the wound has around 70 per cent of the strength of normal skin, but this is principally conferred by the sutures. When these are removed, after 7–10 days, the wound strength drops to 10 per cent of normal; a point to emphasize to patients. Strength then increases rapidly over the next month to reach a maximum at around three months, when a well-healed scar will have 70–80 per cent of the tensile strength of uninjured skin. Interestingly, the strength does not correlate with the amount of collagen but may be related to the type, with type I being stronger than the type III deposited early in the repair process. Abnormal regulation of this process is responsible for the development of keloid scars.

The processes involved in healing by secondary intention are the same as those for primary intention, but the amount of scar tissue generated is greater. One feature that helps to speed up the healing process, and that is not seen in relation to healing of incised wounds, is wound contraction. Because scar contraction is so effective, even a 6-cm gash like Edward's will reduce to about half the diameter or less once it has scarred. Whilst not a problem on his thigh, in a wound at a more strategic site – over a joint, for instance – scarring of this degree could interfere with function and an alternative approach, such as skin grafting, may have to be employed. Wounds of this size can alternatively be closed in a two-stage operation – first the wound is cleaned by washing and debridement, and left to granulate for 5–7 days. When it is clear that it is healing well, the surgeon will then scrape the wound base and sides until there is pinpoint bleeding, indicating good vascularity, and the edges, now under less tension due to diminished tissue oedema, can be apposed and sutured together. (This will still result in healing by secondary intention, with the production of moderate scar tissue, since there has been appreciable tissue loss.)

Most wounds, whether of skin or internal organs, will heal in this way but an interesting exception is bone. This breaks the rules and does not heal with a fibrous scar. Even if the 'scaffold' is completely distorted, as with a traumatic fracture, it will remodel to resemble the original structure and function. If it did not, the bone would remain flexible at the breakpoint.

Healing in bone

We have not forgotten Edward's fractured femur. The femur is a tubular bone, which means that it is formed of a hollow sheath of lamellar bone, which is filled with fat, bone marrow and a delicate mesh-work of bony trabeculae. The tubular shaft imparts the strength of the bone, and the lamellae (or layers) indicate the direction in which the bone has been laid down – in line with the direction of stress. The direct trauma imparted on the femur by the car crash caused it to fracture transversely across its shaft. About a litre of blood will have oozed from vessels damaged at the site, causing a localized haematoma. Early bruising and swelling of the thigh was evident by the time he reached hospital, since extracting him from the car crash took well over an hour. The two free fracture ends grated together when the leg was moved, which caused Edward great pain and produced the sensation of crepitus at the fracture site, as noted in the A&E department.

The fracture was reduced, i.e. pulled back into alignment, and maintained in this position by traction. The site was immobilized in a plaster cast to allow optimal conditions for healing. Inside the leg, the body is beavering away at much the same thing. At the fracture site a kind of internal splint is formed by the haematoma, formed from clotted blood, and also the localized tissue swelling, secondary to the

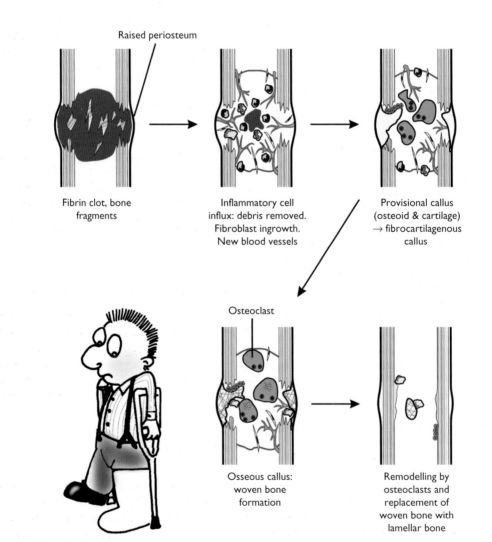

Figure 4.32 Bone healing

release of inflammatory mediators. Polymorphs and macrophages from the blood and surrounding tissues appear within hours and increase in number over the next 2 days. They phagocytose the debris: bony fragments, blood clot and damaged connective tissue. Under the influence of inflammatory mediators, fibroblasts invade the wound site and the ingrowth of new capillaries is stimulated, carrying nutrients to the site. If pressed, the site is still slightly mobile at this stage, but is 'sticky', and is still tender. As the healing process progresses, fibrous tissue and cartilage is laid down, and this ossifies to form woven bone. In Edward's case, this takes 6 weeks.

At this point the fracture is considered to be united, and is no longer tender or mobile under pressure, although it remains swollen. Radiologically there is a clear difference between the original tubular lamellar bone, still obviously sundered but linked by a cuff of woven bone around the wound site, which appears as a loose bony meshwork on X-ray. Several factors influence the rate at which fractures heal, particularly the type and site of the fracture (upper limb heals quicker than lower, oblique or spiral fractures more quickly than transverse) and the age and nutritional state of the patient. For instance a child with a simple spiral fracture of the humerus may heal in 3 weeks, whereas an elderly patient, an adult with a comminuted fracture or any patient with a fracture at a poor-healing site, such as the lower leg, may take 24 weeks to achieve union.

It will take several weeks/months more for the woven bone to be remodelled by osteoclasts within the bone, and for osteoblasts to lay down lamellar bone along the lines of stress, and the patient must be gently mobilized as soon as possible to assist this process. Once union has occurred and the patient is bearing weight, the lumpy new cortical bone gradually becomes resorbed and smoothed out and the excess medullary new bone is removed, restoring a normal medullary cavity. Woven bone, which is quite rapidly formed and which is much less efficient at weight bearing, is resorbed completely and is replaced by lamellar bone. This restoration to normality may take up to a year.

Fortunately, Edward is young and well nourished, and heals quickly. He is back on the rugby ground nine months later. He returns to his supermarket job rather more quickly than is sensible, and develops a small incisional hernia in his abdominal scar. It is causing him no problem at present and he has decided to put up with it.

Healing in nervous tissue

Other specialized tissues heal in specific ways.

CENTRAL NERVOUS SYSTEM

Cerebral infarction is a typical example of neuronal loss. Neurons are a 'permanent' tissue, and in general, once lost they are gone forever. Encouragingly there is now some evidence to suggest that a limited degree of regeneration can take place in the hypothalamic–neurohypophyseal system. Scarring is not a feature of necrosis within the central nervous system – dead brain tissue liquefies and is gradually cleared, leaving empty spaces often called 'lacunar infarcts'. The process elicits the proliferation of glial cells which, together with the ingrowth of capillaries, may constitute a physical barrier to the regeneration of new neuronal fibres. There is encouraging new work in this field, particularly involving the use of bone marrow stem cells.

PERIPHERAL NERVOUS SYSTEM

Severed axons can regenerate. New fibrils sprout from the proximal end of the severed axon, each invaginating the surrounding Schwann cells as they grow, at a rate of about 1 mm per day. If a fibril grows down an existing endoneurial sheath, its function may be recovered. Often, this does not happen and instead the regenerative efforts result in a tangle of fibres embedded in fibrous scar, a 'traumatic neuroma'.

What can go wrong with the healing processes?

When it comes to wound healing, it is not any one thing but rather a complex and dynamic interplay between many factors within an intricate network that determines the final outcome. Failure to heal satisfactorily can be the result of either systemic or local factors.

SYSTEMIC FACTORS

Nutrition

Deficient protein intake may inhibit collagen formation and so inhibit the regaining of tensile strength. Sulphur-containing amino acids such as methionine seem to be particularly important. Vitamin C deficiency has been found to inhibit the secretion of collagen fibres by fibroblasts and adversely affects the deposition of chondroitin sulphate in the extracellular matrix of granulation tissue. Vitamin A has important functions in relation to epithelial proliferation and epithelial differentiation, important in wound healing. A role for zinc in wound healing was discovered more or less by accident. In the course of a study on the effects of certain amino acids on wound healing, a phenylalanine analogue that had been expected to impair healing, instead accelerated it. Careful study of this analogue revealed that the sample used had been contaminated by zinc. Zinc deficiency, such as is found in patients who have been on parenteral nutrition for long periods and in patients with severe burns, is associated with poor healing.

Steroid treatment, chemotherapy and radiotherapy

It is well known that steroids damp down the inflammatory response and are of great use in diseases where the inflammatory response is causing more harm than good. The effect on healing may be a secondary phenomenon related to this effect on inflammation. This is probably due to a reduction in macrophages entering the wound and, hence, a reduction in macrophage-derived factors important in healing. There may also be a direct effect on fibroblasts to reduce collagen production. Steroids are therefore administered in situations where inappropriate scarring is taking place, such as in interstitial fibrosis in the lung.

Chemotherapy and radiotherapy also reduce the number of circulating monocytes and so probably cause a reduction in wound macrophages.

LOCAL FACTORS

Foreign material and/or infection

The presence of infection or of a foreign body will increase the intensity and prolong the duration of the inflammatory response to injury. It is worth remembering that fragments of dead tissue, such as bone, and other elements of the patient's own tissues which have become misplaced, such as hair or keratin, act as foreign bodies.

Poor immobilization of wound edges

Excess mobility in any tissue will impair healing and prolong the time to full recovery. In bones, this may cause non-union or the development of pseudarthrosis.

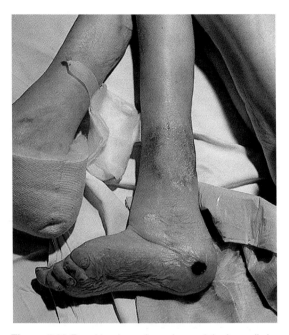

Figure 4.33 Poor blood supply, oedema of the lower limbs, poor nutrition and infection may all contribute to the failure to heal of a pressure sore in a bed-ridden patient

Vascular supply

If the arterial perfusion of the wound site is compromised by stenosis or occlusion, as for instance in atherosclerosis, healing may be delayed or completely inhibited. Adequate venous drainage is also important, and impairment of this may play a part in the genesis of chronic ulcers, which often occur on the anterior surface of the legs in elderly patients. Poor oxygenation of adequately perfused tissue, for instance in severe anaemia, will also impair healing.

PROBLEMS SPECIFIC TO BONE HEALING

- Non-union often as a result of excess movement in the fracture ends, the gap is bridged by fibrous scar tissue instead of the usual bone-forming process. This can result in a useless bone, which cannot resist the pull of attached muscles. If the fibrous segment is extremely short, a good union may be achieved, at the cost of bone strength.
- Pseudarthrosis This is analagous to non-union, but here a joint develops, sometimes with a synovial space and cartilagenous lining. Obviously this creates a useless bone.
- Mal-union The bony ends are poorly apposed, and may overlap. Mal-union may result in a

shortened, deformed bone with a degree of normal function. In other forms of mal-union, adhesions may form between adjacent muscle and the bone, as a result of scarring following inflammation.

- Osteomyelitis A focus of infection may persist following a compound fracture. However, osteomyelitis more commonly results from blood-borne spread of bacteria.

How can wound healing be improved?

The discussion of factors modifying wound healing emphasizes that a clean, uninfected, immobile wound with the sides closely apposed in a healthy patient is most likely to heal quickly and neatly. There are several new approaches to wound healing currently under investigation. For example, wound healing may be improved by the local use of ultrasound or laser therapy, which are thought to increase vascular permeability. Synthetic growth factors, applied topically, may stimulate the healing of chronically ulcerated sites and there has been particular interest in the topical application of keratinocyte growth factor and transforming growth factor beta. Stubborn bone fractures may be persuaded to unite by the passage of electrical currents through the bone.

Before we finish, we should not forget the complications of healing. While a cleanly incised wound from an appendicectomy may only cause minor embarrassment to the vain, scarring resulting from severe burns may limit movement across joints due to contractures. A scar in the heart, following the death of muscle fibres from a myocardial infarction, may dilate to produce an aneurysm. This may become the site of thrombus formation and may also produce cardiac arrhythmias, both of which may cause death. Repeated inflammation of the liver because of alcohol ingestion or viral infection, may produce scar tissue that distorts the normal architecture and produces cirrhosis.

CHAPTER 5

The immune response

THE LYMPHATIC SYSTEM IN INFLAMMATION

Before we go on to discuss the other types of inflammatory response, we must consider the role of the lymphatic system in inflammation.

The lymphatic system comprises the collections of organized lymphoid tissues and interconnecting networks of vessels called the lymphatics. Lymphocytes are produced and mature in the bone marrow and thymus. They migrate in the blood to populate and proliferate in the lymph nodes, the spleen and the lining of the gut and respiratory tract, the so-called mucosa-associated lymphoid tissue or MALT. The lymphatic vessels comprise a one-way circulatory system linked to, but separate from, the blood circulation. Lymphocytes which have returned to the bloodstream via the thoracic duct re-enter the tissues. The recirculation of lymphoid cells is important, as it allows information about invading organisms to be shared with other areas of lymphoid cell production. A lymphocyte that has come from a specific area, such as the gut, recognizes particular surface molecules on the endothelial cells of that area (addressins) that allow it to 'home' back to the same tissue.

Lymphatic channels begin as blind-ended sacs, with ultra-thin walls. They consist of little more than endothelial lining cells supported by delicate collagen fibres initially, but as these vessels drain into larger ones they start to resemble veins, eventually developing a muscularized wall. The lymph is all eventually channelled into one large vessel, the thoracic duct, which empties into the venous system at the junction of the left subclavian and internal jugular veins. Like the venous system, lymphatic channels have valves and rely on the pumping action of adjacent muscles to create flow. A distinctive feature of the lymphatic system is the presence of a chain of lymph nodes, stationed at strategic points within the body – these form checkpoints at which the contents are filtered and screened for miscreants.

In tissue capillary systems, more fluid moves out of capillaries due to the pump pressure within the system (hydrostatic pressure) than is returned to the bloodstream due to the pull of plasma proteins (plasma oncotic pressure). This is especially so if there is nearby inflammatory activity, causing plasma proteins to leak out of the excessively permeable vascular endothelium. The tissue fluid is termed lymph and it drains into the lymphatic channels that are present in all tissues. In addition to the fluid, lymph also contains a variety of inflammatory cells, particularly lymphocytes and cells of monocyte/macrophage lineage. The actual number of cells is very variable and increases if the tissue is inflamed. Foreign antigens and particles can also enter the lymph, sometimes loose but often within specialized cells of the monocyte/macrophage lineage.

Let us consider the case of a 10-year-old boy complaining of a severe sore throat which is making it painful to swallow. Examination of his pharynx shows red, swollen tonsils with a purulent exudate on the surface. He also complains of painful lumps in his neck – these are the lymph nodes on either side of the sternomastoid muscle which have enlarged in response to the throat infection.

A swab taken from the tonsil grows *Streptococcus pyogenes*, Lancefield group A. Streptococci, along with other Gram-positive bacteria, have peptidoglycan in their outer wall, which stimulates the inflammatory response. This is the cause of the boy's throat symptoms and the enlargement of the local lymphoid defences in the pharynx. But why are the lymph nodes swollen too? If, for the sake

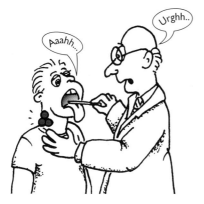

Tonsillar swelling with an overlying purulent discharge is often seen in a sore throat caused by bacterial infection. The draining neck lymph nodes are often swollen and painful

Patrolling and fixed macrophages, circulating lymphocytes and the components of the innate immune system perform 'sentry duty' against invaders

Lymphoid tissue in the body is organized into lymph nodes, mucosa-associated lymphoid tissue (MALT) and the spleen

Figure 5.1a Lymph node enlargement occurs when an antigen, carried in the lymph from the site of infection, stimulates an immune response

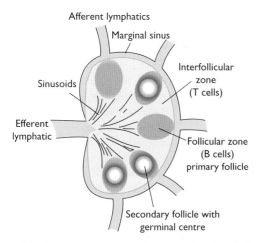

Lymph fluid collected from the interstitial space in the tissues trickles into the marginal sinus of a lymph node via several afferent lymphatics

Lymph contains macrophages, lymphocytes and foreign antigens. It percolates through the lymph node cortex (peripheral region containing B cell follicles), paracortex (T cell rich zone) and medulla and exits via a single efferent lymphatic

The lymph will pass through several more lymph nodes before it empties into the venous system via the largest lymphatic vessel, the thoracic duct

Figure 5.1b Diagram of a lymph node to show location of afferent and efferent lymphatics, B zone (cortex), T zone (paracortex) and medulla

Key components of the lymph node

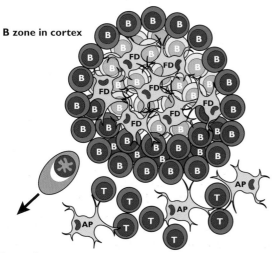

The follicle dendritic cells in the B zones (follicles) and the antigen-presenting cells in the T zones form a mesh resembling a sieve. They catch and present antigen to B and T lymphocytes

A highly specific immune response is generated. B cells produce antibody and T cells produce helper and suppressor/cytotoxic cells

B and T memory cells are generated and guard against another infection by the same agent

Figure 5.1c Higher power view of a secondary follicle and adjacent paracortex to illustrate the anatomical relationship between B cells and FDCs, and T cells and APCs

of illustration, one of the nodes were to be excised for microscopical examination, it would show a number of changes. These arise because lymph fluid, with cellular and particulate matter containing foreign bacterial antigens, drains into lymph nodes of the neck and initiates a specific adaptive immune response inducing proliferation and differentiation of T and B cells.

The responses of T and B cells require help from other cells. T cells cannot recognize foreign antigens unaided and B cells are inefficient at it. These helper cells are called accessory cells and fall into two broad categories, both of monocyte/macrophage lineage.

The first group is called dendritic antigen presenting cells (APC) – dendritic, because they have branch-like processes that increase their surface area. After engulfing a foreign antigen, they can break it into smaller fragments (epitopes) and present different aspects of the antigen to T cells. They express high levels of cell surface co-stimulatory molecules, which help to drive the T cell response. T cell activation requires both antigen presentation and the engagement of co-stimulatory molecules. Cells other than APCs can also stimulate T cell activation – for example B cells, macrophages and epithelial and endothelial cells, all of which can express co-stimulatory molecules.

T cell activation requires both antigen presentation and the engagement of co-stimulatory molecules. Although dendritic cells are the most efficient cells for presentation of antigen, there are other cells which can perform this function. These include B cells, macrophages, epithelial and endothelial cells.

The dendritic APCs should not be confused with follicular dendritic cells (FDC), the second type of accessory cell. FDCs are confined to the lymphoid follicles. They are possibly not of macrophage/monocyte lineage but nevertheless express Fc and complement receptors. FDCs cannot phagocytose or process antigen, but can trap and display it on their surface as whole molecules and they are potent stimulators of B cell differentiation.

The APCs carrying the antigen reach the lymph node through afferent lymphatics and filter through the paracortex where they meet the army of T cells ready for the response. The T cells, recognizing the antigenic epitopes presented by APCs, proliferate and differentiate into helper T cells, which coordinate key aspects of the immune response and

initiate the B cell response. FDCs stimulate B cells to produce antibodies tailored to fit a particular antigen. These changes lead to enlargement of the lymph node, which can be palpated in the neck as in this case.

As we discussed, APCs can trap organisms (in this case, streptococci) to prevent their dissemination into the blood. They do this by grabbing opsonins – attached portions of immunoglobulin (Fc component) or complement (C3b). The opsonins are fixed to the surface of the bug itself or to any soluble antigenic fragments that it may have released. You already know that bacterial wall fragments can directly stimulate the complement cascade to produce C3b. Since at this stage the adaptive immune response has not yet been stimulated and antibody production is a function of the immune response, you may have wondered how there can be any immunoglobulin around for the phagocyte to adhere to? Like any good general anticipating a possible attack, the body prepares itself during the early months of a baby's life. At this time the bone marrow generates millions of different B cell clones, each capable of secreting an antibody likely to be of use in combating infection, and these cells patrol the body. If an antibody is a reasonable 'fit' with an antigen, it can stick to it well enough to opsonize the particle.

The type of agent responsible for an inflammatory reaction determines the most appropriate host immune response. The lymph node is organized into zones to fulfil this function: B lymphocytes, which can develop into plasma cells that produce antibodies, are gathered into aggregates called follicles. These are situated in the cortex of the lymph node; T lymphocytes reside outside the follicles in the interfollicular zone. Bacterial infections, such as the streptococcal infection suffered by our patient, are characterized by the enlargement of the B cell areas (follicular hyperplasia). If, as is more usual, a virus had caused the sore throat, then the T cells would be more important and there would be paracortical hyperplasia.

With any luck, the defences initiated in our 10-year-old patient's lymph nodes will stop the infection from spreading further. If it fails, the streptococcal infection may reach the blood. Infection of the blood (septicaemia) can also occur if organisms that have invaded tissues can directly enter blood vessels instead of lymphatics. The septicaemic patient is gravely ill with fevers, shivering attacks (rigors) and a dangerous lowering of the blood pressure ('shock'). The spleen is all-important here; its structure and functions are analogous to those of the lymph node: it has sinusoids lined by macrophages and specific B and T cell areas, but the fluid percolating through is blood rather than lymph. It exists to trap organisms, debris and particulate matter and to promote immune cell proliferation.

THE ADAPTIVE IMMUNE RESPONSE

The adaptive immune response can be split into humoral immunity and cell-mediated immunity. Humoral immunity occurs as a result of B cells transforming into plasma cells that produce immunoglobulin (which is the same as antibodies). Cell-mediated immunity occurs through T cells. There are several subsets of T cells, but the two most important are the T suppressor/cytotoxic cells, capable of direct attack and lymphokine production and the T helper cells, which act to regulate the immune response and interact widely with other immune-reactive cells.

We start life with an army of B and T cells, raw recruits perhaps, but willing to go into action at the press of a button. Both originate from stem cells in the bone marrow, but early on the T cells are lured away to the thymus by an attractant substance, thymotaxin. The 'action' buttons, or cell surface receptors, have been prepared by an intelligence service that has attempted to anticipate every eventuality. Each cell has a unique receptor, generated after the B cells have undergone a series of rearrangements in their immunoglobulin genes whilst in the bone marrow, and the T cells have similarly rearranged their T cell receptor genes during their maturation in the thymus.

Humoral immunity

HOW DOES A B CELL PRODUCE THE CORRECT ANTIBODY FOR A NEW ANTIGEN?

Surprisingly, it is the antigen which chooses the B cell best equipped to fight it, rather than the other way round! The B cell has no choice in the matter! Mother Nature equips the body with an enormous number of B cells, each armed with a receptor for a unique antigen. Imagine the B cells, lined up around the wall of a dance hall, waiting for the right antigen to ask them to dance! Each B cell has the genetic code for a single antibody and it displays this

antibody on its own cell surface. This 'B cell receptor complex' consists of immunoglobulin M (IgM, see below), which is stuck to the membrane and binds antigen. The IgM is unique to that B cell. The IgM is complexed with other proteins that traverse the cell membrane and are essential for signal transduction, after antigen binding. Only B cells with an antibody that matches the antigen will bind it and thus be stimulated to proliferate. Of course, it requires an enormous number of B cells with different genetic codes to ensure that the body has a B cell equipped to fight any new foreign antigen. (There are at least 10^8 different immunoglobulin molecules in the serum.) Nature discovered a brilliant way of producing this variety of codes, and then used a similar approach for T cell receptor molecules (see page 129).

Whilst we are discussing the receptors displayed on the surface of a B cell, we should mention CD40, which binds to the CD40 ligand present on helper T cells. Without CD40, B cells cannot mature to form plasma cells or secrete IgG, IgA or IgE antibodies. B cells also express a number of co-stimulatory cell surface molecules such as CD80 and CD86 which interact with CD28 on T cells and are critical in development of T cell/B cell interaction. B cells, like macrophages, express MHC class II molecules and carry receptors for complement and the Fc component of immunoglobulin molecules, although they do not phagocytose. You will probably have come across glandular fever (infectious mononucleosis), caused by Epstein–Barr virus (EBV). The virus infects B cells with ease, since its antigen is the same as the complement receptor (CD21), so it has a key to the door.

At the first encounter between a B cell and an appropriate antigen, there is a proliferation of immunologically identical B cells, called clones, together with memory cells. However the 'fit' between the antibody and the antigen can be improved considerably by a bit of adjustment – the difference you might say between an off-the-peg and a tailored garment. The tailoring is achieved through interactions between B cells and antigen presented by follicle dendritic cells. The follicle dendritic cell is a potent inducer of hypermutation in the hypervariable region of the antibody.

A large population of daughter B cells is produced through cloning and these differentiate to form plasma cells; a population of circulating memory B cells is also generated. Plasma cells secrete huge quantities of antibody into the bloodstream

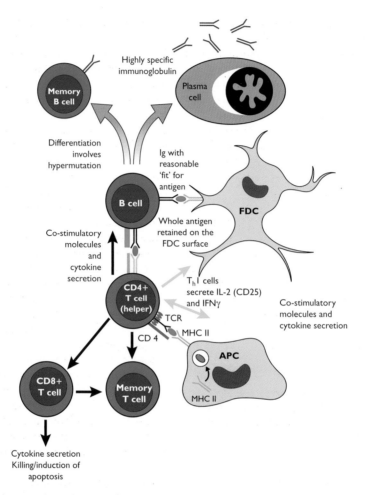

Arrows indicate direction of stimulation

Follicle dendritic cells (FDC) trap bound antigen in the lymph using complement or Fc receptors. The antigen is not processed, but is presented to the B cell and is a potent stimulator for B cell maturation, including hypermutation of the immunoglobulin antigen recognition site to create high affinity antibodies

Antigen-presenting cells (APC) process phagocytosed antigen and combine it with MHC II, which moves to the cell surface and interacts with T (helper) cells in conjunction with CD4 and the T cell receptor complex (TCR) Helper T cells are of two types:

- T_h1 cells secrete IL-2 and interferon gamma. IL-2/IL-2 receptor interaction is the target of much current interest, since if it can be 'mopped up' by administration of antibody, the stimulus for cell proliferation may be reduced or removed, with implications for inflammation-driven disease

- T_h2 cells stimulate antibody production and activate eosinophils and mast cells

Figure 5.2 Interactions between antigen-presenting cells and T and B lymphocytes

and tissues, deluging the antigen. Initially, the antibody is of IgM type and later the B cell clone switches to produce IgG. This 'heavy chain switch' is useful clinically – the presence of IgM antibody indicates a recent infection, of no more than a few weeks' duration. Finding IgG antibody is less useful, as it can indicate that the patient has been exposed to the antigen at almost any time in the past, from weeks to years. If the particular antigen is encountered again, the memory cells will quickly undergo clonal proliferation and swamp it with specific antibody.

It is worth stating that a B cell inflammatory reaction will lead to the generation of numerous different antibodies, all directed at different antigenic sites. This is therefore a 'polyclonal' response, i.e. several different B cell clones are stimulated and each will produce its own particular antibody. This is an important concept since certain cancers that affect the lymphoid system (e.g. multiple myeloma) may be difficult to differentiate from an inflammatory condition when a patient first presents to the doctor. Multiple myeloma is a tumour of bone marrow caused by a malignant proliferation of plasma cells. Since all malignancies originate in a single mutated cell, it follows that all the antibodies secreted by a malignant proliferation of plasma cells will be identical. Compare the two electrophoretic strips shown in Fig. 5.3.

This is probably a good moment to think about antibodies! What do they look like and exactly how do they bind to antigen? What are these subtypes? – we have come across only IgM and IgG so far! And how can such a large number of diverse antibodies have been generated from cells with a common ancestor?

WHAT ARE ANTIBODIES AND HOW DO THEY WORK?

Immunoglobulins are collectively known as 'gamma globulins' because of their motility on electrophoresis, and although this is an historical term you may still hear it used. For instance, an immunodeficient

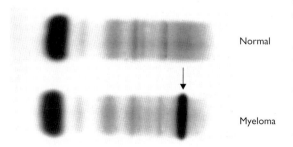

An extra band is present in an electrophoretic strip from a patient with myeloma, due to very large quantities of a single type of immunoglobulin secreted by a malignant clone of plasma cells. The control strip shows no significant bands in the gamma region

Figure 5.3 Myeloma: M band (arrowed)

patient is likely to be treated with 'pooled gamma-globulin', i.e. concentrated immunoglobulins derived from blood from a number of different donors.

Each immunoglobulin molecule is formed from two identical heavy chains and two identical light chains joined by interchain disulphide links. There are two types of light chain (kappa and lambda) and five types of heavy chain (G, A, M, D, E). The light chains can combine with any type of heavy chain and do not influence biological function, whereas each heavy chain type supports different biological functions (Table 5.1). IgG is the most prevalent and exhibits the most basic immunoglobulin structure, referred to as a monomer. IgM is the largest: five monomeric units are joined by a J chain to make a massive pentamer. A key feature of this molecule is that it is too large to cross the placenta (see Fig. 2.11, Rhesus incompatibility). IgA is most important as a mucosal protector (e.g. in gut secretions). At these sites it exists as a dimer, linked by a J chain and a 'secretory component' derived from the gut epithelial cell. In the gut there are 20–30 times more IgA-producing than IgG-producing cells. IgA defends both the luminal and subepithelial zones. In addition, intestinal B lymphocytes can be stimulated by antigens and then migrate via the lymphatics and blood to localize in other areas, such as breast or salivary glands, so that specific IgA defends these sites also. In the blood IgA exists in a monomeric form. IgD is a slightly mysterious monomeric immunoglobulin; it is found in mucosa-associated lymphoid tissue (MALT), particularly in the wall of the gut, but its precise role is not clear. IgE binds mast cells and has a major role in the defence against parasites, but can be a nuisance in type I hypersensitivity reactions.

Most importantly, immunoglobulin recognizes antigen through the variable regions on the molecule. After that, the constant regions initiate the biological functions, such as complement fixation and opsonization, appropriate for the immunoglobulin class. Although diagrams generally depict antibody molecules as simple bent dinner forks (Fig. 5.4), they actually have a complex three-dimensional structure with many 'folds'.

Binding of antigen to antibody can lead to a variety of effects. Cross-linking of antigenic particles or cells will produce precipitation or agglutination, while binding of antibody to an active site on a virus or toxin can result in neutralization. Other components of the immune response can become involved, as when antibody fixes complement to

Table 5.1 Immunoglobulin types

	Complement fixation by		Macrophage/ polymorph binding	Mast cell/ basophil binding	Cross placenta	Function
	Classical pathway	Alternative pathway				
IgG	++	−	++	−	++	Combats microorganisms and toxins. Most abundant Ig in blood and extravascular fluid
IgA	−	+−	+−	−	−	Most important immunoglobulin for protecting mucosal surfaces. Combines with secretory component to avoid being digested
IgM	+	−	−	−	−	Important in early response to infection as it is a powerful agglutinator
IgD	−	−	−	−	−	?Function. Present on the surface of some lymphocytes and may control lymphocyte activation/suppression
IgE	−	−	+−	+−	−	Involved in mast cell degranulation, thereby protecting body surfaces. Important in allergy and parasitic infections

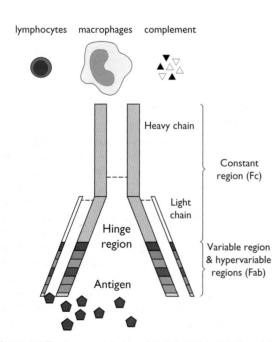

lymphocytes   macrophages   complement

Heavy chain

Constant region (Fc)

Light chain

Hinge region

Variable region & hypervariable regions (Fab)

Antigen

Functions of Fc portion:
- Opsonization for phagocytosis
- Complement activation
- Stimulation of B and T and NK cell response

Functions of Fab portion:
- Bind antigen on microorganisms, prime for killing or immobilize and prevent entry into gut
- Bind and neutralize toxins

Figure 5.4 The immunoglobulin molecule is active at both ends! The antigen-binding site is a three-dimensional structure, with three key sites at which bonds are made. Through a process of hypermutation, low-affinity binding sites can mutate to show high affinity

produce lysis or enhanced phagocytosis. Antibody can also promote cell-mediated cytotoxicity involving NK cells, so-called antibody-dependent cell-mediated cytotoxicity (ADCC).

Antigen binds to the variable region, in which there are three hypervariable regions forming a potential 'pocket' for antigen attachment. The shape of the pocket is dependent on the outer electron clouds of its atoms – which of course determines the antigen shape that it recognizes. The important point is that this interaction depends on the antigen and antibody having complementary profiles; no covalent bonding is involved, so the chemical composition is not crucial. The shapes do not have to be a perfect fit but a close fit gives the strongest binding. As mentioned above, fine-tuning can be undertaken by a B cell in conjunction with follicle dendritic cells in the germinal centre, and the genetic make-up governing the three hypervariable regions in each pocket can be adjusted for a better antigen fit, before the clonal expansion of the B cell population is undertaken. This generates a population of antibodies with excellent binding properties.

Nature has found this approach so useful that a common structure, the immunoglobulin homology unit, is the basic building block for a range of molecules involved in cell–cell recognition, the so-called immunoglobulin gene superfamily. Some of these are shown in Fig. 5.5. CD4, expressed on helper T cells, binds to major histocompatibility complex (MHC) II and CD8, on suppressor/cytotoxic T cells, binds MHC I. These interactions are essential, in fact T cell activation requires there to be both antigen binding by the T cell receptor and T cell stimulation by the binding of either CD4 or CD8 to their respective MHC receptors. There are also several 'co-stimulatory molecules' that are important in cell–cell interactions.

THE MHC SYSTEM

The human MHC (major histocompatibility complex) system, also called the HLA (human leukocyte antigen) system, is coded for on chromosome 6 where there are six loci, three for class I antigens (A, B and C) and three for class II antigens (DP, DQ and DR). Class I molecules are expressed on virtually all nucleated cells while class II molecules are restricted to antigen-presenting cells, other macrophages and B cells, but can be expressed on many other cell types, if they are stimulated with γ-interferon.

Each person has an (almost) unique set of MHC molecules that are present on most cells and are inherited. This is relevant to transplantation, where it is essential to have a good 'match' between the donor and the recipient to minimize the risk of rejection. An identical twin will provide an excellent match, some siblings are a good match but other people's organs carry MHC antigens that will be identified by the recipient's immune system as foreign and the tissue will be rejected.

The MHC molecules are important because T cells cannot react with free, native antigens (that is a job for the immunoglobulin molecules). T cells can only bind to antigens that have been processed by special antigen-presenting cells or macrophages and are then displayed on the cell surface alongside MHC molecules.

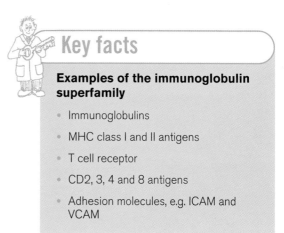

Key facts

Examples of the immunoglobulin superfamily

- Immunoglobulins
- MHC class I and II antigens
- T cell receptor
- CD2, 3, 4 and 8 antigens
- Adhesion molecules, e.g. ICAM and VCAM

GENERATION OF DIVERSITY IN THE IMMUNE SYSTEM

If you have forgotten what genes are made of and how they can be translated to form proteins, refer to Fig. 2.27. You will be aware that much of our DNA appears to code for nothing, and that the important sections that encode sequences of amino acids are called exons and the in-between stuff consists of introns. A similar mechanism exists for the generation of multiple unique antigen-recognition sites in T cells and B cells, for the chains that make up the T cell receptor and those that make up the immunoglobulin molecule, respectively. For the sake of simplicity we will consider, in a little detail, only the processes involved in generating diversity in the B cell heavy chains.

The immunoglobulin heavy chain is constructed from four building blocks, the variable (V), diversity

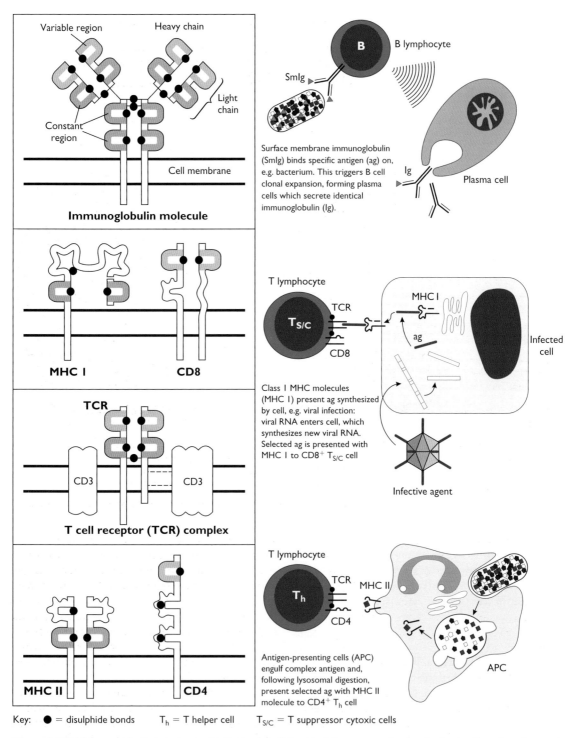

Key: ● = disulphide bonds T_h = T helper cell $T_{S/C}$ = T suppressor cytoxic cells

Figure 5.5 The immunoglobulin homology unit is the basic building block for a range of molecules involved in cell–cell recognition, the 'immunoglobulin gene superfamily'. The T cell receptor complex is one such molecule, as are the co-stimulatory molecules CD4 and CD8, and the MHC molecules with which they interact and several other molecules that play an important role in immune reactions, such as intercellular adhesion molecules (e.g. ICAM-1) and lymphocyte function antigen (e.g. LFA-3)

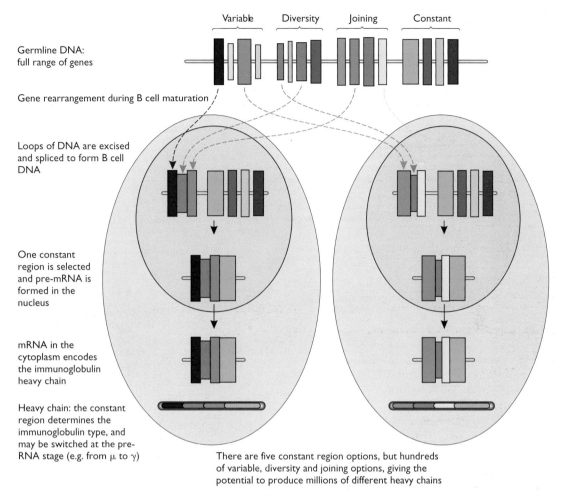

Figure 5.6 Gene rearrangement in the B cell heavy chain. This example shows two different heavy chains being produced

In the figure the following labels appear:

Variable   Diversity   Joining   Constant

Germline DNA: full range of genes

Gene rearrangement during B cell maturation

Loops of DNA are excised and spliced to form B cell DNA

One constant region is selected and pre-mRNA is formed in the nucleus

mRNA in the cytoplasm encodes the immunoglobulin heavy chain

Heavy chain: the constant region determines the immunoglobulin type, and may be switched at the pre-RNA stage (e.g. from μ to γ)

There are five constant region options, but hundreds of variable, diversity and joining options, giving the potential to produce millions of different heavy chains

(D), joining (J) and constant (C) regions. These are four groups of exons separated by introns and, in lymphoid cells during maturation, one gene from each of three of the groups is rearranged by creating loops of DNA, so that they lie adjacent to each other. The genes coding for each chain are not a continuous structure in non-lymphoid cells but are groups of exons separated by long non-coding introns.

There is great diversity within the V, D and J groups but the constant region genes are limited in number, with only a single gene for each subclass of molecule – thus for immunoglobulin heavy chains these are Cμ, Cγ, Cα, Cδ, Cε, which code for Ig's M, G, A, D and E respectively.

Once the chosen V, D and J regions have been aligned satisfactorily, the intervening DNA is snipped away and the contiguous segments are joined (excising and splicing). The process is rather like cutting

and pasting using a computer. Immunoglobulin heavy chain gene rearrangement is a two-stage process. Having rearranged the V, D and J regions satisfactorily within the nucleus, the cell must make its choice of heavy chain. V, D and J are separated from the five C genes by a long intron. Just as the mRNA is formed, the constant region selection is made, the intron is excised and the mRNA leaves the nucleus for the cytoplasm, to be translated into protein by the ribosomes.

Why is the C region treated differently? Probably because a lymphocyte that has recognized an antigen with the variable region on its surface molecule may need to produce molecules with different constant regions. Each immunoglobulin molecule has slightly different functions. For example IgG is better in activating the complement complex, whereas IgA is designed to neutralize microbes

Table 5.2 T lymphocyte subsets

	CD4+			CD8+	
	Suppressor/inducer	Helper/inducer		Suppressor cells	Cytotoxic cells
		Th1	Th2		
Genetic restriction (MHC)	II	II	II	I	I
Suppressor activity	+ + (provide help)	−	−	+ +	−
Cytotoxic activity	−	+	−	−	+ +
Help for immunoglobulin	−	+	+ + +	−	−

MHC = major histocompatibility complex.

T cells are important against infections, in graft rejection, in graft-versus-host disease, in some hypersensitivity reactions and in tumour immunity. Th1 cells assist macrophages in stimulating cell-mediated immunity. Th2 cells assist B cells by stimulating immunoglobulin production and regulating immunoglobulin class.

in the mucosal surfaces. The switch of constant region occurs during the germinal centre reaction before differentiation to plasma cells. The antigen-recognition site and the variable region remain the same; the constant region has changed.

It is easy to see how an enormous variety of molecules can be produced in this way. For example, the mouse immunoglobulin heavy chain molecule genome is produced from a choice of 500 V gene segments, 15 D gene segments and 4 J gene segments. This gives a possible repertoire of $500 \times 15 \times 4$ combinations for the heavy chain. That chain will be combined into an immunoglobulin molecule and, in humans, approximately 10^8 different immunoglobulins are produced in this way.

Although exactly the same type of process is undertaken for the generation of diversity in the T cell receptor and other similar molecules, it must be emphasized that the V, D, J and C groups of genes are different for each type of molecule (i.e. heavy chain, light chain, TCRα, TCRβ, etc.). Also, the genes for each chain are rearranged independently. Only the genes on one of a pair of chromosomes is rearranged, the locus on the paired chromosome is inhibited (allelic exclusion).

Cell-mediated immunity

Cell-mediated immunity is achieved by T cells. There are several types of T cell that differ in their biological roles. Some act as helper cells, some as cytotoxic cells, some as killer cells and some as suppressor cells. A population of null lymphocytes, which are neither T nor B, are called natural killer (NK) cells.

Small Print

CD (cluster designation) numbers indicate that a particular cell has a surface antigen that can be detected with a specific antibody. This has proved very useful for identifying leukocytes.

Some CD antigens useful in leukocyte identification:

Antigen	Principally expressed on
CD3	Mature T cells
CD4	'Helper/inducer' T cells
CD8	'Suppressor/cytotoxic' T cells
CD15	Monocytes and granulocytes
CD16 and CD56	Natural killer cells
CD20	Most B cells
CD68	Monocytes/macrophages

T cells bear a variety of surface molecules, some of which are common to many T cell types (e.g. CD3), while others are specific to the various subtypes (e.g. CD4, CD8). These molecules are involved in antigen recognition by combining with the T cell receptor.

HOW IS ANTIGEN RECOGNIZED BY T CELLS?

We have mentioned already that T cell recognition of antigen is similar to that of B cells, though it is a bit more complicated. The T cell receptor (TCR) on the surface of the majority (about 95 per cent) of T cells is composed of an α-chain and a β-chain with constant and variable regions analogous to those of immunoglobulins. The remaining minority of T cells have a receptor made up of γ- and δ-chains; these T cells tend to migrate to epithelial surfaces, such as the gut or respiratory epithelial lining cells.

Antigen binds to a receptor site on the TCR. The TCR is linked to a cluster of polypeptide chains, collectively named the CD3 molecules; together TCR and CD3 make up the T cell receptor complex. In fact, the similarities between the TCR and immunoglobulin structure go even deeper, as the genetic mechanisms for producing the necessary enormous diversity are almost identical. As in the immunoglobulin molecule, rearrangement of germ-line DNA during the T cell maturation process (in the thymus, rather than the bone marrow, where B cells mature) generates a series of somatic mutations such that every T cell has a unique receptor. As with B cells, self-reacting cells are deleted at an early stage. Like the immunoglobulin molecule, the T cell antigen receptor site depends on a three-dimensional fit to form non-covalent bonds with antigen. However, the hypermutation mechanism, so important in the generation of high-affinity immunoglobulin molecules, does not affect the T cell receptor genes.

WHAT IS THE DIFFERENCE BETWEEN HELPER AND SUPPRESSOR/CYTOTOXIC T CELLS AND NK CELLS?

Helper cells, which have the molecule CD4 included in the T cell receptor complex, make up about 60 per cent of the body's mature T cells. They will only recognize processed antigen if the CD4 receptor combines with class II MHC molecules. By a combination of releasing interferon, interleukins and binding co-stimulatory molecules, helper T cells stimulate other T cells, NK cells, macrophages and B cells. In AIDS, the immune system is devastated because the human immunodeficiency virus (HIV) has a receptor for CD4, and thus enters and destroys the function of the cell most centrally placed in co-ordinating cell-mediated immunity and much of humoral (antibody-mediated) immunity.

Cytotoxic or suppressor T cells, with CD8 included in the TCR complex, make up about 30 per cent of mature T cells. They bind to processed antigen associated with class I molecules. In fact, they cannot recognize any antigen which is not presented in conjunction with MHC class I molecules, which are expressed by every nucleated cell in the body. One of their most important roles is that of recognizing viral-infected cells. When viruses replicate within cells, viral antigen is expressed on the cell surface. When this viral antigen is presented, together with MHC class I, to a cytotoxic T cell, it springs into action, and lyses the cell membrane, destroying the infected cell. CD8$^+$ T cells are also thought to be pivotal in the generation of peripheral tolerance (see later) and in tumour immunity; both the cytotoxic cells, which can lyse other cells, and the suppressor cells, which just induce anergy, are important in this process.

Natural killer (NK) cells are neither T nor B cells and make up 10–15 per cent of the circulating blood lymphocytes. They contain cytoplasmic granules and have three important membrane receptors: one for the Fc component of IgG, one antigen receptor and a non-CD8 type receptor for MHC I receptor (present on all normal nucleated cells). Cells coated with antibody will be recognized via the Fc receptor and lysed by NK cells (this process is known as antibody-dependent cell-mediated cytotoxicity or ADCC). The lysis is achieved by molecules such as perforin and granzyme contained within the cytoplasmic granules. Other cells whose antigen binds with the NK cell antigen receptor are saved from death by possession of their MHC I molecule, which represses NK cell lysis. If the NK cell cannot 'see' the MHC I receptor because it has been altered (e.g. by tumour, viral infection or drug binding), the target will be lysed.

TOLERANCE

The ability of the body to mount an immune response against foreign antigens raises a very important question. How does the immune system distinguish between an antigen that is foreign and one that is normally present on the cells in the body?

This process, known as tolerance, can be acquired at two stages: the first occurs during lymphopoiesis (lymphoid cell maturation) and is known as central tolerance. The second occurs once the mature B and T cells have been released into the peripheral tissues and is referred to as peripheral tolerance. Tolerance is achieved by a mixture of cell deletion or the generation of anergy in self-reacting cells. These mechanisms induce tolerance such that antigens exposed to the immune system during fetal life are not capable of eliciting a response in later life. Hence nature has devised a neat system of differentiating self from non-self. Or has it?

AUTOIMMUNE DISEASE

As the heading suggests, the body can, on occasion, turn on itself and begin to react with self antigens to destructive purpose. Autoimmune diseases are estimated to affect up to 7 per cent of the population. Mostly this is due to a breakdown in tolerance, but occasionally new antigens are generated which cross-react with the body's cells.

It is thought that this loss of tolerance can occur in several ways: exposure of the immune system to sequestered (hidden) antigens is the most easily explained. Parts of the body that are not exposed to the immune system during fetal life can produce a response later on – lens protein and spermatozoa are just two examples. A person who has suffered severe trauma to one eye, with the release of lens protein into the blood, runs the risk of forming antibodies to the protein. A few weeks later, the other eye may be severely damaged by an antibody-mediated inflammatory reaction (a condition known as sympathetic opthalmitis). Mumps may give rise to inflammation of the testis (orchitis), which causes sperm antigens to be released into the blood circulation. As a result, anti-sperm antibodies may develop and these can cause infertility.

Occasionally, there is cross-reaction between a microbial antigen and normal body cells, due to a similarity in shape or structure between the self and microbial antigens – unthinkingly the body develops an antibody or cell-mediated reaction against itself as it expunges the microbe. A person at risk of such a complication would be our 10-year-old patient who presented at the start of this chapter with a sore throat due to a Lancefield group A streptococcal infection. This bacterium is notorious for carrying antigenic determinants which mimic the endocardium of the heart so closely that the patient develops inflammatory foci in the wall of the heart. This life-threatening condition, which can lead to long-term cardiac damage, is known as rheumatic fever. The incidence of rheumatic fever has plummeted in recent years, possibly due to early eradication of the infection by prompt antibiotic therapy.

Following on from this point it is obvious that defects in any of the immune system's regulatory molecules may lead to aberrations in tolerance. It is thought that much of the peripheral tolerance mechanism relies on anergy on the part of self-reacting immune cells, easily lost if the system controls are tampered with.

Lastly, even anergic T or B cells may be induced to behave against their will by outside forces. An example of this is infection by Epstein–Barr virus, which can stimulate an infected B cell to produce antibodies. If an anergic self-reacting B cell happens to become infected, it will be switched on despite its best intentions.

The autoimmune diseases include many clinically important and potentially life-threatening conditions. They are generally divided up into those diseases that affect a single organ (organ-specific) and those that affect several organs or tissues (non-organ-specific) (Table 5.3). You will come across some of these diseases elsewhere – for instance, the antibodies in Graves' disease stimulate the thyroid-stimulating hormone receptor to secrete thyroxine and thus cause thyrotoxicosis – an example of a type II hypersensitivity reaction.

We will briefly describe systemic lupus erythematosis (SLE) to illustrate the wide-ranging effects of a non-organ-specific autoimmune disease.

Systemic lupus erythematosus is a systemic disorder in which there is chronic, relapsing and remitting damage to the skin, joints, kidneys and almost any organ. Like most immune disorders, it has a higher incidence in women. In the USA, it is also more common in black populations and it tends to occur in the second and third decades. Patients may present with a characteristic 'butterfly' rash on the face, or with more subtle symptoms. Many present after their kidneys have been damaged beyond repair, i.e. chronic renal failure. The fundamental feature of the disease is inflammation of the small arterioles and arteries, i.e. a vasculitis, often related to the deposition of antigen–antibody complexes in the vessel walls. Involvement of the glomerular capillaries in the kidney produces a variety of types of glomerulonephritis. The other sites of involvement are joints (synovitis), heart (non-infectious endocarditis – named after Libman Sacks, and pericarditis), lungs (pleuritis and effusions) and CNS (focal neurological symptoms due to vasculitis). The course of the illness is extremely variable and unpredictable and may range from mild skin involvement to severe renal disease leading to death.

In the autoimmune disorders, the immune response is well controlled but the initiating event of antigen recognition is wrong. There is another group of disorders in which antigen recognition proceeds normally but the body's response is exaggerated. These are called hypersensitivity reactions (page 40).

TRANSPLANTATION

We have already mentioned the role played by the MHC type I and II antigens, displayed on cell membranes, in governing the body's response to

Table 5.3 Autoimmune diseases and autoantigens

Disease	Antigen(s)
Organ-specific diseases	
Hashimoto thyroiditis	Thyroid peroxidase, thyroglobulin/T4
Pernicious anaemia	Intrinsic factor
Insulin-dependent diabetes mellitus (IDDM)	Beta-cells in the pancreas (tyrosine phosphatase)
Addison disease	Adrenal cortical cells (ACTH receptor and microsomes)
Autoimmune haemolytic anaemia	RBC membrane antigens
Graves' disease	TSH receptor on thyroid cells
Pemphigus	Epidermal keratinocytes
Bullous pemphigoid	Basal keratinocytes
Guillain–Barré syndrome	Peripheral nerves (gangliosides)
Polymyositis	Muscle (histidine tRNA synthetase)
Non-organ-specific diseases	
Systemic lupus erythematosus	Double-stranded DNA, nuclear antigens
Chronic active hepatitis	Nuclei, DNA
Scleroderma	Nuclei, elastin, nucleoli, centromeres, topoisomerase 1
Primary biliary cirrhosis	Mitochondria (pyruvate dehydrogenase complex E2)
Rheumatoid arthritis	IgG (rheumatoid factor, connective tissues, collagen)
Multiple sclerosis	Brain/myelin basic protein
Sjögren syndrome	Exocrine glands, kidney, liver, thyroid
Several organs affected	
Goodpasture syndrome	Basement membrane of kidney and lung (type IV collagen)
Polyendocrine	Multiple endocrine organs (hepatic – cytochrome p450; intestinal – tryptophan hydroxylase)

From Lydyard *et al.*, 2000: *Pathology Integrated: An A–Z of Disease and its Pathogenesis.* London: Arnold.

transplanted tissue or cells. You will realize, from reading the hypersensitivity sections, that the body may generate a type IV, cell-mediated, response against any tissue that fails to give the right MHC signals to the T cells. The host may already carry antibodies against a tissue (e.g. blood) transplanted into him – hence the requirement for cross-matching red blood cells and checking that the host's serum does not carry antibodies that can react with the donor's T lymphocytes. Thus type II hypersensitivity reactions are also important in tissue transplantation.

It is obvious but worth mentioning that, for patients who require a bone marrow transplant, it is the donor cells that react against the host, sparking off graft-versus-host disease if there is a mismatch.

For reasons that are unclear, some organs need far more precise tissue matching than others – the most stringent requirements are for kidney and bone marrow grafts. Surprisingly, the heart and liver require little more than ABO compatibility (i.e. matching blood types).

IMMUNIZATION

The immune system is a natural defence mechanism but it can also be manipulated so that it will respond more quickly to a new antigen and so, hopefully, reduce the impact of the infection. This is called immunization. Immunization may be active or passive. Active immunity involves using inactivated or attenuated live organisms or their products and the effect is reasonably long lasting and calls up an adaptive immune response. Passive immunity results from injecting human immunoglobulin; the effect is immediate but only lasts 1–2 weeks.

It would be a crime to consider immunization without pausing for a moment to think about its history and the man responsible for developing its use. The man is Edward Jenner (1749–1823), a pupil of John Hunter. Jenner lived with Hunter for his first 2 years in London and the friendship they developed continued after Jenner left London to start general practice in Berkeley, Gloucestershire. Jenner was

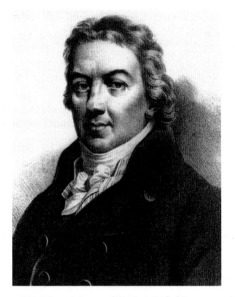

Figure 5.7 Edward Jenner (1749–1823) (Courtesy of the Wellcome Institute for the History of Medicine)

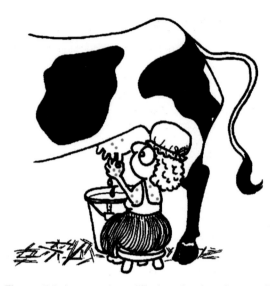

Figure 5.8 Jenner successfully inoculated against smallpox with cowpox (From Lakhani, S. 1992: Early clinical pathologists: Edward Jenner. *J Clin Pathol* 45. Reproduced with kind permission of the BMJ Publishing Group)

profoundly influenced by Hunter's interest in natural history and in his methods of scientific investigation. To one of Jenner's questions, Hunter is said to have replied, 'I think your solution is just; but why think? Why not try the experiment?'.

Even before Jenner, it had been noticed that an attack of smallpox protected against further disease. It was known that the epidemics varied in severity and that it was best to contract a mild form of smallpox as this resulted in lifelong protection. This knowledge was widespread; in India, children were wrapped in clothing from patients with smallpox; in China, scabs from smallpox patients were ground and the powder was blown into the nostrils; in Turkey, female slaves were injected under the skin with dried preparations of pus from smallpox patients. Inoculated slaves fetched a high price while pock-marked slaves were worth nothing! Lady Mary Wortley Montagu, the wife of the British Ambassador in Constantinople, was aware of these techniques and she took the risk of having her own children inoculated. When she returned to England in 1718, she tried to convince her friend, the Prince of Wales that he should do the same. He was worried about experimenting on the royal children but, when six orphan children were successfully immunized against smallpox, he consented and the royal children were inoculated. Some advances in medical ethics have been made since those days!

Jenner and others had noticed that cows suffered from a pustular disease resembling smallpox called 'variolae vaccinae' – cowpox. It was known that this disease could be transmitted to humans and that, apart from local symptoms, there were no lasting ill-effects. There was a widespread belief that those who had suffered from cowpox became immune to smallpox. The idea of using the cowpox virus to induce immunity to smallpox thrilled Jenner but, rather than jumping to conclusions, he followed Hunter's example and experimented. On 14 May 1796, Jenner inoculated a boy of eight named James Phipps with cowpox. The boy's illness took a predictable course and he recovered. On 1 July, he inoculated the boy with smallpox and no reaction occurred, either on this occasion or on a subsequent occasion a few months later.

Jenner described this experiment to the Royal Society but it was rejected. He continued to make his observations and, in 1798, published his work entitled *An Inquiry into the Causes and Effects of the Variolae vaccinae*. Hence inoculation with smallpox was replaced by inoculation with cowpox. The word 'vaccination' came into use and smallpox cases dropped in the UK as a series of laws (Vaccination Acts of 1840, 1841, 1853, 1861, 1867 and 1871) made vaccination free and compulsory, with parents liable to repeated fines until their children were vaccinated. Compulsion was withdrawn in 1948 and smallpox was eradicated globally by 1980, with the last naturally occurring case recorded in Somalia in October 1977.

Active immunization

First exposure to an antigen provokes a primary response in which IgM is the major antibody. Further exposure to the antigen produces a secondary response that occurs faster, produces higher levels of antibody and the class is predominantly IgG. In addition to humoral immunity, cell-mediated immunity is also induced. The aim of active immunization is to give sufficient doses of antigen to ensure that,

after completing the course of immunization, the person can mount a rapid effective response if exposed to the disease. The number of doses, time intervals and need for booster doses varies with the vaccine, the natural history of the disease and the likelihood of encountering the infection.

The present immunization schedule for children in the UK and the recommendation for adults who are unimmunized or in a high-risk group is given in Table 5.4.

Table 5.4 The British National Vaccination Schedule

At birth
Tuberculosis (BCG) for those with infected or previously infected family members; immigrants from countries with a high prevalence of tuberculosis and their children and infants
Hepatitis B for babies born to mothers who are chronic carriers of hepatitis B virus or to mothers who have had acute hepatitis B during pregnancy plus their close family members

2nd, 3rd and 4th months
Diphtheria, tetanus, pertussis and poliomyelitis (DTP + P).
Haemophilus influenzae type b (HiB)
Meningococcal serogroup C (MenC)

12–15 months
Measles, mumps and rubella (MMR)

Pre-school
Diphtheria, tetanus, acellular pertussis and poliomyelitis boosters (DTaP + P)
Measles, mumps, rubella booster (MMR)

10–14 years
Tuberculosis (BCG) if PPD skin test negative

14 years
Rubella (girls only). Once the cohort of children who have been immunized at 12–15 months and again pre-school reaches this age this extra dose is unlikely to be necessary
Diphtheria, tetanus and poliomyelitis boosters (DT and P)

Adults
Tetanus and poliomyelitis boosters 10 yearly only for those at risk of soil contaminated wounds (tetanus), or health care workers (poliomyelitis). Travellers may warrant 10-yearly toxoid boosters when they are going to countries where post-exposure tetanus immunoglobulin will not be available
It was decided as an interim measure, during the academic term for 1999–2000, to offer polysaccharide meningococcal vaccine (serogroups A and C) to students in colleges and universities of higher education and conjugate meningococcal (serogroup C) to those at secondary school. Eventually, as the new childhood vaccination schedules become established these 'catch-up' campaigns should become unnecessary

All ages
Hepatitis B for those likely to be in close contact with carriers or at occupational risk, e.g. healthcare workers.
Influenza for those at risk of serious disease or complications, including travellers in these risk categories going to epidemic areas
Pneumococcal for those at risk of serious disease or complications, including travellers in these risk categories going to epidemic areas

This is based upon advice from the 'UK Joint Committee for Vaccination and Immunisation' (JCVI). The final decision on whether to receive these vaccines is dependant upon agreement between the patient, parent and the administering doctor or nurse.

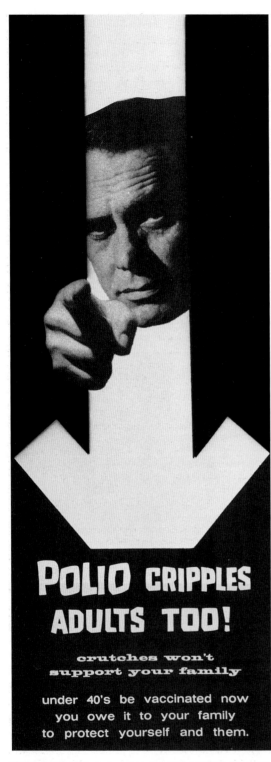

Figure 5.9 Bookmarks have been a popular method of advertising and in the 1940s they were used to convey public messages on subjects such as health and road safety (Courtesy of Kirkdale Bookshop, London)

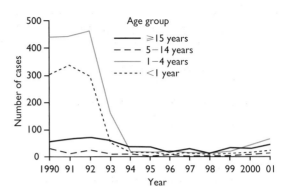

Figure 5.10 *Haemophilus influenzae* type b disease in England and Wales by age group (1990–2001) (PHLS and CDSC data) (From Public Health Laboratory Service (2002) Continuing surveillance of invasive *Haemophilus influenzae* disease. *CDR weekly* **12**(26)

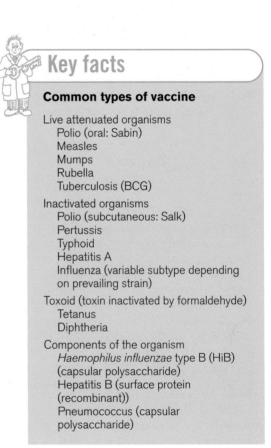

Key facts

Common types of vaccine

Live attenuated organisms
    Polio (oral: Sabin)
    Measles
    Mumps
    Rubella
    Tuberculosis (BCG)

Inactivated organisms
    Polio (subcutaneous: Salk)
    Pertussis
    Typhoid
    Hepatitis A
    Influenza (variable subtype depending on prevailing strain)

Toxoid (toxin inactivated by formaldehyde)
    Tetanus
    Diphtheria

Components of the organism
    Haemophilus influenzae type B (HiB) (capsular polysaccharide)
    Hepatitis B (surface protein (recombinant))
    Pneumococcus (capsular polysaccharide)

Clinicopathological case study – lobar pneumonia

Clinical

A 60-year-old man presented to the casualty department complaining of a productive cough, fever, rigors and general malaise. The onset of symptoms was sudden and he had been perfectly well two days previously. He had no past medical history of note and he was not on any medication.

Systemic enquiry:
Respiratory system – he was coughing up rusty-coloured sputum and also complained of chest pain on inspiration.

Allergies – nil known.

Examination:
Temperature – 39.40°C (normal 37°C)
Pulse 90/min regular (normal approx 70/min).
Respiratory rate 30/min (normal approx 14/min).

Examination also revealed a dull percussion note in the right lower zone and auscultation confirmed decreased air entry and bronchial breathing. There was also a pleural rub over the affected area.

Investigations:
Full blood count – white cell count 18×10^9/L (95% neutrophils) (normal $4–11 \times 10^9$/L with approx 65% neutrophils).
Chest X-ray – opaque right lower lobe.

Sputum culture – *Streptococcus pneumoniae*.

A diagnosis of lobar pneumonia was made and he was started on a course of penicillin. He did not have a history of allergy to this drug.

Pathological

The symptoms are due to local respiratory irritation from the inflammatory process and the fever is secondary to the production of pyrogens.

Inflammation causes vasodilatation, followed by margination and emigration of cells. Together with increased permeability, this leads to a purulent exudate within alveoli which is coughed up as sputum.

The chest pain is due to friction between two inflamed pleural surfaces which are roughened and adherent due to the inflammatory exudate. This is also responsible for the pleural rub heard on auscultation.

Pyrogens cause a rise in body temperature by resetting the thermoregulatory centre in the hypothalamus. A rise in temperature will also increase the metabolic rate and therefore an increase in cardiac output. Decreased gas transfer plus the rise in temperature will lead to an increase in the respiratory rate.

The decreased air entry due to the inflammatory exudate within alveoli is responsible for the dull percussion note and the findings on auscultation.

Cytokines cause bone marrow stimulation and hence a leukocytosis.

Airless alveoli full of exudate appear white on X-ray.
This is the most common organism causing lobar pneumonia.
With effective treatment, there will be complete reversal of all the clinical and radiological signs as the exudate is cleared away from the alveoli.
This ideal process may not occur and healing may take place by scarring. Lobar pneumonia differs from the more common bronchopneumonia in that the latter tends to be patchy and caused by a variety of organisms, e.g. H. influenzae.

Live attenuated viral vaccines, such as polio, measles, mumps and rubella, generally produce the most long-lasting immune responses and oral polio vaccine has the advantage of having maximal effect on local gut immunity, the natural portal of entry for wild polio. Non-live vaccines may be more effective when combined with adjuvants to enhance the immune response. For example, aluminium phosphate and aluminium hydroxide are used in DTP vaccine.

Passive immunization

Passive immunity relies on using either pooled plasma containing a variety of immunoglobulin to local infectious agents or specific immunoglobulin obtained from convalescent patients or recently immunized donors. Specific immunoglobulins are available for tetanus, hepatitis B, rabies and varicella zoster. They are most commonly used for post-exposure prophylaxis.

Key facts

Important pathogens for which there are no vaccines

(*trials of possible vaccines in progress)

- Rhinoviruses (colds)
- HIV/AIDS*
- Cytomegalovirus (CMV)
- Epstein–Barr virus (EBV)
- Gonorrhoea
- Syphilis
- Leprosy
- Trachoma
- Malaria*
- All parasitic and protozoal infections

QUESTIONS

What are the key defences against infectious diseases?

- Public health measures (page 82)
- Natural barriers, e.g. skin and mucosal surfaces (page 75)
- Innate immunity
- Adaptive immunity and immunization (pages 125 and 135)
- Healing and repair of wounds to restore defences (page 115)

What are the main elements of the immune response?

Describe cell-mediated and humoral immunity, including:

- Cell types: T and B lymphocytes, macrophages, other antigen-presenting cells
- Location and transport of immune cells (reticuloendothelial system) (Fig. 5.1)
- Antigen recognition, processing and cellular response (Fig. 5.2)

What is inflammation?

Describe acute and chronic inflammation including:

- Clinical features (page 87)

- Cell types involved (Table 4.1; Fig. 4.2)
- Tissue changes (Figs 4.4 and 4.8)
- Possible outcomes (Fig. 4.7)

How do wounds heal? How is the process altered in specialized tissues?

- Describe healing by primary and secondary intention (Figs 4.30 and 4.31)
- Discuss the process in bone (Fig. 4.32) and nervous tissue (page 123), including the distinction between labile, stable and permanent cells (Fig. 4.29)

Describe the immunization recommendations in your area of clinical practice and the important pathogens for which no effective vaccine exist?

- Immunization schedule for UK (page 137)
- Recommendations for travellers available on the internet at www.immunisation.nhs.uk
- Pathogens without an effective vaccine (page 140)

FURTHER READING

Cotran, R.S., Kumar, V. and Collins, T. (1999) *Robbins Pathologic Basis of Disease*, 6th edition. W.B. Saunders, Philadelphia.

Davidson, A. and Diamond B. (2001) Advances in immunology: autoimmune diseases. *New England Journal of Medicine* 345, 340–50.

Gabay, C. and Kushner, I. (1999) Mechanisms of disease: acute-phase proteins and other systemic responses to inflammation. *New England Journal of Medicine* 340, 448–54.

Kamradt, T. and Mitchison, N.A. (2001) Advances in immunology: tolerance and autoimmunity. *New England Journal of Medicine* 344, 655–64.

Luster, A.D. (1998) Mechanisms of disease: chemokines – chemotactic cytokines that mediate inflammation. *New England Journal of Medicine* 338, 436–45.

Lydard, P.M., Whelan, A. and Fanger, M.W. (2000) *Immunology*. BIOS Scientific, Oxford.

Medzhitov, R. and Janeway, C. (2000) Advances in immunology: innate immunity. *New England Journal of Medicine* 343, 338–44.

Underwood, J.C.E. (2000) *General and Systematic Pathology*, 3rd edition. Churchill Livingstone, London.

Walport, M.J. (2001) Advances in immunology: complement part 1 and 2. *New England Journal of Medicine* 344, 1058–66, 1140–4.

PART 3
Circulatory Disorders

Introduction

When I first applied my mind to observation from the many dissections of Living Creatures as they came to hand, that by that means I might find out the use of the motion of the Heart and things conducible in Creatures; I straightwayes found it a thing hard to be attained, and full of difficulty, so with Fracastorius I did almost believe, that the motion of the heart was known to God alone.

William Harvey (1578–1657)

It is extraordinary to think that diseases whose effects are as diverse as those of gangrene, strokes, heart attacks and divers' 'bends' are all disorders of the circulatory system. The general features of circulatory disorders are almost the opposite of the cardinal features of inflammation that we learnt about in Chapter 4 – for 'calor (heat), rubor (redness), tumor (swelling) and dolor (pain)' read 'coldness, pallor/cyanosis, pain and loss of sensation'.

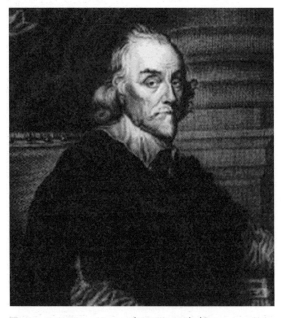

Figure 1 William Harvey (1578–1657) (Courtesy of the Wellcome Institute for the History of Medicine)

Why is this? The drop in temperature and change in colour are easily understood, since blood carries body heat from the core and dissipates it in the extremities and it is the red colour of the oxygenated haemoglobin pigment in the red blood cells that makes pale-skinned persons look pink. Anything that decreases blood flow to a finger or toe will decrease the tissue perfusion by warm blood, making it cold and pale, and any delay in delivery of red blood cells to the affected digit will mean that more of the haemoglobin will have given up its oxygen load, leaving blue-coloured deoxyhaemoglobin (cyanosis).

Pain is a variable phenomenon, depending on the tissue affected and the type of injury; for example a 'heart attack', or myocardial infarction, caused by sudden blockage of a coronary artery, is usually associated with intense central chest pain, often radiating down the left arm, while a gradual 'furring up' of the arteries supplying the legs causes severe pain on walking, which disappears when the demand for oxygen by the leg muscles is removed by rest (intermittent claudication). By comparison, a 'stroke', in which the blood supply to part of the brain is suddenly interrupted, will generally cause weakness or paralysis, but no pain.

Loss of sensation also varies according to the type of vascular disease and the tissue or organ affected: a stroke may destroy a sensory pathway to the brain, leading to a large area of numbness that may involve half the body, while blockage of the blood flow to a toe would cause numbness in just the area supplied by the vessel because of ischaemic damage to the local sensory nerves.

You will have gathered from the preceding discussion that the term 'circulatory disorders' encompasses a spectrum of symptoms and signs related to an abnormality in the blood supply. Circulatory disorders may be 'local' or 'systemic' and may gradually develop over months or years or strike suddenly and catastrophically. They may result from a problem in the vessels, in the blood or in the heart. Perhaps the easiest way to look at these diseases is to relate them to a domestic plumbing system, the main components of which are the pipes and the pump. Pipes may gradually 'fur up' (atherosclerosis), or become blocked (vascular occlusion). In plumbing the blockage may be water freezing in the winter while our cardiovascular equivalent is thrombosis. Sometimes small fragments of thrombus may break off and be carried around the system until they lodge in a pipe with a diameter too small to let them through (embolism). Burst pipes (haemorrhage) are a nuisance and can be extremely damaging. Sometimes one can spot the area at risk, because the pipe may bulge alarmingly before it bursts (aneurysm). Pump failure for whatever reason is fairly disastrous and in the heart, this may be due to valve disease, myocardial infarction, infection, congenital abnormality, etc.

Some solutions to these problems have been found. Thus affected segments of piping can be replaced (arterial bypass grafts), pumps can be tinkered with (valve grafts) or replaced (heart transplants), high pressure causing strain on the system can be relieved (antihypertensive drugs) and sometimes it is possible to remove some of the 'scale' that furs up the pipes (reaming out of arteries using balloon catheters or, more recently, lasers). Of course these are usually only partial solutions and there is no doubt that prevention is the best medicine.

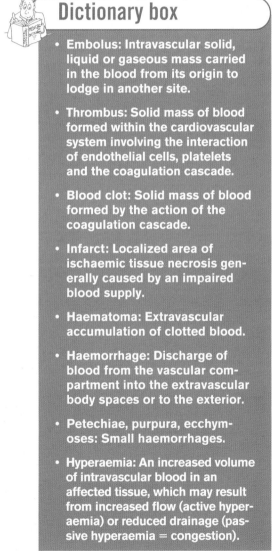

Dictionary box

- **Embolus: Intravascular solid, liquid or gaseous mass carried in the blood from its origin to lodge in another site.**

- **Thrombus: Solid mass of blood formed within the cardiovascular system involving the interaction of endothelial cells, platelets and the coagulation cascade.**

- **Blood clot: Solid mass of blood formed by the action of the coagulation cascade.**

- **Infarct: Localized area of ischaemic tissue necrosis generally caused by an impaired blood supply.**

- **Haematoma: Extravascular accumulation of clotted blood.**

- **Haemorrhage: Discharge of blood from the vascular compartment into the extravascular body spaces or to the exterior.**

- **Petechiae, purpura, ecchymoses: Small haemorrhages.**

- **Hyperaemia: An increased volume of intravascular blood in an affected tissue, which may result from increased flow (active hyperaemia) or reduced drainage (passive hyperaemia = congestion).**

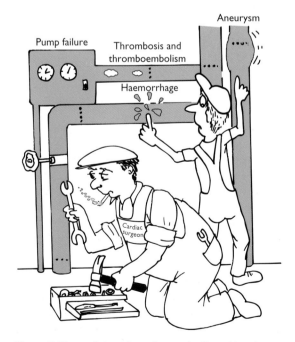

Figure 2 The cardiovascular system can be likened to a domestic plumbing system

It would be unjust to discuss circulatory disorders without a brief mention of the historical figures involved. If you had been alive in the sixteenth century, you would have been taught that blood was produced by the liver and then carried in the veins to the organs where it was consumed; this was Galen's theory of the regeneration of the blood. The portion of blood from the liver that entered the right side of the heart divided into two streams. One route was through the pulmonary artery to bathe the lungs and the other route was across the heart through 'inter-septal pores'. The left ventricle received this blood, which mixed with the 'pneuma' (air) coming to the heart through the pulmonary veins. The blood, fortified by the 'pneuma', was then ejected via the aorta towards the peripheral organs.

In 1628, this theory was challenged when Dr William Harvey published his famous work, *De Motu Cordis*, describing the dual circulation of the blood; but even in the sixteenth century people were starting to doubt Galen's theory. There were several problems with the theory. First, nobody had managed to identify 'inter-septal' pores, so Michael Servetius, the Spanish theologian and physician, suggested that blood travelled from the right to the left ventricle by circulating through the lungs, an idea for which he died a martyr's death after being denounced by John Calvin for holding heretical opinions! Secondly, Galen's theory proposed a mixture of air and blood in the left side of the heart, which was a difficult concept to accept once the structure of the heart valves was established. Leonardo da Vinci had drawn these accurately but it was Andrea Caselapino who described the valves' actions correctly, in 1571, and went on to use the term 'circulatio'. Thus Harvey, who studied in Padua from 1600 to 1602, would have been familiar with the Italians' ideas and was able to reach his own conclusions by 'standing on the shoulders of these giants'. Even Harvey was left with a problem, he could not demonstrate the connections between the arterial and venous sides of the circulation. The discovery of the capillaries had to wait for Marcello Malpighi's microscopical analysis of frog lung in 1661.

CHAPTER 6

Vascular occlusion and thrombosis

VASCULAR OCCLUSION

To return to the present day, we shall first consider the problems of vascular occlusion.

Vascular occlusion may be arterial or venous and the effect of any occlusion will depend on:

- the type of tissue involved
- how quickly the occlusion develops
- the availability of collateral circulation.

Collateral vessels provide an alternative route for the blood and they are sometimes able to compensate completely, especially if the occlusion develops slowly. The venous system has more collaterals than the arterial system. For example, there are anastomoses between the portal and systemic veins, around the lower end of the oesophagus and also linking veins between the deep and superficial venous plexuses in the leg. This means that occlusion of a deep vein in the calf does not produce haemorrhagic infarction of the foot but only a mild oedema of the tissues and congestion of the superficial veins because of their increased flow. Unfortunately, not all veins have a collateral system. If the central vein of the retina is occluded, as may happen in thrombosis of the cavernous sinus due to local infection, the tissue of the orbit becomes oedematous and congested so that the eye is pushed forward (proptosis) and there may be local haemorrhage as the small vessels rupture because of the increased pressure. In the worst cases the venous pressure rises until it exceeds the arterial pressure and prevents arterial flow. This produces infarction, i.e. death of the tissue, and the infarcted tissue is red or purple and swollen because of the haemorrhagic oedema. The word 'infarction' actually comes from the Latin *farcire*, meaning 'to stuff', and it is thought to have originally been used for the appearance of venous infarcts stuffed with blood.

Arterial collaterals exist in various areas such as the gut, circle of Willis and, to some extent, in the heart (Fig. 6.11). Arterial occlusion without the benefit of collaterals will produce ischaemic infarction where the tissue is pale without any swelling. Occasionally arterial infarcts are haemorrhagic because there is reperfusion or some limited arterial flow leading to leakage of blood from necrotic small vessels. In incomplete arterial occlusion the effects depend on the tissue's demand for metabolites. Brain and heart tissue are highly susceptible to ischaemic injury, while bone and skeletal muscle are quite resistant. It is possible to reduce a tissue's demand by cooling the tissue as is done in some types of surgery.

Vascular occlusion can result from:

- thrombosis
- embolism
- atherosclerosis
- external compression
- spasm.

We shall discuss the first three of these causes in some depth in this chapter, starting with thrombosis.

THROMBOSIS

Patients presenting with an arterial thrombus are generally middle-aged or elderly and may have circulatory problems due to atherosclerosis. Many will be smokers and some may suffer from diabetes. Their symptoms and signs will depend entirely on which vessel is affected. In contrast, a patient with venous thrombosis may be any age but generally will be rather immobile or forced to be immobile, such as after an operation. Such patients frequently complain of pain in a calf muscle and often swelling of the foot and ankle.

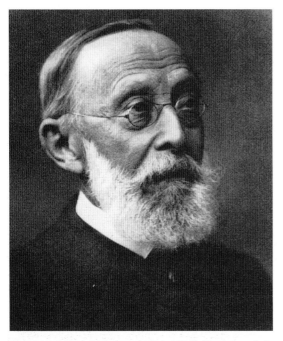

Figure 6.1 Rudolf Virchow (1821–1902) (Courtesy of the Wellcome Institute for the History of Medicine

But why should such people suddenly develop a thrombus? Much is known now about normal haemostatic mechanisms, but the most important factors influencing thrombus formation were described more than a century ago by Rudolf Ludwig Karl Virchow.

Virchow was born on 13 October 1821. As a child he excelled at school and his examination reports were rather monotonous as they contained only three terms – 'excellent', 'very good' and 'most satisfactory'! Virchow attended medical school in Berlin in 1839 and, even before the existence of platelets and clotting factors was known, had suggested that the development of a thrombus depended on:

- alteration to the constituents of the blood
- damage to the endothelial layer of the blood vessel
- changes in the normal flow of blood.

These three factors are known as Virchow's triad and they are the clues that allow us to understand what has happened to our patients with venous and arterial thrombosis (page 149). But first we must revise the body's normal haemostatic mechanisms.

Normal haemostatic mechanisms

Blood and the blood vessels perform an incredibly complex set of tasks. The blood vessels provide a conduit and the blood transports nutrients, waste products and components to defend against infection. However, the vessels are not a simple tube because it is crucial that substances can diffuse between the blood in the vessel and the surrounding tissues. This means that the small vessels (capillaries) must be permeable, i.e. they are designed to leak. The trick is to ensure that the leakage is under control. For larger vessels that do not need to be permeable, a potential problem occurs because the vascular system is a closed, pressurized system and so at risk of rupture. We must also remember that the network of blood vessels is vast and many are superficial and so susceptible to traumatic damage.

All of this means that the normal haemostatic mechanisms are crucial for stopping blood from leaking but they must also be finely controlled so that thrombus does not form under normal circumstances. There are three main components to the maintenance of haemostasis:

- platelets
- soluble blood proteins of the coagulation pathway
- the vessel wall.

Briefly, the sequence of events in thrombus formation is as follows. Injury to the vessels causes an initial vasoconstriction, which helps to slow the blood flow. The damaged endothelium of the vessel exposes the subendothelial connective tissue, which attracts platelets and causes them to adhere to the damaged area to form the primary haemostatic plug. The adhesion of the platelets alters their physiology and causes them to release soluble factors which, together with tissue factors, results in the formation of fibrin via the coagulation pathway. The fibrin acts to stabilize the platelet plug and the process is termed secondary haemostasis.

If this was all that was involved in maintaining haemostasis, could we really survive the assault on our circulation? Of course not! If the above system was set in motion with nothing to check its progress, soon the whole circulation would come to a standstill and become one big mass of thrombus. This is avoided by clearance, inhibition and inactivation of the coagulation factors as well as by digestion of fibrin.

Now if we return to Virchow's triad, we can consider both the normal physiology and pathology of each component in more detail.

BLOOD CONSTITUENTS IN NORMAL HAEMOSTASIS

The most important blood constituents involved in normal haemostasis and thrombosis are platelets and the numerous components of the coagulation pathway.

Platelets

Platelets are small (2 μm) cytoplasmic fragments produced by megakaryocytes in the bone marrow. They survive for 8–12 days in the peripheral circulation and contain a variety of granules (see later).

Their role in thrombosis can be divided into three phases:

* adhesion
* secretion
* aggregation.

When the endothelium is damaged and collagen is exposed, the first event is adhesion of platelets. This is achieved via platelet surface membrane receptors:

* gpIa/IIa, which binds to collagen
* gpIb/IX, which binds to von Willebrand's factor (vWF or factor VIII-related antigen)
* gpIIb/IIIa, which binds to fibrinogen and vWF.

Following adhesion, the platelets release the contents of their granules. There are two main types of granules: the alpha granules and dense bodies (Fig. 6.2). The most important secretory products are calcium, which is needed for the coagulation pathway, and adenosine diphosphate (ADP) and thromboxane (TxA$_2$), which induce platelet aggregation. Platelet aggregation involves the gpIIb/IIIa receptor complex mentioned above. This is expressed after activation and is most important in binding fibrinogen, which acts as a bridge to the adjacent platelet (Fig. 6.2). Not surprisingly, there are 'loops' in this process to amplify the reaction. Most importantly, activated platelets express platelet factor 3, which stimulates the intrinsic pathway of the coagulation cascade (see below), resulting in the production of thrombin. Thrombin acts to stimulate platelets and so enhances the reaction.

The platelet has another important facet to its character: it has mechanical properties. An unstimulated platelet has a disc shape maintained by microtubules and actin and myosin filaments at the periphery. On activation, the platelet is transformed into a sphere with long pseudopods that spread over the damaged surface and then, after aggregation, the internal filaments slide so that the platelet plug contracts to stabilize and anchor it.

Small Print

Some diseases caused by platelet abnormalities

* von Willebrand's disease: lack of vW factor
* Bernard–Soulier syndrome: lack of gpIb
* 'Grey platelet' syndrome: lack of alpha granules
* Wiskott–Aldrich syndrome: lack of dense granules

All these conditions are rare but they illustrate the consequences of platelet granule abnormalities.

Platelet granule contents

Alpha granules	fibrinogen
	von Willebrand factor
	thrombospondin
	platelet-derived growth factor (PDGF)
	fibronectin
	platelet factor 4 (an antiheparin)
Dense granules	ADP/ATP
	calcium
	histamine
	adrenaline
	serotonin

Coagulation components

The components and pathway involved in coagulation are shown in Fig. 6.3. This is the same system as the one we mentioned in Chapter 4 when discussing inflammatory mediators. Then we were particularly interested in fibrin degradation products, now our interest focuses on fibrin, which is the final product of the pathway and acts to stabilize the plug of aggregated platelets.

The coagulation pathway has been divided traditionally into the extrinsic and intrinsic pathways, although a complex interplay occurs between them and few people now make the distinction. The

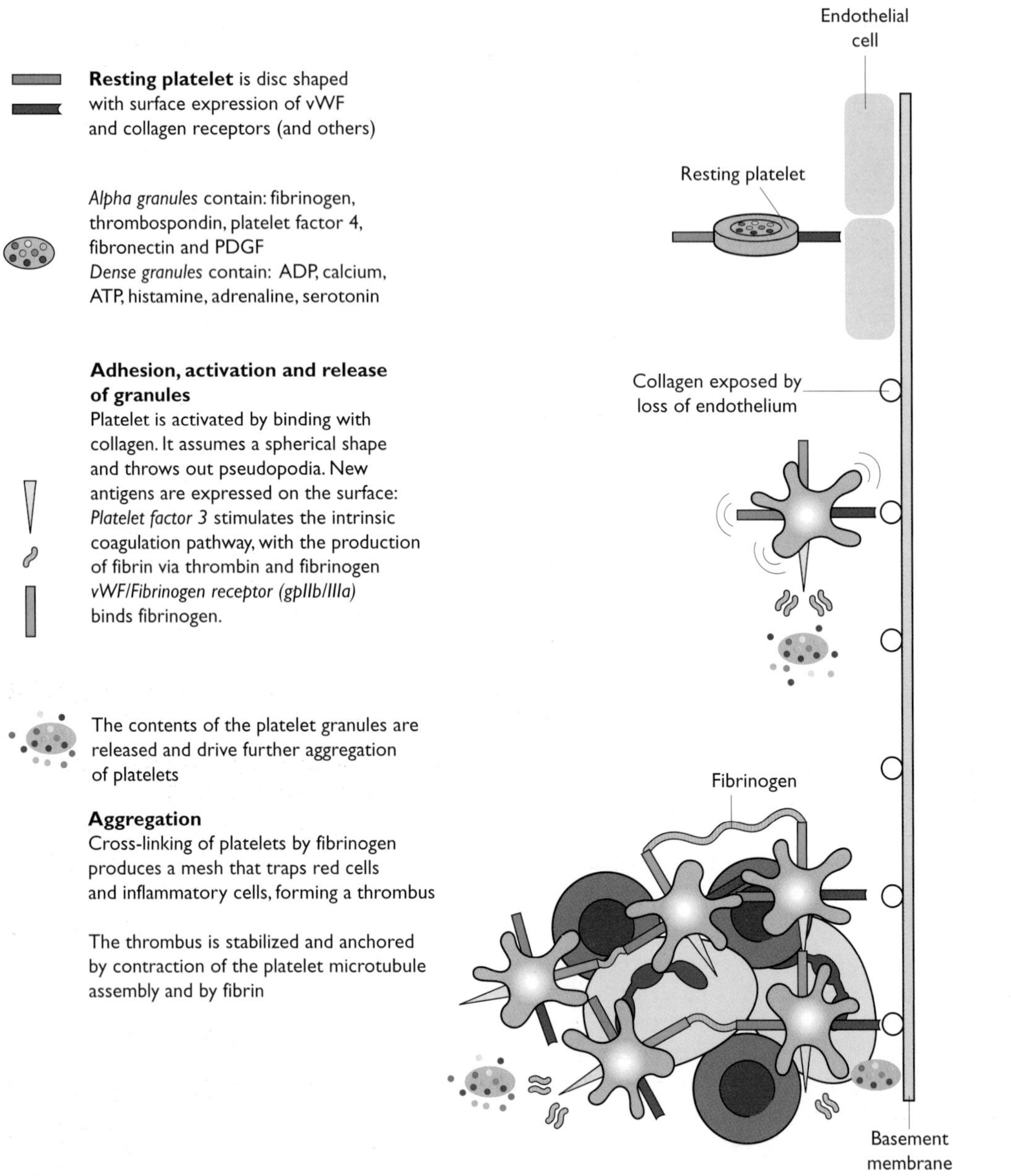

Endothelial
cell

Resting platelet is disc shaped
with surface expression of vWF
and collagen receptors (and others)

Resting platelet

Alpha granules contain: fibrinogen,
thrombospondin, platelet factor 4,
fibronectin and PDGF
Dense granules contain: ADP, calcium,
ATP, histamine, adrenaline, serotonin

**Adhesion, activation and release
of granules**
Platelet is activated by binding with
collagen. It assumes a spherical shape
and throws out pseudopodia. New
antigens are expressed on the surface:
Platelet factor 3 stimulates the intrinsic
coagulation pathway, with the production
of fibrin via thrombin and fibrinogen
vWF/Fibrinogen receptor (gpIIb/IIIa)
binds fibrinogen.

Collagen exposed by
loss of endothelium

The contents of the platelet granules are
released and drive further aggregation
of platelets

Aggregation
Cross-linking of platelets by fibrinogen
produces a mesh that traps red cells
and inflammatory cells, forming a thrombus

Fibrinogen

The thrombus is stabilized and anchored
by contraction of the platelet microtubule
assembly and by fibrin

Basement
membrane

Figure 6.2 Platelet adhesion, activation and aggregation

common pathway begins at factor X, which acts on
prothrombin to produce thrombin, which itself has
a variety of actions but most importantly converts
fibrinogen to fibrin. Generally each step in this cascade involves:

- an activated enzyme
- a substrate for a coagulation factor
- a co-factor
- calcium ions (factor IV)

- phospholipid surface.

Some feedback loops are included in the figure
but, for simplicity, the control mechanisms that
inhibit or inactivate reactions have been omitted.
These mechanisms include:

- depletion of local clotting factors
- clearance of activated clotting factors by the
liver and mononuclear phagocyte system

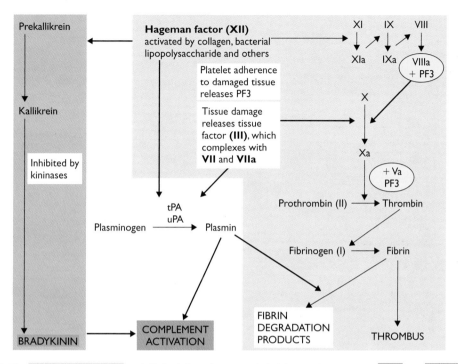

Figure 6.3 The coagulation cascade and fibrinolytic pathways and their interactions with the kinin and complement systems. Heavy arrows ➔ denote activation of other systems. Inhibition pathways are not shown. ○, co-factor

- neutralization of activated coagulation factors by forming a complex, e.g. antithrombin III, α_2-macroglobulin
- proteolytic degradation of active coagulation factors, e.g. protein C
- fibrinolysis – this is of major importance.

The most important enzyme capable of digesting fibrin is plasmin. This is produced from plasminogen either by a factor XII-dependent pathway, by therapeutic agents such as streptokinase, or by tissue-derived plasminogen activators. There are two types of plasminogen activator (PA):

- urokinase-like PA (uPA)
- tissue-type PA (tPA).

They differ in that uPA activates plasminogen in the fluid phase, whereas tPA (principally produced by endothelial cells) is active only when attached to fibrin. Conveniently, some plasminogen is bound to fibrin as a thrombus is formed and so is perfectly situated for conversion by the tPA to plasmin, which can then digest the thrombus. Compounds capable of breaking down thrombi have enormous therapeutic potential for restoring blood flow before significant myocardial or cerebral infarction has occurred.

VIRCHOW POINT 1: ALTERATION IN THE CONSTITUENTS OF THE BLOOD

Blood that clots more readily than usual is termed hypercoaguable. This may be caused by a variety of different mechanisms including:

- an increase in blood cells (polycythaemia)

Dictionary box

Polycythaemia: An increase in red cells which occurs as a normal compensatory mechanism if the person has chronic hypoxaemia because of chronic cardiorespiratory problems or because they live at high altitudes. It can also occur because of uncontrolled erythropoietin production by various tumours (e.g. renal cell carcinoma). or uncontrolled proliferation of the haematopoietic cells. This neoplastic proliferation is called polycythaemia rubra vera and patients often present with thrombosis.

- loss of the plasma fraction of the blood (severe burns)
- increased numbers of platelets
- increased amount or aggregation of plasma proteins (myeloma, cryoglobulinaemia)
- severe trauma
- disseminated cancer
- late pregnancy.

Presumably, hypercoagulability results from either an increase in activated coagulation proteins, an increased risk of platelet aggregation or a decrease in antithrombotic proteins, however, the actual sequence of events leading to this state is not clear at present. Some mechanisms have been elucidated such as deficiencies of protein C and hereditary lack of antithrombin III.

VIRCHOW POINT 2: CHANGES IN THE ENDOTHELIUM

Normal endothelium

The fact that the vascular tree is lined by endothelium means that the endothelial surface must be resistant to thrombus formation. The endothelium is quite remarkable, for it is capable of initiating both thrombogenic and antithrombogenic stimuli (Fig. 6.4). Normally these two groups of actions are finely balanced in favour of preventing thrombus formation. Damage to the endothelium, however, will tip the balance towards thrombosis. The endothelium also has another very important role which is to prevent the elements of blood from coming into contact with the subendothelial connective tissue, which is highly thrombogenic. This tissue normally comprises collagen, elastin, fibronectin and

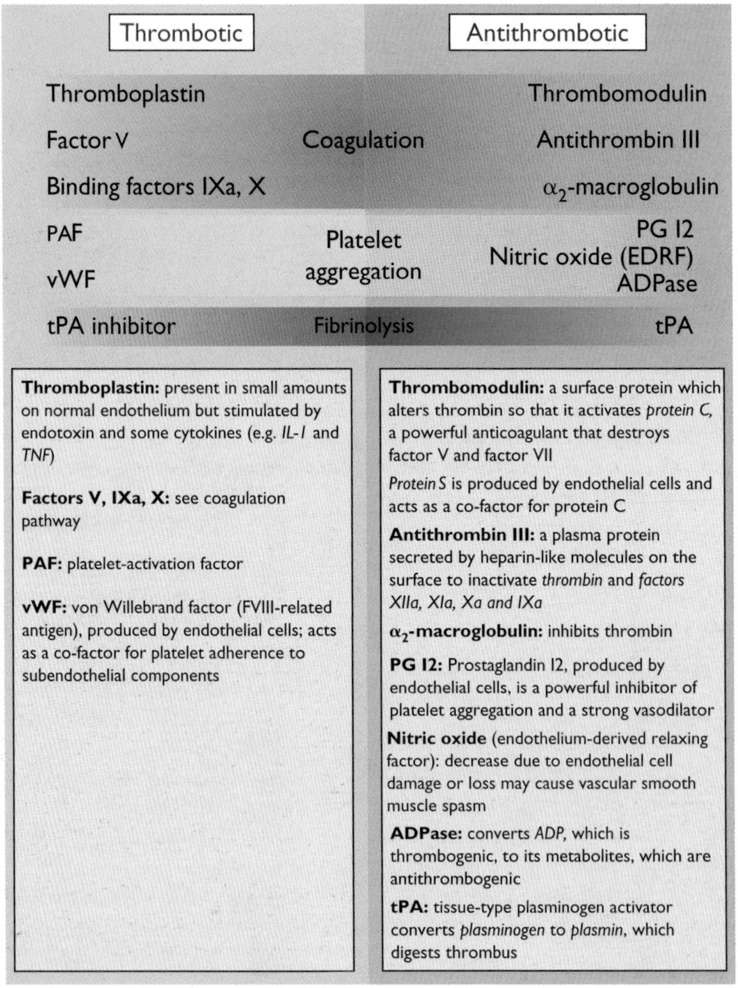

Thrombotic		Antithrombotic
Thromboplastin		Thrombomodulin
Factor V	Coagulation	Antithrombin III
Binding factors IXa, X		α_2-macroglobulin
PAF	Platelet aggregation	PG I2 Nitric oxide (EDRF) ADPase
vWF		
tPA inhibitor	Fibrinolysis	tPA

Thromboplastin: present in small amounts on normal endothelium but stimulated by endotoxin and some cytokines (e.g. *IL-1* and *TNF*)

Factors V, IXa, X: see coagulation pathway

PAF: platelet-activation factor

vWF: von Willebrand factor (FVIII-related antigen), produced by endothelial cells; acts as a co-factor for platelet adherence to subendothelial components

Thrombomodulin: a surface protein which alters thrombin so that it activates *protein C*, a powerful anticoagulant that destroys factor V and factor VII

Protein S is produced by endothelial cells and acts as a co-factor for protein C

Antithrombin III: a plasma protein secreted by heparin-like molecules on the surface to inactivate *thrombin* and *factors XIIa, XIa, Xa and IXa*

α_2-**macroglobulin:** inhibits thrombin

PG I2: Prostaglandin I2, produced by endothelial cells, is a powerful inhibitor of platelet aggregation and a strong vasodilator

Nitric oxide (endothelium-derived relaxing factor): decrease due to endothelial cell damage or loss may cause vascular smooth muscle spasm

ADPase: converts *ADP*, which is thrombogenic, to its metabolites, which are antithrombogenic

tPA: tissue-type plasminogen activator converts *plasminogen to plasmin*, which digests thrombus

Figure 6.4 Endothelial thrombotic/antithrombotic mechanisms

glycosaminoglycans. Collagen is by far the most important of these constituents and it activates the coagulation pathway as well as being a strong stimulator of platelet aggregation. In vessels affected by atheroma, not only is the endothelium more readily damaged but the subendothelial tissue consists of the components of atheroma which are extremely thrombogenic.

Damage to the endothelium

Endothelial damage is of most significance in arterial thrombosis. There may be obvious loss of endothelial cells or more subtle metabolic damage to the cells. Endothelial cells may be lost where an atheromatous plaque has ulcerated or when vessels are damaged by surgery, infection, immune-mediated damage (arteritis), indwelling vascular catheters or infusion of sclerosing chemicals in the treatment of varicose veins and haemorrhoids. Haemodynamic stress is believed to be important in producing metabolic damage to arterial endothelial cells in areas where there is turbulent flow or in patients with prolonged high blood pressure. Other potentially damaging agents include derivatives of cigarette smoke, bacterial toxins, immune complex deposition, transplant rejection and radiation.

In the heart, the endocardial surface is covered by endothelium, which can be damaged in a myocardial infarction. Also the valve surface endothelium may be damaged by inflammatory endocarditis, which promotes thrombus formation on valve leaflets resulting in altered function, a variety of heart murmurs and the danger of throwing emboli into the systemic circulation. Clinically, the most important change is the endothelial damage related to atherosclerosis (see pages 173).

VIRCHOW POINT 3: CHANGES IN THE NORMAL FLOW OF BLOOD

There are two principal ways in which the normal flow can be disturbed: the normal lamellar flow pattern can be altered (turbulence) or the speed may be reduced (stasis), but both lead to similar changes.

During normal flow, red and white blood cells concentrate in the central, fast-moving stream, while platelets flow nearer to the periphery, and the layer closest to the endothelium is usually devoid of cells and platelets. If the blood flow slows down or turbulence produces local counter-currents, several factors increase the likelihood of thrombus formation:

- platelets come into contact with the endothelium
- turbulence may damage endothelial cells
- there is no inflow of fresh blood containing clotting factor inhibitors
- there is no clearance of blood containing activated coagulation factors.

As you see, both turbulence and stasis operate in thrombosis but turbulence is most important in arteries whereas stasis is more important in veins.

Arterial thrombosis

Turbulence tends to occur where arteries branch and over the irregular surface of an atheromatous plaque. It also occurs when cardiac valves have been damaged by inflammation, as may occur with

Key facts

Causes of endothelial damage

- Haemodynamic forces
- Hyperlipidaemia
- Cigarette smoke
- Immune and infective attack
- Bacterial toxins
- Irradiation
- Direct trauma
- Various mutagens

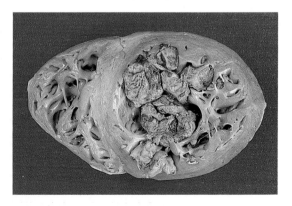

Figure 6.5 Apical section of heart with thrombus in left ventricle following myocardial infarction

Key facts

Factors influencing thrombus formation

Virchow's triad:

Altered blood	increased cells increased platelets increased protein decreased fluid
Altered wall	endothelial loss (atheroma) endothelial damage (smoking)
Altered flow	stasis turbulence

rheumatic fever and infective endocarditis, or have been replaced by artificial valves.

Stasis is generally only important in arterial thrombosis if the heart or arteries have been damaged. Abnormal dilatations of large vessels (aneurysms) will produce pockets of stagnant blood which will thrombose, and myocardial infarction may result in a localized area of damaged heart muscle, which does not move, or in an arrhythmia that will affect the contraction of a whole chamber.

Venous thrombosis

Thrombus formation, related to stasis of blood, is more common in the venous circulation and particularly occurs in the legs or pelvic veins of immobile individuals. Why is stasis common in the leg vessels when the patient is immobilized? If you remember the physiology of venous return from the legs, you will recall that it is contraction of skeletal muscles that pushes blood along the veins and it is the presence of valves that ensures the direction of flow. Understanding this has influenced patient management. Patients are encouraged to move their legs regularly when confined to bed, leg muscles are stimulated to contract during long operations and it is no longer common to have patients bed-bound for weeks.

Thrombus formation often begins within the venous valve pockets. The initial cluster of platelets activates the clotting cascade to produce a small

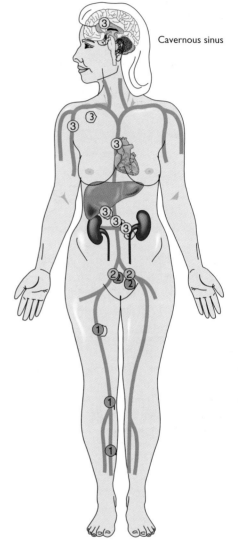

Cavernous sinus

In order of frequency:	Clinical setting
1. Leg veins	Immobility, post-surgery and hyper-coagulability states
2. Pelvic veins	Post-childbirth, puerperal sepsis, pelvic surgery and tumours
3. Others:	
Inferior vena cava	Extrinsic compression by tumour, extension from leg or iliac veins
Renal vein	Tumour extension from kidney
Portal/hepatic veins	Local sepsis, tumour compression
Cavernous sinus	Facial sepsis
Superior vena cava	Extrinsic compression by mediastinal tumour
Axillary vein	Trauma from rucksack, local surgery

Figure 6.6 Sites and clinical setting of venous thrombosis

thrombus. A second phase of platelet aggregation then occurs to cover the original thrombus and promote a further wave of coagulation. This process is repeated again and again to extend the thrombus, so-called propagation. The resultant thrombus has alternate layers of platelets and a red cell/white cell/fibrin mixture, which produces a rippled effect, termed 'lines of Zahn'. The direction of the lines relates to the pattern of blood flow in the vessel. These platelet layers anchor the thrombus to the adjacent endothelium, helping to stabilize it.

Once a vessel is completely occluded by thrombus, blood flow ceases and the stagnant column of blood clots without the production of any 'lines of Zahn'. This is called 'consecutive' clot and it is particularly dangerous because it is only adherent to the vessel wall through its attachment to the original focus of thrombus. This makes it especially likely to break off and embolize to another area (see later).

If the blood flow is slowed in the entire limb, then a very large consecutive clot is formed along the length of the limb's venous system. Alternatively, the consecutive clot only extends to the point where the next venous tributary enters the main vessel. Here the blood may be flowing at a reasonable speed, but the presence of activated clotting factors will promote the adherence of a layer of platelets which may result in a fresh wave of thrombosis from this point. The involvement of platelets, however, does mean that the clot will be anchored at the points at which the tributaries enter and be slightly less likely to embolize. Lines of Zahn can also be seen in arterial thrombus. These processes are illustrated in Figs 6.7 and 6.8.

It is also worth emphasizing at this point that, like most phenomena in the body, the three major factors of Virchow's triad rarely work in isolation. In myocardial infarction, ischaemia damages the endocardium but the affected myocardium also fails to move normally, hence causing local stasis of blood, which is also important in formation of the thrombus within the ventricle. So, while it is imperative that one knows the basis for Virchow's triad, it is also important to remember that many factors interact to produce the final picture in any one patient.

Natural history and complications of thrombosis

Once a thrombus has formed, what are the possible outcomes? As you know, the body possesses many effective systems for regulating thrombus formation during normal haemostasis. The ideal solution is that these systems halt the thrombotic process and remove the debris to leave a normal blood vessel. This process is termed resolution. If the thrombus cannot be removed, it may be organized or recanalized. Alternatively, it may be cast off into the circulation i.e. it may embolize.

Resolution is thought to occur commonly in the small veins of the lower limb. Interestingly, venous intima contains more plasminogen activator than arterial intima, which may be the reason. Drugs with a thrombolytic action, such as streptokinase, can be given to patients early after thrombosis to promote dissolution of the clot and, hence, resolution. It is important that this drug is given within

Key facts

Arterial and venous thrombosis compared

	Arterial	Venous
Clinical setting	Person with atheroma	Immobile person
Pathogenesis	Turbulent flow	Stasis
	Damaged endothelium	Hypercoagulable blood
Symptoms	Sudden onset	Slow onset
Complications	Infarction	Pulmonary embolus
	Arterial embolism	

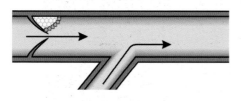

Decreased blood flow or increased coagulability
Thrombus forms in valve pocket. Platelets adhere to surface of thrombus

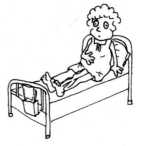

Lines of Zahn

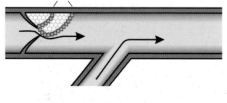

Platelet layer propagates further thrombus formation
'Lines of Zahn' formed by alternating red and white cell and platelet deposits, orientated along blood flow.
Fibrin contracts

Consecutive clot

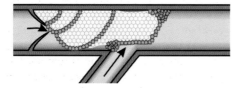

Once lumen occluded, 'consecutive' unstable, clot forms
No lines of Zahn, slow flow and no new platelets. Weakly attached to wall and easily dislodged

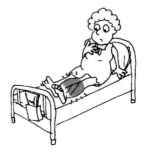

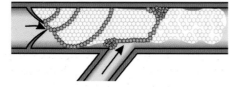

Entry of tributary
i. may stabilize thrombus by re-attaching to wall

ii. permits further propagation

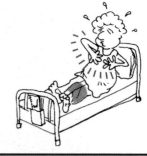

iii. may carry fragments of thrombus into general circulation: embolization

Figure 6.7 Venous thrombosis: development, propagation and embolization

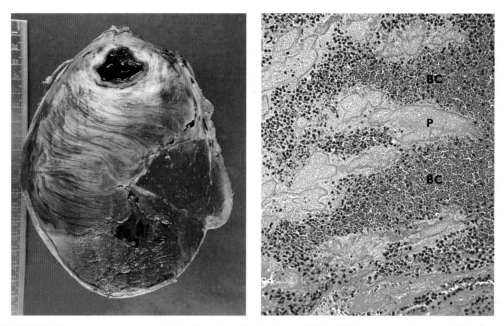

Figure 6.8 Splenic artery aneurysm containing thrombus showing lines of Zahn. Photomicrograph shows alternating layers of platelets (P) and blood cells (BC) trapped in a fibrin mesh

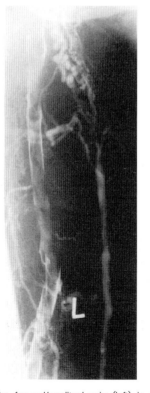

Figure 6.9 The femoral/popliteal vein (left) is occluded by thrombus so that the contrast medium only fills the edge of the vessel

hours because the drug has much less effect on polymerized fibrin, which predominates later.

Organization of a thrombus involves similar processes to the organization of inflammation described in Chapter 4. When the thrombus has formed, polymorphs and macrophages begin to degrade and digest the fibrin and cell debris. Later, granulation tissue grows into the base of the thrombus so that the thrombus is converted into a mass of small vessels separated by connective tissue. These vessels originate from the vasa vasorum of the adventitia of the blood vessel and it is unlikely that the blood flowing through these is of much clinical importance (but see below for collateral circulation).

Alternatively the thrombus may occlude only part of the vessel, so that on cross-section it is attached to one side of the lumen. Organization of this mural thrombus also involves digestion by inflammatory cells, but differs in that small vessels grow in from the luminal surface rather than from the outer layers. Ultimately, the thrombus shrinks and is covered by endothelial or smooth muscle cells which produce platelet-derived growth factor (PDGF). As we shall see, this is of interest because of its potential role in the formation of atheromatous plaques (page 174).

Recanalization is a term used by clinicians to indicate that there is useful flow through a previously occluded vessel. Obviously, if streptokinase treatment has been successful, the thrombus will be dissolved, the original intimal lining will still exist and the clinician will see flow on the arteriogram; the clinician will call this recanalization but we will not!

A similar situation occurs if the clot retracts so that it is obstructing only part of the flow (Fig. 6.10). The blood flow is, at least partially, restored but through the original lumen and not through new channels.

To a pathologist, recanalization involves the production of *new* endothelial-lined channels that convey blood through the occlusive thrombus. This

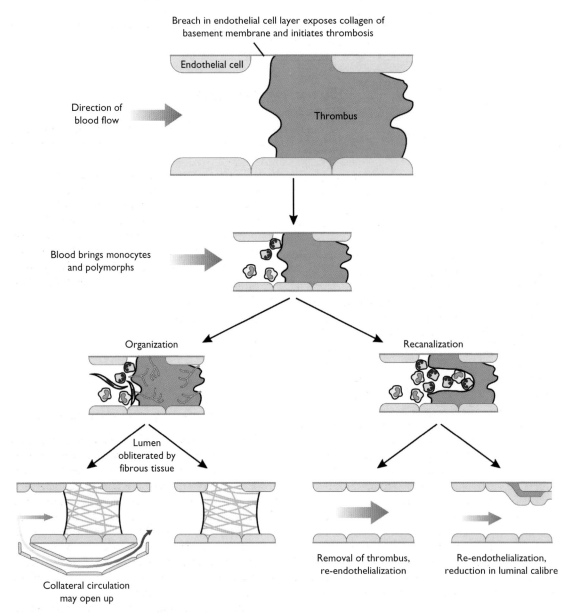

Figure 6.10 Thrombotic obstruction of an artery or vein may be overcome by a variety of mechanisms. In some instances the vessel remains obliterated and new channels must be found for flow, or the affected tissue will die. Alternatively, thrombus may break off and embolize to distant sites. An arterial thrombus will impact in small arterioles or capillary beds and usually causes tissue infarction; a venous embolus will generally lodge within the pulmonary vasculature and may cause shock

is thought to occur by the production of clefts within the thrombus, resulting from a combination of local digestion and shrinkage. The clefts extend through the clot and become lined by endothelial cells derived from the adjacent intima. This can produce several channels separated by loose connective tissue. The amount of flow through such a segment will depend on the number and size of the conduits but the vessel will not be 'as good as new'.

This is a convenient moment to digress and discuss the way in which the cardiovascular system tries to compensate for a reduced flow through a vessel. Just as you might try to avoid a traffic jam by driving through the back roads, so the blood will search for alternative routes. The availability of such routes depends on the local anatomy. In the venous circulation, there are specific anastomoses between the systemic and portal systems around the rectum, oesophagus, umbilicus and the retroperitoneal vessels, but the penetrating veins linking the deep and superficial lower limb venous plexuses are of more relevance to our patient with a deep vein thrombosis. Thus, if a segment of the deep veins is occluded, the blood will bypass it by moving into the superficial plexus.

The arterial system has some well-characterized alternative routes, such as the arterial roundabout of the circle of Willis and the dual arterial supply of the lung. However, most organs do not have a dual supply and must rely on collateral vessels opening up if the main supplying vessel is occluded. If we take the heart and coronary arteries as an example, then we can often see a collateral arterial circulation in a patient who has suffered a coronary artery thrombosis, as is demonstrated in the arteriogram shown in Fig. 8.3 (page 188). The apparently new network of small vessels has always existed but little blood would flow through these channels because it was easier to flow down the larger artery. Once thrombosis occurs, the resistance to flow increases in the main vessel, making the small channel route attractive and, hence, visible on arteriograms.

Where are these vessels? This is an area of great interest because, theoretically, any patient with a large network of connecting vessels would have some protection from suffering a large myocardial infarction. There are three main possibilities. In probable order of clinical importance, these are:

- small arterioles within the myocardium
- side branches from the large coronary arteries
- vasa vasorum.

John Hunter carried out an elegant experiment to demonstrate collateral circulation. He tied one of the carotid arteries in a stag from Richmond Park and observed the effect on the corresponding antler. The carotid pulse on that side disappeared and the antler went cold and stopped growing. Within a few weeks, however, the warmth returned and the antler started to grow again. Hunter demonstrated the collateral circulation by sacrificing the stag and injecting the carotid artery. Elegant as it was, such an experiment would not go down a bundle nowadays!

EMBOLISM

One of the complications of thrombosis is embolism and we will now go on to consider the different types of emboli and their complications.

An embolus is solid, liquid or gaseous material that is carried in the blood from one area of the circulatory system to another area. Almost all (circa 99 per cent) of emboli arise from thrombi and, thus, there is a tendency to use the term thromboembolism as synonymous with embolism. This is not strictly accurate as there are many other, though admittedly rarer, causes of emboli. These include:

- fragments of atheromatous plaques
- bone marrow
- fat
- air or nitrogen
- amniotic fluid
- tumour
- foreign material, e.g. intravenous catheter.

Since the majority of the emboli come from thrombi, we shall start our discussion with this particular type. Where emboli lodge depends on their size, origin and the relevant cardiovascular anatomy. Those that arise in the venous system can travel through the right side of the heart to end up in the pulmonary circulation. Those that arise in the left side of the circulation will block systemic arteries and the clinical effect will depend on the organ involved, be it brain, kidneys, spleen or the periphery of limbs.

Emboli to the lungs from venous thrombosis represent an important preventable cause of morbidity in hospitalized patients and we shall consider this first.

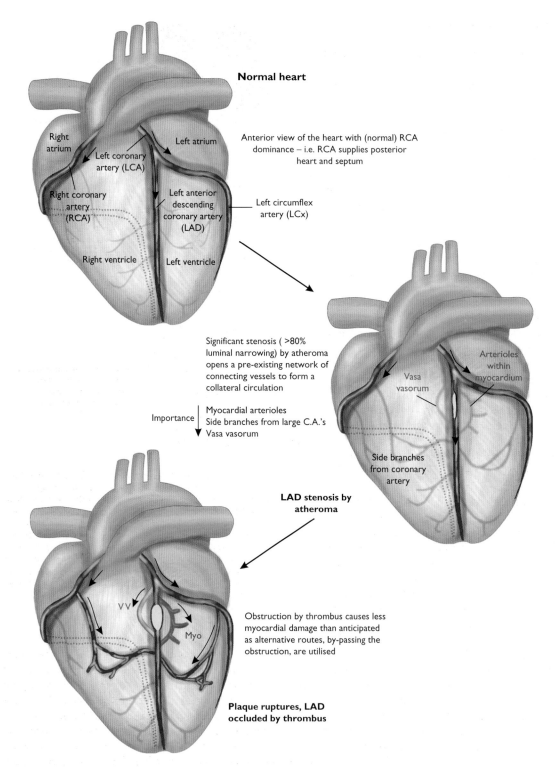

Normal heart

Right atrium

Left atrium

Left coronary artery (LCA)

Right coronary artery (RCA)

Left anterior descending coronary artery (LAD)

Left circumflex artery (LCx)

Right ventricle

Left ventricle

Anterior view of the heart with (normal) RCA dominance – i.e. RCA supplies posterior heart and septum

Significant stenosis (>80% luminal narrowing) by atheroma opens a pre-existing network of connecting vessels to form a collateral circulation

Importance
Myocardial arterioles
Side branches from large C.A.'s
Vasa vasorum

Vasa vasorum

Arterioles within myocardium

Side branches from coronary artery

LAD stenosis by atheroma

v v

Myo

Obstruction by thrombus causes less myocardial damage than anticipated as alternative routes, by-passing the obstruction, are utilised

Plaque ruptures, LAD occluded by thrombus

Figure 6.11 The development of a collateral circulation in the heart. In many patients with coronary artery atherosclerosis, luminal narrowing occurs gradually enough for the heart to adapt, by opening alternative circulatory paths. This leads to less than the expected amount of damage should a by-passed segment of coronary artery undergo sudden complete obstruction by thrombosis

Pulmonary embolism

The lungs are very interesting organs because they have a dual blood supply. Not only does the lung receive deoxygenated blood via the pulmonary arteries, but it also receives oxygenated blood from bronchial arteries feeding directly from the aorta. Hence, the lungs have an established collateral arterial circulation. This means that occlusion of a branch of the pulmonary artery rarely causes infarction of the lung parenchyma and, because the alveolar walls are intact, resolution is possible. The effects of a pulmonary embolus will depend on three factors:

- the size of the occluded vessel
- the number of emboli
- the adequacy of the bronchial blood supply.

THE SIZE OF THE OCCLUDED VESSEL

If a large embolus occludes a main pulmonary artery or even sits astride the bifurcation of the pulmonary trunk, a so-called saddle embolus, the patient's blood pressure will suddenly drop and there may even be instant death. If the patient survives and reaches the hospital, it may be possible to lyse the embolus using medical therapy or remove it surgically (embolectomy). It is tempting to postulate that the circulatory collapse is due to acute strain put on the right heart by sudden obstruction to the outflow tract. However, this cannot be the whole story because patients tolerate ligation of the pulmonary artery during removal of a lung at surgery. Possibly the left ventricular outflow drops because the left atrial filling has been reduced or perhaps there is a reflex vasoconstriction of the entire pulmonary vasculature.

Around 95 per cent of emboli originate in the ileofemoral venous system with a small number coming from the pelvic veins, calf muscle veins and superficial veins of the legs. Obviously, the diameter of these emboli will correspond with the diameter of the vessel of origin, which is less than the size of the major pulmonary arteries. So how does an embolus block a vessel larger than itself? The answer is that it becomes coiled, as illustrated in Fig. 6.12.

Not infrequently, a long single embolus may fragment in the circulation to produce numerous small emboli. These may reach the small pulmonary arteries as a 'shower' to occlude several vessels at the same time, producing similar sudden, severe clinical effects similar to those of a single large embolus.

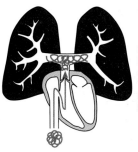

Large P.E.
Large embolus coils within major pulmonary artery. "Saddle" embolus blocks both pulmonary arteries. This produces circulatory collapse

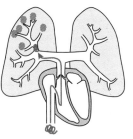

Medium P.E.
Dual blood supply protects lung from effects of pulmonary arterial obstruction

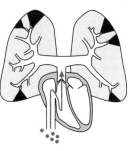

Multiple emboli combined with poor bronchial blood supply
Leads to pulmonary infarction Bronchial artery not shown

Figure 6.12 The effects of pulmonary embolism range from catastrophic shock with circulatory collapse, through moderate or mild respiratory impairment with pleuritic chest pain, to virtually no symptoms at all. The size, number and timing of the emboli and the quality of the bronchial artery circulation all influence the outcome. If small embolic events are sufficiently separated by time, thrombolytic mechanisms may clear them and restore normal circulation. The type of embolus also influences the sites affected and the clinical outcome. Here we illustrate three patterns of pulmonary thromboembolism

If a medium-sized pulmonary artery becomes blocked, this may produce no clinical effect because the bronchial circulation is able to supply the lung parenchyma. Generally there will be local haemorrhage but no damage to the framework of the lung and so complete resolution can occur. If the haemorrhage is small, the patient may be asymptomatic, but if it is large, the patient may have some shortness of breath or haemoptysis.

If the small peripheral pulmonary arteries are involved, there may be infarction because the area is beyond the territory of the bronchial collateral supply so the pulmonary arteries are, in effect, end arteries. Generally the area affected will be quite small but may produce symptoms, especially if there are multiple emboli.

Dictionary box

- **Dyspnoea: Sensation of shortness of breath. When associated with cardiac failure, it may be due to pulmonary oedema interfering with gaseous exchange and lung stretch reflexes. If worse on lying flat, it is called** orthopnoea.

- **Haemoptysis: Coughing up blood from the respiratory tract.**

THE NUMBER OF EMBOLI

Multiple emboli may be thrown into the lungs as a single event or there may be successive embolic episodes. The first situation occurs when a single large embolus fragments into smaller emboli before reaching the lungs. The second scenario happens when initially only part of the thrombus breaks off but, hours or days later, a second piece follows. If a patient survives the initial pulmonary embolus, there is a 30 per cent risk of suffering from a further embolus. This makes it extremely important that the patient receives prompt and effective anticoagulant therapy to reduce the risk. However, the anticoagulant therapy will not remove the existing embolus; that requires fibrinolytic treatment as described earlier. Sometimes a patient will remain in 'shock' despite complete lysis of the embolus and this is possibly due to intense vasoconstriction of the peripheral pulmonary vessels.

THE ADEQUACY OF THE BRONCHIAL BLOOD SUPPLY

If a patient suffers from heart failure or has pre-existing pulmonary disease, the bronchial blood supply will be impaired and emboli lodging in medium-sized pulmonary arteries will result in infarction. Since the blockage is relatively proximal, the infarct will be large, extending as a cone with the apex at the blocked vessel and the base on

the pleura (see Fig. 6.12). Initially, the area will be firm and purple because of the haemorrhage and congestion but later it will be replaced by pale fibrous tissue and the area will shrink. Infarcts are most common in the lower lobes of the lungs and are multiple in 50 per cent of cases.

These patients tend to get chest pain related to inflammation of adjacent pleura and shortness of breath due both to a reduction in lung volume and humoral and neural factors leading to vasoconstriction and bronchoconstriction.

A typical clinical scenario is that of an elderly patient in hospital who has cardiac failure and a fractured neck of femur following a fall. The combination of recumbency, cardiac failure and postoperative dehydration combine to create an ideal situation for the formation of a deep vein thrombosis in the leg veins. A moderate sized embolus, over a background of an inadequate collateral supply due to cardiac failure, results in significant ischaemia of the lung parenchyma and infarction.

THE FATE OF THE EMBOLUS

In some ways this is similar to that of a thrombus. Ideally it will be lysed by the fibrinolytic system to restore patency of the vessel. If not, organization takes place and the mass will be incorporated into the wall with possible recanalization of the vessel. Spontaneous lysis is often very good so it is important to support the patient to allow 'nature' to do the healing.

If there are multiple emboli or repeated episodes of embolization and organization, the pulmonary vessel wall will thicken, resulting in a rise in pulmonary arterial pressure (pulmonary hypertension). This in turn means an increased workload for the right ventricle, which tries to compensate by becoming thicker (hypertrophy). Eventually, the right ventricle may not be able to compensate and cardiac failure will ensue. Right ventricular enlargement due to pulmonary disease is called cor pulmonale.

Systemic embolism

Systemic emboli travel in the internal circulation and commonly originate in the left side of the heart from thrombi forming on areas of myocardial infarction or thrombus forming on an atheromatous aorta. Other causes include fragments of atheromatous plaques which result from fissuring or ulceration of a plaque which releases its fibrin, lipid and cholesterol mixture into the circulation.

Arterial emboli, unless very small, nearly always cause infarction. Emboli to the lower limbs may produce gangrene of a few toes or of the entire limb. Cerebral emboli cause death or infarction unless the embolus lodges in an area which receives adequate collateral supply through the circle of Willis. Alternative sites are the upper limb and the vessels supplying the gut, kidney and spleen. A special type of systemic embolus is the infected material from vegetations on the heart valves in infective endocarditis. These produce septic infarcts and large abscesses in the affected tissues.

Key facts

Sources of thromboemboli

Heart

- Left ventricle secondary to myocardial infarction
- Left atria secondary to fibrillation
- Rheumatic heart disease
- Cardiomyopathy
- Infective endocarditis
- Valve prosthesis

Vessels

- Ulcerated arteriosclerotic plaques
- Aortic aneurysm
- Arterial prosthesis

Dictionary box

Paradoxical embolus: This forms when a venous thrombus passes through a right to left congenital cardiac anomaly.

Other types of emboli

The other types of emboli generally enter veins rather than arteries because veins have thinner walls and a lower pressure. Therefore, most are venous emboli which lodge in the lungs.

BONE MARROW EMBOLI

Bone marrow emboli are occasionally seen in histological sections of lungs at autopsy. This is especially likely if the patient has suffered major trauma, such as a road traffic accident, but can even occur with the 'trauma' of attempted cardiac resuscitation, particularly in elderly people whose costal cartilages have ossified. Anything which fractures bone can release bone and bone marrow into the venous circulation with resultant pulmonary emboli but the clinical significance of this type of embolization is unclear.

FAT EMBOLI

Fat from the marrow cavities of long bones or from soft tissue also can enter the circulation as a result of severe trauma. However, they even form without any trauma and so alternative mechanisms must operate. Fortunately, although fat globules are found in the lungs of most victims of severe trauma, less than 5 per cent will suffer from the 'fat embolism syndrome', which is characterized by respiratory problems, a haemorrhagic skin rash and mental deterioration 24–72 hours after the injury. The syndrome is unlikely to result merely from mechanical blockage of vessels but probably involves chemical injury to the small vessels of the lungs, producing pulmonary oedema and activation of the coagulation pathway to cause disseminated intravascular

Key facts

Causes of fat embolism

- Severe trauma
- Diabetes mellitus
- Sickle cell disease
- Pancreatitis
- Hyperlipidaemias

coagulation (DIC). However, the exact mediators have not been identified. The origin of the fat in the non-trauma cases may be chylomicrons and fatty acids in the circulation coalescing to form droplets; the emulsion instability theory.

AIR AND NITROGEN EMBOLI

Large quantities of air within the circulation can act as emboli by forming a frothy mass that can block vessels or become trapped in the right heart chambers to impede its pumping. Air can either enter the circulation from the atmosphere or it can be produced within the circulation by alteration of pressure.

Severe trauma to the thorax may open large vessels (e.g. internal jugular veins), allowing air to be sucked in during inspiration, or air may be forced into the uterine vessels during badly performed abortions or deliveries. Fortunately, small quantities of air, as may be introduced during venesection, dissolve in the plasma and it probably takes about 100 mL to produce problems.

A special type of air embolism occurs in deep sea divers. Normally insoluble gases, such as nitrogen or helium in the diver's breathing mixture, will dissolve in the blood and tissues at the high pressures that occur deep beneath the sea surface. As the diver surfaces, the pressure is reduced and the gas begins to come out of solution as minute bubbles. If the reduction of pressure is rapid then these bubbles form emboli that are particularly likely to lodge in the skeletal and cerebral circulation. The situation is slightly more complicated because platelets adhere to the nitrogen bubbles, activate the coagulation system and produce disseminated intravascular coagulation (see below). The acute form of decompression sickness or 'bends' involves pain around joints and in skeletal muscle, respiratory distress and, sometimes, coma and death. In the early stages, it can be treated by putting the victim in a 'decompression' chamber where the high pressure will redissolve the bubbles and allow a slow, controlled decompression. The chronic form, or caisson disease, produces multiple areas of ischaemic necrosis in the long bones. (A caisson is a high-pressure underwater chamber.)

AMNIOTIC FLUID EMBOLI

This is an uncommon, but life-threatening form of embolization. Basically, amniotic fluid is forced into the circulation due to tearing of the placental

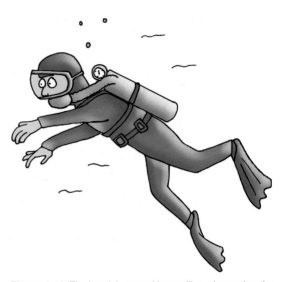

Figure 6.13 'The bends', caused by capillary obstruction due to intravascular nitrogen bubble formation in divers who depressurize too rapidly, is one of the less common types of embolization encountered in routine practice

membranes and rupture of the uterine or cervical veins. These emboli are a mixture of fat, hair, mucus, meconium and squamous cells from the fetus and they most commonly lodge in the mother's alveolar capillaries. Clinically, there is sudden onset of respiratory failure, often followed by cerebral convulsions and coma. There is also excessive bleeding as a result of disseminated intravascular coagulation (DIC) and the consumption of clotting factors. Over 80 per cent of the patients who develop amniotic fluid emboli will die. The exact mechanism is still unclear but it is not due simply to blockage of the pulmonary vasculature; it is postulated that some factor, such as prostaglandin $F_{2\alpha}$, in the amniotic fluid may be involved.

TUMOUR EMBOLI

Embolization of tumour is an important mechanism of tumour spread but it is unlikely to have any immediate cardiovascular effects. The mechanisms involved in this process are discussed in Chapter 13.

DISSEMINATED INTRAVASCULAR COAGULATION

This is a convenient moment to discuss DIC. We have just mentioned amniotic fluid embolism and we are about to move on to 'shock'; both are

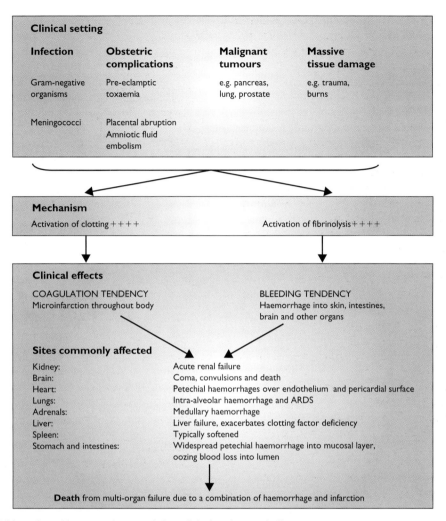

Figure 6.14 Disseminated intravascular coagulation: clinical settings and effects

conditions that can produce DIC. Furthermore, DIC results from a loss of control in the clotting and fibrinolytic systems, which should still be fresh in your memory!

DIC has no typical clinical presentation because any organ may be affected and the major problem may be excessive clotting, which blocks numerous vessels, or inadequate clotting resulting in haemorrhage. As a general rule, sudden-onset DIC presents with bleeding problems, is particularly associated with obstetric complications and may resolve once the obstetric situation improves. In contrast, chronic DIC is more common in patients with carcinomatosis and the thrombotic manifestations dominate.

Small thrombi form anywhere in the circulation and produce microinfarcts. In the brain this may

result in convulsions and coma, lung damage produces dyspnoea and cyanosis and renal changes cause oliguria and acute renal failure. Fibrin deposition not only produces thrombi but also results in a haemolytic anaemia as the red cells fragment whilst squeezing through the narrowed vasculature (microangiopathic haemolytic anaemia).

The fundamental problem is that there is excessive activation of coagulation, which ultimately is complicated by consumption of the coagulation factors and overactivity of the fibrinolytic system. Clotting activation occurs through the extrinsic pathway, initiated by tissue thromboplastin, and the intrinsic pathway, commencing with activated factor XII, but it should be remembered that clotting activation will also stimulate the fibrinolytic pathways, particularly through the factor XII path, and fibrin-degradation products inhibit fibrin production. These latter mechanisms will predominate in haemorrhagic DIC.

Many of the diseases mentioned produce DIC via the extrinsic pathway. For example, the placenta is believed to release tissue thromboplastin in obstetric problems, mucus from some adenocarcinomas can activate factor X and bacterial endotoxins can prompt the release of thromboplastic substances contained in endothelial and inflammatory cells. However, nothing involving bacterial endotoxins is simple! They can also activate the intrinsic pathway directly through factor XII and indirectly by damaging endothelial cells. They even inhibit the anticoagulant activity of protein C.

Not surprisingly, the prognosis is very variable and the management extremely difficult because one is trying to balance a see-saw that is out of control. If you inhibit the clotting system too much with heparin or antithrombin III, the patient will bleed, but any bleeding tendency may require fresh frozen plasma, which may contribute to microthrombus formation.

CHAPTER 7

Atherosclerosis and hypertension

So far we have concentrated on thrombosis and embolism, both of which are conditions that may suddenly affect healthy people of any age. Now we will move on to the major cardiovascular problems of later life, namely arteriosclerosis, hypertension, myocardial infarction and aneurysms. These are overwhelming causes of morbidity and mortality in developed countries but they are not an inevitable consequence of ageing and so it is of great importance to try to identify the causative and risk agents.

ATHEROSCLEROSIS

The arteriopath

Let us briefly consider a possible clinical picture in a patient debilitated by vascular problems. A 48-year-old man complains of blurring of his vision. He is known to suffer from diabetes, which is a complex metabolic disorder characterized by hyperglycaemia (raised blood glucose). At the age of 14 years, he presented with the typical diabetic symptoms of tiredness, weight loss, polyuria (increased urine production) and polydypsia (increased thirst). The blood glucose was raised, glucose was found in his urine and he has been on insulin therapy since that time.

His present complaint of blurred vision started three months ago. On questioning, he also complained of shortness of breath, especially on exertion, and cramps in his calf muscles on exercise. On examination, he was found to have a raised blood pressure, a mild degree of cardiac failure with pulmonary oedema, small haemorrhages and small blood vessel proliferation in his retina and systolic bruits in his neck (abnormal sounds, heard through the stethoscope, caused by turbulent blood flow). His blood tests showed a small rise in urea and creatinine, indicating a degree of renal impairment.

This unfortunate man is an 'arteriopath', i.e. he has widespread disease related to arterial pathology. The arterial pathology comes under the general heading of arteriosclerosis, commonly referred to as 'hardening of the arteries', although this does not relate to a specific pathologically recognized entity. His large and medium-sized arteries are likely to be narrowed by fibrolipid atherosclerotic lesions and his small arteries and arterioles will show the proliferative or hyaline changes of arteriolosclerosis. Atherosclerosis is principally a disease of the intima and may result in narrowing of the vessel, obstruction or thrombosis. Arteriosclerosis, on the other hand, affects the media, with a resultant increase in wall thickness and decreased elasticity that may lead to hypertension.

Let's look at his symptoms to see if we can suggest a cause for each problem.

- His long-standing diabetes makes him much more likely to develop atherosclerosis than non-diabetic people of the same age.
- Fibrolipid atheromatous plaques in his coronary arteries will reduce the perfusion of the cardiac muscle, resulting in chronic ischaemia, which damages the heart muscle so that it pumps less efficiently. Because the left side of the heart generally fails first this will result in pulmonary oedema.
- Atheroma in the carotid arteries produces the bruit heard on auscultation and may lead to cerebral infarction.
- The combination of poor cardiac function and atheromatous plaques in the abdominal aorta and femoral vessels will explain the pain and cramp in his calf muscle, which is secondary to poor perfusion.
- Hyaline arteriolosclerosis will affect small renal vessels, leading to glomerular damage, which will induce hypertension through a

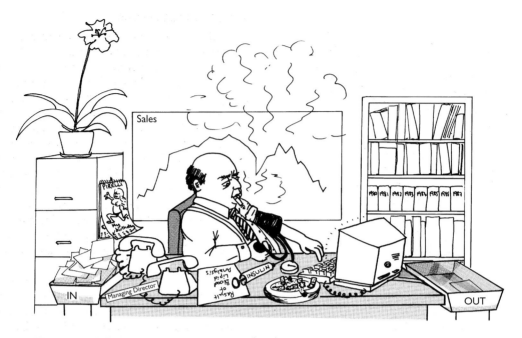

Figure 7.1 The arteriopath. Risk factors include: age, gender (male), obesity, smoking, diabetes, lack of exercise, hypertension, hyperlipidaemia and type 'A' personality (impatient, workaholic)

complicated mechanism involving the hormones renin and angiotensin. This exacerbates the atheroma and worsens the cardiac failure.

- The cause of his blurred vision may be of vascular origin as the retina is frequently damaged by small haemorrhages, microaneurysms and new vessel formation, although diabetes can also produce a host of other ocular changes.

The next stage in understanding this man's disease is to consider the actual appearance of his vessels.

What does the atherosclerotic vessel look like?

The lesion of atherosclerosis is not one specific entity but a spectrum of arterial changes including:

- atheromatous fibro-lipid plaques
- fatty streaks
- intimal cushion lesions.

Inevitably there is controversy over whether the different lesions are stages in the evolution of an atheromatous plaque and we shall review the evidence when describing each lesion. Different authors use different terminology, which can be

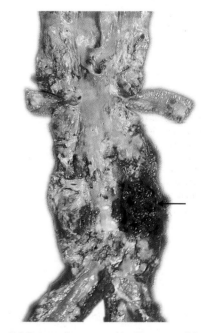

Figure 7.2 Descending aorta with atheroma and thrombus in an aneurysm (arrow)

confusing, so we summarize them in the box below. From the clinical point of view, it is the atheromatous fibrolipid plaque that is to blame for producing occlusive vascular disease.

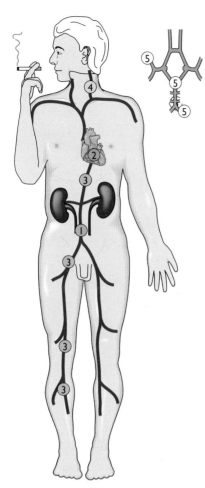

Sites in order of frequency
1. Abdominal aorta
2. Proximal coronary arteries
3. Descending thoracic aorta, femoral and popliteal arteries
4. Internal carotid artery
5. Vertebral/basilar/middle cerebral arteries

Figure 7.3 Distribution of atheroma

Key facts

Terms used in atherosclerosis

- Atheromatous plaque = fibrolipid plaque = fibroatheroma

- Fatty streak = Intimal xanthoma

- Intimal cushion lesion = intimal mass lesion

ATHEROMATOUS PLAQUE

The atheromatous plaque, also referred to as a fibrous or fibrolipid plaque, is raised above the surrounding intima and protrudes into the lumen. It is whitish-yellow in colour and varies in size from 0.5 to 1.5 cm and may even become bigger if adjacent plaques coalesce. On slicing, the plaque is composed of a fibrous cap covering a soft, yellow, lipid centre, which reminded the early pathologists of porridge or gruel and so was termed atheroma. The intima is greatly thickened by the fibrofatty deposition and the media may be thinned due to a loss of smooth muscle cells, resulting in both a loss of elasticity and a weakening of the wall. The adventitia may show new vessels budding off the vasa vasorum and providing the potential for a collateral circulation if obstruction occurs.

In general, the fibrous cap is composed of smooth muscle cells, collagen, elastin and proteoglycans. Beneath this there is a more cellular region of macrophages, T lymphocytes and smooth muscle cells covering the soft gruel-like mass of lipid, cellular debris, cholesterol clefts, plasma proteins and lipid-laden cells (foam cells) derived from macrophages and smooth muscle cells. At the edges of the lesion, there may be new vessel formation.

These plaques are commoner in the aorta, femoral, carotid and coronary arteries, where they may produce clinical problems by causing partial or complete occlusion, thrombosis, embolism or aneurysm formation. Areas of turbulent flow are worst affected so that lesions often occur around the ostia of vessels. The abdominal aorta is more liable to atheroma than the thoracic aorta, but the explanation for this is unknown.

From the clinical standpoint, it would be nice to know which lesions are fairly stable and which are liable to cause problems. This has led to the classification of plaques as fibrous or lipid-rich depending on the predominant feature, i.e. a thick fibrous cap or a large lipid pool. Also the plaque can be concentric or eccentric, with the eccentric plaque retaining some active media capable of responding to vasomotor signals. About 12 per cent of atherosclerotic plaques in coronary arteries are both eccentric and lipid rich, and it is these that are most likely to undergo acute thrombosis because of plaque injury. In around 25 per cent of cases of plaque injury, the damage is superficial, involving only surface endothelium and superficial collagen. Some believe that these result from vasospasm and are more common in cigarette smokers. In the remainder, there is deep plaque fissure leading down to the lipid pool, which is a powerful stimulant for platelets and the clotting cascade.

There is much interest in the 'unstable' plaques and whether it is possible to make them more stable. Unstable plaques are known to have fewer smooth muscle cells, less extracellular matrix, more extracellular lipid and many lipid-filled macrophages. Plaque stability is seen as a balance between damage and repair in the intima. The damage is due to inflammation mediated by macrophages and T cells and the repair involves smooth muscle cells producing matrix and fibres. It is hoped that influencing the macrophage activity might reduce the incidence of acute coronary events. A number of proteases have been implicated in thinning of the fibrous cap, in particular the matrix metalloproteinase (MMP) stromelysin 3. Other important factors may be γ-interferon through its action inhibiting collagen synthesis, and increased macrophage apoptosis.

As well as improving the stability of the plaques, the reduction of thrombus formation is likely to be important, and so stopping smoking or taking low-dose aspirin is beneficial.

To summarize, plaques are not static lesions but can change in a gradual or abrupt way and can also be influenced by changes in other layers of the vessel wall. In the coronary arteries, if there is a slow increase in plaque volume it is likely to lead to stable angina. Deep plaque fissuring will produce acute thrombosis and episodes of unstable angina, myocardial infarction or sudden death. Endothelial dysfunction or superficial plaque injury may lead to inappropriate vasoconstriction. Atrophy of the media can result in aneurysm formation and vessel proliferation in the adventitia can provide a network of collateral vessels. Ruptured plaques can heal and plaques, in general, may remodel or calcify.

FATTY STREAKS

Fatty streaks, like atheromatous plaques, occur in large muscular and elastic arteries but differ in that they are commonest in the region of the aortic ring and the thoracic aorta. They do not affect blood flow but could represent a precursor lesion for atheromatous plaques. They first appear as tiny, round or oval flat yellow dots that become arranged in rows and finally coalesce to form a streak. The earliest streak is composed of just lipid-laden macrophages and T cells without any smooth muscle proliferation or extracellular lipid. Later,

extracellular lipid and smooth muscle cells are found together with collagen, elastin and proteoglycans. Thus, the components are similar to those of an atheromatous plaque but there is far less fat and no necrotic centre. However, some people would only use the term 'fatty streak' for the earliest stage, with the other forms representing a progression towards a fibrolipid plaque.

The aortic surface area covered by streaks increases up to the third decade but then declines as atheromatous plaques occupy the intima. Interestingly, they occur proximal to branch points and ostia in areas of low haemodynamic stress and so are not correctly sited to be forerunners of fibrolipid plaques. The population distribution is also very different, with fibrolipid plaques commoner in males in developed countries, whereas fatty streaks are found from a very early age and are independent of sex, race or geography.

INTIMAL CUSHION LESIONS

An intimal cushion is a white thickening at a branching point or ostium due to an increase in extracellular matrix and smooth muscle cells. There is almost no lipid and the suggestion that this is a precursor lesion for fibrolipid plaques is based on the similarity in their distribution and the presence of smooth muscle proliferation. Even in early infancy, smooth muscle cells have entered the intima, raising the possibility that humans are predestined to atheroma if suitable additional factors are present later. The initiating factors for intimal cushion formation are unknown but likely to involve endothelial dysfunction. The smooth muscle cell proliferation has been shown to be clonal.

Risk factors for atherosclerosis

Now that we have a mental image of the appearance and distribution of atherosclerosis, we shall consider the risk factors that are believed to be important.

AGE

Deaths from ischaemic heart disease increase with advancing age. Interestingly, initial involvement by atheroma affects different vessels at different ages. Thus, small aortic lesions appear in the first decade, coronary artery lesions in the second decade and cerebral arterial lesions in the third decade.

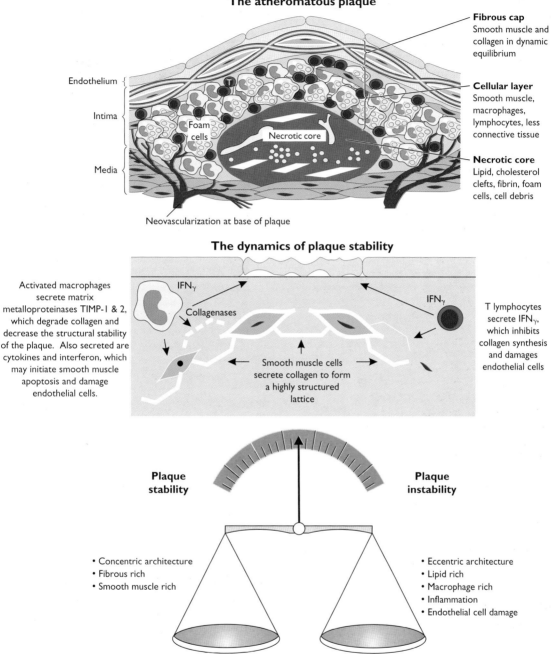

Figure 7.4 The atheromatous plaque and the dynamics of plaque stability

GENDER

The death rate from ischaemic heart disease is higher in males than in females up to the age of 75 years, after which the incidence is similar.

Myocardial infarction is extremely rare in premenopausal women, suggesting that endocrine differences may be important and that the effect of oestrogens on lipid metabolism is a possible

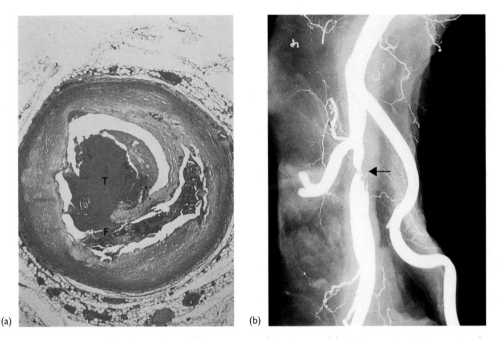

Figure 7.5 (a) Atheromatous plaque with fissuring (F) and thrombus (T) formation. (b) Angiogram showing narrowing (arrow) of the coronary artery corresponding to (a)

mechanism. However, initial evidence suggesting that hormone replacement therapy (HRT) protects against cardiovascular disease has not been confirmed and HRT may increase the risk of venous thrombosis, like the contraceptive pill.

GENES

As our knowledge of the genome increases, we find more associations with particular diseases and can try to unravel the likely mechanism in order to consider possible interventions. Genetic influences on cardiovascular disease include:

- genes affecting cholesterol levels through changes to LDL receptor, apolipoprotein B and apolipoprotein C
- variants in angiotensinogen associated with hypertension
- predisposition to type 2 diabetes
- altered inactivation of nicotine, which decreases the likelihood of smoking
- altered ion channel proteins influencing rare causes of arrhythmias.

Racial differences exist but these are thought most likely due to socio-economic, dietary and 'lifestyle' effects, with only sporadic genetic factors.

SMOKING

Smoking one packet of cigarettes a day increases the likelihood of having a myocardial infarction by 300 per cent. Traditionally, more men than women have smoked, but as women have taken up the habit, their risk has risen. Fortunately, giving up smoking reduces the risk, which means it is likely that smoking does not only promote atheroma but may also cause occlusion of vessels. This could be due to an increased local clotting tendency because of altered platelet function. Stopping smoking for 1–2 years reduces the risk of myocardial infarction to 'only' twice that of non-smokers. So-called 'safer' cigarettes, which have a lower tar and nicotine content, reduce the risk of bronchial carcinoma but do not appear to reduce the risk of coronary heart disease.

How smoking damages vessels is not known, but suggestions include increased free radical activity, raised carbon monoxide levels or a direct effect of nicotine.

HYPERTENSION

Hypertension significantly increases the risk of ischaemic heart disease and 'strokes'. The diastolic blood pressure level is considered more important than the systolic level and a diastolic pressure consistently greater than 95 mmHg is deemed harmful. Drug treatment to reduce the blood pressure decreases the risk in patients with moderate to severe hypertension but it is unclear whether it benefits patients with mild hypertension. Most of the evidence suggesting the role of hypertension as a risk factor involves complex multifactorial analysis of large studies, which, although the proper method for assessing the evidence, is not as easy to grasp as some simpler observations. Evidence of the direct role of hypertension in producing atheroma comes from two examples of congenital abnormalities of the cardiovascular system. Patients with congenital narrowing of part of the aorta (coarctation) develop atheroma in the proximal hypertensive segment but not in the distal region, where the pressure is lower. The other example is the rare abnormality of having one coronary artery originating from the low-pressure pulmonary artery. The coronary artery linked to the aorta develops atheromatous changes with age but the artery linked to the pulmonary supply remains atheroma-free.

HYPERLIPIDAEMIA

Evidence for the role of fats in atheroma comes from a variety of sources and the literature on the role of lipids in atherosclerosis would fill a library, so we shall just highlight some of the more important points.

- Atheromatous lesions contain far more lipid than the adjacent intima.
- Atheromatous plaques are rich in cholesterol and cholesterol esters (65–80 per cent), derived from blood lipoproteins.
- Intimal lesions can be produced in some animals by increasing the plasma concentration of certain lipids through drug or diet manipulation.
- Macrophages accumulate cholesterol (LDL) and this is increased if there is endothelial damage.
- In populations with a high incidence of atherosclerosis there are high plasma concentrations of certain lipids. Low-density lipoproteins (LDL) rich in cholesterol appear most harmful, very low density lipoproteins (VLDL) do some harm but high-density lipoproteins (HDL) appear cardioprotective.
- In families with genetic disorders causing hypercholesterolaemia or in groups with acquired hypercholesterolaemia (e.g. hypothyroidism and nephrotic syndrome), atherosclerosis is increased.

- Cardiovascular mortality can be reduced by lowering the plasma cholesterol with diet or drugs (e.g. cholestyramine).

DIABETES

The risk of a myocardial infarction in a diabetic patient is twice that in a non-diabetic patient and their arterial disease is widespread. Arterial disease accounts for around 70 per cent of the deaths of diabetics in Western countries. A possible mechanism is change in lipids so that HDL may be decreased and LDL increased because receptor-mediated catabolism is reduced.

OTHER POSSIBLE RISK FACTORS

These include:

- lack of regular exercise
- obesity
- low weight at one year of age
- high carbohydrate intake
- 'type A' personality/stress

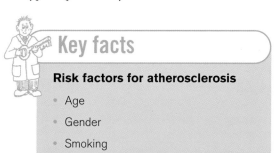

Key facts

Risk factors for atherosclerosis

- Age
- Gender
- Smoking
- Hypertension
- Hyperlipidaemia
- Diabetes

CAN 'LIFESTYLE' CHANGES PREVENT CARDIOVASCULAR DISEASE?

This is what your patients really want to know! Should they be losing weight, taking regular exercise, stopping drinking, stopping smoking and altering their diet? The epidemiological studies suggest that these are risk factors but does intervention make a difference and who should do it?

First, what is the ideal diet? You should be a reasonable weight because in patients who are very overweight, weight reduction of about 10 kg reduces LDL cholesterol by 7 per cent and raises HDL cholesterol by 13 per cent. Regular exercise appears to enhance this effect. The standard teaching is that diets should restrict total fat intake to less than 30 per cent of all calories with no more than 10 per cent of this fat being from saturated fat, cholesterol intake should be limited to less than 300 mg/day and fibre intake should be increased. Unfortunately, this only produces a drop in total cholesterol of about 2 per cent and, although greater reduction can be achieved with more stringent diets, they are generally too unpalatable. Eating at least one portion of oily fish per week appears to reduce mortality but adding betacarotene, vitamin C or E supplements (i.e. similar to a high fruit and vegetable diet) has not been demonstrated to have an effect.

Moderate alcohol consumption may actually help to reduce strokes, but heavy drinking increases the risk by raising blood pressure. Exercise appears to have a good impact in both primary and secondary prevention, but 30 minutes per day for at least 5 days per week is probably required.

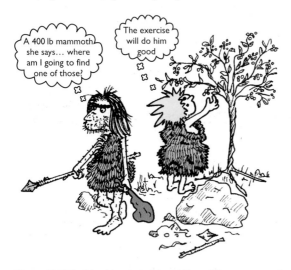

Figure 7.6 Lifestyle changes: a lot could be said to recommend a return to the low-fat, fibre-rich dietary habits of our forbears

The alternative is to use drugs such as statins, which inhibit the enzyme HMG CoA reductase and so reduce endogenous production of cholesterol. The statins also produce some lowering of triglycerides (TG) and a rise in HDL levels. The current recommendation in the UK for the use of statins depends on whether it is primary or secondary prevention (i.e. patients without or with clinically overt atherosclerotic disease). For patients with overt atherosclerotic disease, both lifestyle changes and statin therapy are recommended. For primary prevention, the current approach is to use statins if

the 10-year CHD risk is greater than 30 per cent (approx. equivalent to a cardiovascular disease risk of 40 per cent) so as to lower LDL cholesterol by 30 per cent or to less than 3 mmol/L. Lifestyle changes are recommended even if the risk is less than 30 per cent and may eliminate the need for statins. There are various tables and software available for calculating the 10-year risk of coronary heart disease (CHD = fatal or non-fatal myocardial infarction and angina) or cardiovascular disease (CVD = CHD plus stroke, heart failure and peripheral vascular disease).

How is the atheromatous plaque produced?

Now that we know who is most likely to suffer from atherosclerosis, we need to look at the theory of how atheroma is produced. The 'reaction to injury' theory has its origin deep within the history books as it incorporates the ideas of Virchow, Duguid and Rokitansky.

REACTION TO INJURY THEORY

Virchow believed that leakage of plasma proteins and lipid from the blood to the subendothelial tissue stimulated intimal cell proliferation. He regarded the cell proliferation as a form of low-grade inflammation and termed it the 'imbibition hypothesis', later often called the 'insudation' or 'infiltration' hypothesis. Karl Freiherr von Rokitansky is credited with the 'encrustation' theory, which suggested that thrombi forming on damaged endothelium could become organized to form a plaque. The modern 'reaction to injury' theory was proposed by Russell Ross and John Glomset in 1976. Essentially they suggest that some change or damage to the vascular endothelium causes increased permeability to proteins and lipid and also leads to the aggregation of platelets and monocytes. These leukocytes release various enzymes and growth factors which promote smooth muscle cell proliferation. Monocytes migrate from the blood into the subendothelial layers, where they become macrophages and ingest the lipid. A short, sharp injury can be completely repaired but chronic repeated injury leads to the formation of an atheromatous plaque.

Stable atheromatous plaques may not produce any clinical effect but problems occur if a lipid lesion covered by a thin fibrous capsule is disrupted, releasing material that promotes local thrombosis.

The thrombosis may cause an acute occlusion of the vessel, with potentially devastating effects, or only cause a partial occlusion. Partially occlusive thrombus undergoes organization and becomes incorporated into the plaque to increase its size. The factors involved can be thought of as atherogenic factors important in producing the early plaque and thrombotic factors important in its progression.

Endothelial cell damage is known to be produced by a variety of factors such as haemodynamic forces, hyperlipidaemia, cigarette smoke, immune mechanisms, certain viral antigens, irradiation and various mutagens. This damage plays an atherogenic and thrombogenic role. The next stage required in the 'response to injury' theory is that the aggregated platelets and monocytes release

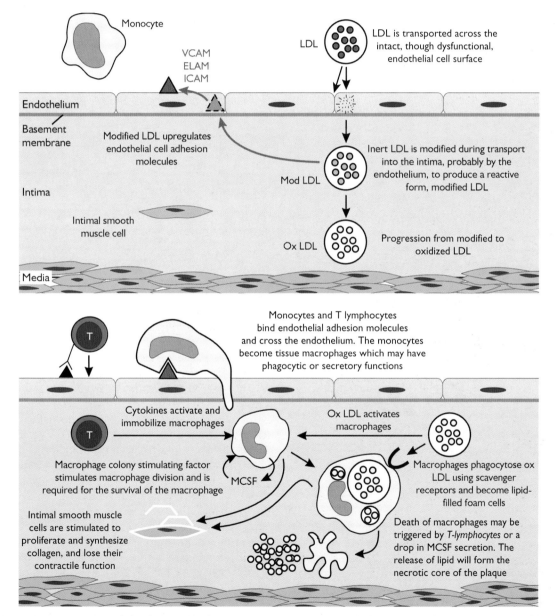

Figure 7.7 The development of the atheromatous plaque: Endothelial cells may be damaged by cigarette smoke, flow disturbances and hyperlipidaemia. This increases their permeability to low-density lipoproteins, which enter the arterial intima by insudation. See Fig. 7.4 for the established plaque

substances to promote smooth muscle proliferation and the influx of more leukocytes.

Platelet-derived growth factor (PDGF) is believed to be important because smooth muscle proliferation is observed *in vivo* in zones where platelets adhere to damaged endothelium and *in vitro* PDGF can promote both proliferation and migration of smooth muscle cells. Interestingly, there are two animal models which provide supporting evidence. In one, the platelets lack alpha granules, which contain PDGF, and the animals do not develop atheroma. In the other, pigs lacking von Willebrand factor, which is necessary for platelet adherence and aggregation, are resistant to both thrombosis and spontaneous atherosclerosis. Other growth factors, such as fibroblast growth factor and endothelial cell growth factor are probably involved, as well as a reduction in the growth inhibitors (TGFβ and endothelial-derived relaxing factor (EDRF)) produced by macrophages and endothelial cells. The end result is that smooth muscle cells migrate from the media to the intima, they proliferate, they accumulate cholesterol and cholesterol esters to become one of the types of foam cells (the other is macrophage-derived) and they also manufacture extracellular matrix.

The influx of leukocytes is apparent from simple observation, i.e. by counting the number of macrophages and lymphocytes in the atheromatous lesions and comparing this with the very small number present in non-atheromatous intima. Once lymphocytes and macrophages are involved, the whole complex army of cytokines can be called into action to promote chemotaxis, cell proliferation, altered permeability, etc.

Oxidized lipoproteins (OLPs) deserve a mention because of the clear association between LDL blood levels and coronary artery disease. It appears that OLPs may be produced by reactive oxygen species, altering the lipoprotein present in plaques. The altered LDL is then recognized by the 'scavenger' receptor on macrophages and phagocytosed so that the macrophage becomes a foam cell. The OLPs may ultimately contribute to the death of the macrophage.

OLPs are thought to be able to cause:

- endothelial cell damage
- smooth muscle cell injury leading to central necrosis of the plaque
- foam cell formation, as the OLPs are taken up by the receptor for modified LDL
- recruitment and retention of macrophages.

What diet will prevent atheroma?

The popular press are fond of reporting the latest diet to prevent atheroma and are then even more delighted to report the contradictions that follow. So what do we really know and what is speculation? Most of the historical evidence on diet comes from comparing populations with distinctly different diets, for instance comparing the fish-eating Eskimos with meat-eating Danes or the butter lovers of Belgium with the olive oil fans of the Mediterranean. Let us digress for a second to consider how we should define a successful diet. Ideally, we would like to prevent the formation of atheromatous plaques, but as we cannot assess the size, number and distribution of plaques in millions of living people in different populations, most researchers opt to monitor the major life-threatening complication of plaques, namely occlusive coronary heart disease (CHD). However, by doing that they are really measuring the outcome of two different pathological mechanisms. The patient must not only suffer from atheroma in their coronary vessels but also undergo an occlusive event such as thrombosis or vasoconstriction, therefore there may be different dietary factors affecting the processes, i.e. 'atherogenic' and 'thrombogenic' dietary factors. Obviously, it is likely that any atherogenic factors operate over decades, and starting on a low-fat diet as you retire will cause little change to your plaques. However, the likelihood of thrombosis could be affected by an alteration of diet in later life.

LIPIDS AND CORONARY HEART DISEASE (CHD)

The first stage in our discussion needs to establish which dietary-derived blood levels correlate with CHD. Then we need to review the biochemical pathways involved so that we can try to understand the complex interplay between dietary intake of a substance and the blood levels. Finally we can consider the observed effects of altering diets.

Risk of coronary heart disease increases with:

- raised serum total cholesterol concentration
- raised LDL cholesterol concentration
- reduced HDL cholesterol concentration.

Of course, it is good to observe the factors that increase the risk, but it is even more important to discover whether manipulating the factor can reduce the risk. We now know that in people with no other specific risk factors (primary prevention studies), the risk of CHD reduces by 10 per cent

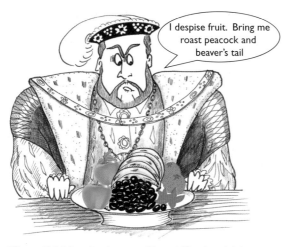

Figure 7.8 Lifestyle changes: Henry VIII enjoyed 14 course banquets, with a vast array of meats and as few vegetables as possible. Henry is thought by some to have developed scurvy in the winter months due to the lack of vitamin C in his diet.

and the risk of non-fatal myocardial infarction reduces by about 20 per cent if a 10 per cent fall in serum total cholesterol is achieved. Similar figures are available for secondary prevention studies (i.e. patients who already have CHD) to support altering the levels of LDL and HDL cholesterol.

LIPID METABOLISM

There are two important pathways for lipid metabolism: the exogenous and the endogenous. Exogenous (i.e. dietary) lipids are digested to release triglycerides (TG) and cholesterol esters. These combine with phospholipids and specific apoproteins to make them water-soluble and are called chylomicrons. The TG component of the chylomicron can move from the circulation into cells by lipoprotein lipase activity on the endothelial surface of cells. Once inside the cell, it may be converted to glycerol and non-esterified fatty acids which are a major energy source.

Once the chylomicron has lost TG, it is called a chylomicron remnant particle (CMR) and it is rich in cholesterol. This particle attaches to liver receptors via ApoB48 and ApoE and enters the hepatocyte.

Endogenous lipid refers to the various lipids produced by the liver. The building blocks are glycerol and fatty acids reaching the liver from fat stores or synthesized from glucose, and cholesterol derived from lipoproteins (such as the CMR) or synthesized locally from acetate and mevalonic acid using the enzyme HMG CoA (hydroxy methyl glutaryl

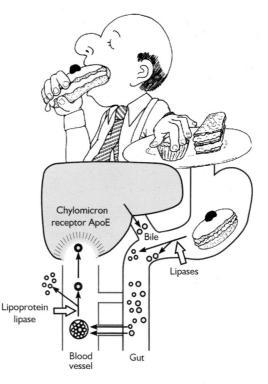

Figure 7.9 Exogenous cholesterol pathway (see key with Fig. 7.10)

coenzyme A). Glycerol and fatty acids combine to produce TG. The liver releases VLDL, rich in TG and with about 25 per cent cholesterol. Loss of some TG produces IDL, and further loss of TG results in cholesterol-rich LDL. This LDL is removed from the

Key facts

Causes of secondary hyperlipidaemia

Nutritional	Obesity
	Alcohol abuse
Hormonal	Diabetes
	Hypothyroidism
Drugs	Beta blockers
	High-dose steroids
Miscellaneous	Stress
	Bile duct obstruction and primary biliary cirrhosis
	Nephrotic syndrome and chronic renal failure

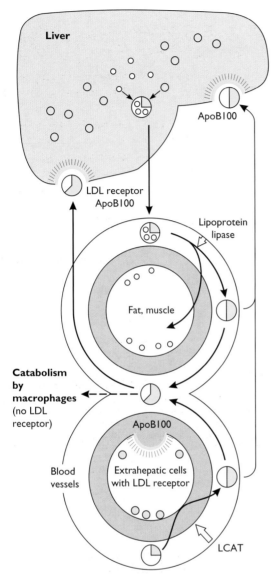

Cholesterol is secreted in very low density lipoproteins (VLDL), which are broken down by lipoprotein lipase in the endothelium of the capillaries in fat and muscle to release triglycerides and form intermediate density lipoproteins (IDL). Some IDL are absorbed by the liver via the LDL receptor, which recognizes apoprotein B100; the remainder are metabolized to low-density lipoproteins (LDL). LDL are taken up by the numerous extrahepatic tissues that bear the LDL receptor, and the remainder is either taken up by the liver or catabolized by macrophages. High-density lipoproteins (HDL), also secreted by the liver, remove cholesterol from the tissues. This is catalysed by plasma lecithin-cholesterol acyltransferase (LCAT). IDL and LDL are formed by a series of metabolic steps

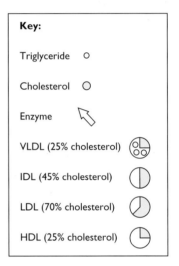

Figure 7.10 Endogenous cholesterol pathway

circulation by attachment to high-affinity LDL receptors via apoprotein B100 on the liver and peripheral cells, and the LDL is broken down to amino acids and cholesterol. The alternative route is through low-affinity LDL receptors and it is these receptors that are thought to be important in atherosclerosis. If there are high levels of LDL, the liver and peripheral cells accumulate some intracellular cholesterol that inhibits endogenous synthesis of cholesterol and suppresses the production of their LDL receptors, so reducing LDL uptake from the blood and probably diverting more LDL to cells with low-affinity receptors.

When we listed the risk factors for atherosclerosis, we had a group labelled 'Other possible risk factors' (page 171). Now that we know something about the relationship between serum lipid levels and CHD, it is educational to compare that list with the causes of secondary hyperlipidaemias.

How do raised altered lipid levels cause coronary heart disease?

So how does it work? How might lowering LDL cholesterol prevent CHD? Now you must appreciate that we are into speculation rather than

Table 7.1 Classification of lipoproteins

Lipoprotein	Site of production	Major lipid	Major apoprotein	Role/fate
Chylomicron	Intestinal mucosal cell	TG	B48	Transport of dietary TG
CMR	Removal of TG from chylomicron	Cholesterol	B48	Transport dietary cholesterol to liver
VLDL	Liver	TG	B100, C11, E	Transport endogenous TG
IDL	Partial removal of TG from VLDL	TG and cholesterol	B100, E	Taken up by liver or converted to LDL
LDL	Further removal of TG from IDL	Cholesterol	B100	Transport endogenous cholesterol to liver and tissues
HDL	Liver and intestinal mucosal cell	Phospholipid	A, D	Complex

CMR = chylomicron remnant particle; IDL = intermediate density lipoprotein; LDL = low-density lipoprotein; TG = triglyceride; VLDL = very low density lipoprotein.

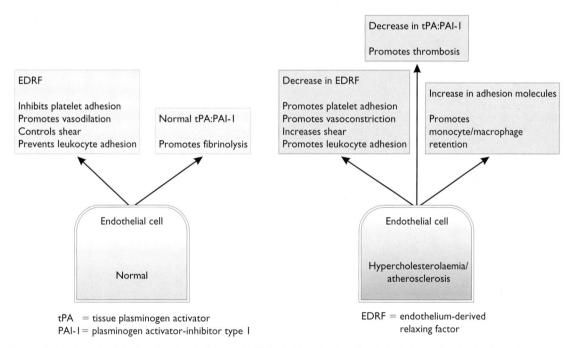

Figure 7.11 Normal and dysfunctional endothelial cells (Adapted from Levine, G. *et al.* Cholesterol reduction in cardiovascular disease. *New England Journal of Medicine* **332**(8), 512–52. Copyright 1995 Massachusetts Medical Society. All rights reserved)

experimentally proven fact. You will remember that acute events in coronary arteries often relate to plaque rupture and plaque rupture is more likely in cholesterol-rich plaques. It is possible, therefore, that there may be a process of 'reverse cholesterol transport' from the plaque to the serum, possibly involving HDL.

Coronary symptoms occur with changes less than full plaque rupture and can relate to small local thrombi or vasospasm of coronary arteries. The link between these is in the multifunctional endothelial cell that is involved in regulating vasomotor tone, inhibiting platelet activity, maintaining a balance between thrombosis and fibrinolysis, and regulating recruitment of inflammatory cells. A crucial mediator of these functions is endothelium-derived relaxing factor (EDRF = nitric oxide, NO), and intracoronary perfusion of acetylcholine (an EDRF agonist) produces vasodilatation of normal coronary arteries but constricts areas affected by atheromatous plaques. This is assumed to be a result of acetylcholine's direct constrictor effect on the underlying smooth muscle in the absence of normal tone regulation by the endothelium, i.e. the endothelial cells are dysfunctional in atheromatous plaques.

The really amazing observation is that the vasoconstriction produced by acetylcholine challenge can be reduced or even converted into slight vasodilatation by a six-month period of lipid-lowering drugs. It is not known quite how the LDL cholesterol causes endothelial dysfunction but there is a suggestion that it is due to increased oxidative stress and some early work raises the possibility that antioxidant drugs may have a beneficial effect.

HYPERTENSION

Many of the circulatory diseases we have discussed are related to hypertension. Atheroma, arteriolosclerosis, myocardial infarction, left ventricular hypertrophy and aneurysms are linked by their association with hypertension, so we should discuss some of what is known about the aetiology and pathogenesis of hypertension.

Hypertension is extremely common, affecting around 25 per cent of adults if a blood pressure of

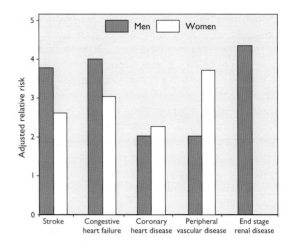

Figure 7.12 Risk of artherosclerotic disease in people with hypertension (From Padwal, R., Straus, S.E. and McAlister, F.A. 2001. Cardiovascular risk factors and their effects on the decision to treat hypertension: evidence based review. *British Medical Journal* **322**: 977–80)

Table 7.2 Causes of secondary hypertension

Renal disease
    Acute or chronic glomerulonephritis
    Vasculitis, e.g. systemic lupus erythematosus
    Renal artery stenosis
    Chronic pyelonephritis
    Diabetic nephropathy

Cardiovascular disease
    Coarctation of aorta (hypertension in upper half of body)
    High cardiac output states

Hormonal
    Phaeochromocytoma – excess catecholamines from tumour
    Cushing's syndrome – excess corticosteroids
        Primary – adrenal cortical adenoma/hyperplasia
        Secondary – pituitary basophil adenoma, corticosteroid therapy or paraneoplastic, e.g. oat cell tumour
    Conn's syndrome – excess aldosterone
        Adrenal cortical adenoma/hyperplasia
        Adrenogenital syndrome
    Acromegaly – excess growth hormone
        Pituitary acidophil adenoma

Neurological
    Raised intracranial pressure
        Haemorrhage
        Tumour
        Abscess
    Hypothalamic or brainstem lesion

Pre-eclampsia in pregnancy

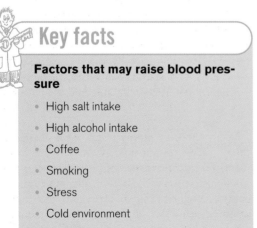

Key facts

Factors that may raise blood pressure

- High salt intake
- High alcohol intake
- Coffee
- Smoking
- Stress
- Cold environment

greater than 140/90 mmHg is regarded as abnormal. Unfortunately, organ damage may be irreversible by the time a patient presents with symptoms so it is important to screen the people who are most susceptible. So you will need to know about the factors influencing blood pressure. Hypertension is predominantly a condition of middle and later life that may be classified as 'benign' or 'malignant'. Fortunately, 'benign' hypertension is much commoner, is relatively stable and is treatable with long-term antihypertensive drugs. 'Malignant' hypertension only affects 5 per cent of hypertensive patients but it is more severe and is liable to affect men under 50 years of age. It is defined as a diastolic pressure of more than 120 mmHg. The major dangers of hypertension are coronary heart disease, cerebrovascular accidents, congestive heart failure and chronic renal failure.

In 95 per cent of cases there is no obvious cause and this is termed primary, essential or idiopathic hypertension. Most of the remainder are due to renal disease, with a small number due to endocrine abnormalities (secondary hypertension).

What mechanisms may operate in hypertension?

We will have to be content with describing some of the theories concerning hypertension, as nobody knows the answers. First it is useful to review the factors influencing the control of blood pressure. In simple terms, the arterial pressure will depend on the cardiac output and the total peripheral resistance. The cardiac output depends on the heart rate, its contractility and the blood volume. It may increase in the early stages of hypertension but is more usually normal. Thus chronic hypertension appears to be a result of increased tone in small arteries and arterioles. The resistance is determined by the arteriolar lumen, which may expand or contract depending on the state of the smooth muscle cells in the vessel wall. This is called local vascular tone and is influenced by a variety of mediators (see list) which may act throughout the body or be produced and have their action locally, i.e. autoregulation. It is suggested that essential hypertension could result from a primary defect in renal sodium excretion, possibly combined with abnormalities in sodium or calcium transport in other cells. Many believe that the salt intake in the Western diet contributes to hypertension and should be reduced

from a daily average of 9 g to 6 g. The normal kidney will increase excretion of salt and water if the blood pressure rises, so that blood volume and hence blood pressure is reduced. It is not known what 'sets' the level at which this occurs but if it is too high, the blood pressure will be raised, although stable. Any defect in sodium or calcium transport that leads to a rise in calcium in vascular smooth muscle would increase vascular tone responses. Vascular tone would also be affected by alteration in any of the mediators already listed. The endothelial-derived mediators are thought to be the most important.

Secondary hypertension is most often related to renal disease and results from abnormalities in the renin–angiotensin system, abnormal salt and water balance and renal vasodepressor substances. Angiotensin II is increased in response to raised renin levels and will increase vascular resistance, by causing vascular smooth muscle contraction, and increase blood volume through aldosterone, which promotes distal tubular reabsorption of sodium. Negative feedback is provided through a lowering of renin levels secondary to the increase in angiotensin II, the raised pressure in the glomerular afferent arteriole and decreased proximal tubule sodium reabsorption, which influences the macula densa. Increased renin secretion occurs in all of the renal causes of hypertension listed in Table 7.2, except for many cases of chronic renal failure. In chronic renal failure, there is sodium and water retention which is probably related to a reduced glomerular filtration rate influencing tubular sodium handling. Theoretically, renal disease might produce hypertension through a reduction in its secretion of vasodepressor substances, such as prostaglandins or platelet-activating factor.

A group of powerful vasoconstrictors are the endothelins. Endothelin I is the most potent vasoconstrictor yet discovered. Its plasma level is not raised in hypertensive individuals but it is produced by endothelium and primarily acts locally on vascular smooth muscle. Production is increased by changes in sheer stress, hypoxia and inflammatory mediators. It may have an important role in maintaining the blood pressure following a myocardial infarction and in endotoxic shock but may be detrimental by producing local ischaemia in heart muscle or in Raynaud's disease. Already antagonists are being tried in clinical trials. It is also mitogenic for smooth muscle cells and so may have a role in the formation of atheroma.

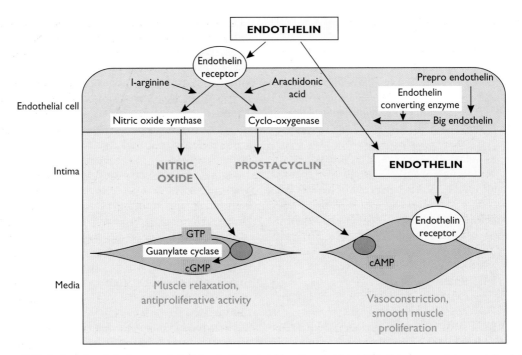

Figure 7.13 Action of endothelin on endothelial cells (Adapted from Brown, M.J. 1997: Science, medicine and the future: hypertension. *British Medical Journal* **314**. With kind permission of the BMJ Publishing Group)

Key facts

Mediators that influence vascular tone

Constrictors	Angiotensin 1
	Endothelin 1
	Catecholamines
	Thromboxane
	Leukotrienes
Dilators	Prostaglandins
	Kinins
	Platelet-activating factor
	Endothelium-derived relaxing factor (nitric oxide)

It is interesting to note the overlap between substances that vasoconstrict and substances that promote growth. Vasoconstrictors, such as nor-adrenaline and angiotensin II, promote smooth muscle growth, while growth factors, such as platelet-derived growth factor and epidermal growth factor, can cause vasoconstriction.

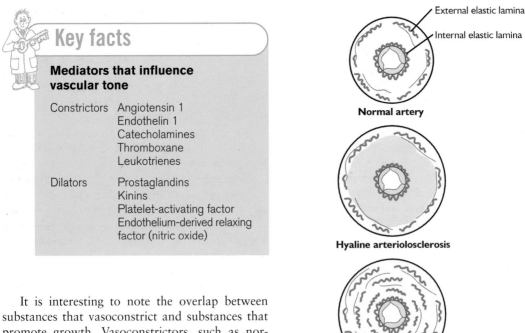

Figure 7.14 Hyaline and hyperplastic arteriosclerosis

What do the vessels look like?

Hyaline and hyperplastic arteriolosclerotic changes are very different to atheromatous damage. They only affect small vessels, do not have any increase in lipid and primarily affect the media, whereas atheroma is initially an intimal problem. Both are very important because of their strong association with hypertension.

Hyaline arteriolosclerosis generally occurs in elderly or diabetic patients and involves the deposition of homogeneous, pink material that thickens the media, resulting in a narrowed vessel. This material is probably a combination of increased extracellular matrix, produced by smooth muscle cells, and plasma components that have leaked through a damaged endothelium.

Hyperplastic arteriolosclerosis is found in patients who have a rather sudden or severe prolonged increase in blood pressure. The media of the vessel wall is thickened by a concentric proliferation of smooth muscle cells and an increase in basement membrane material. In the worst cases (malignant hypertension), there may be fibrinoid necrosis of the vessel walls.

Does wall thickness return to normal if blood pressure is lowered? This is an important question because if vascular resistance was the result of morphological change, then reversal of these changes might produce a normotensive patient who did not require continuous antihypertensive therapy. At present, it is not possible to give a complete answer but, in humans, some antihypertensive drugs do produce some reduction in wall thickness. In animals, the angiotensin-converting enzyme (ACE) inhibitors are clearly effective, while thiazide and hydralazine-like vasodilators have only a minor effect. Thus, simply lowering the blood pressure is not enough and, maybe, some antihypertensives are achieving the morphological changes through other actions on smooth muscle cells.

ANEURYSMS

An aneurysm is a localized dilatation in a blood vessel. It may produce no symptoms, may cause problems through pressing on adjacent structures, may become occluded by thrombus or may rupture with potentially devastating effects.

Let us start with berry aneurysms. As the name suggests, these are more than just a dilatation and look like a cherry stuck on the side of a vessel. Berry aneurysms are usually small, less than 1.5 cm in diameter and are globular in shape. Although referred to as congenital, they are not present at birth but develop because there is a defect in the media of the blood vessels at sites of bifurcation. These occur most commonly around the circle of Willis. Patients with berry aneurysms generally present with a sudden severe headache and some lose consciousness because the aneurysm has leaked. Occasionally, a patient will have ocular problems or facial pain because of pressure on the cranial nerves by an unruptured aneurysm. Frequently, these patients are young or middle-aged and are not normally hypertensive, but are assumed to have raised their blood pressure by acute exertion.

The other important type of aneurysm affecting cerebral vessels is the microaneurysm or Charcot–Bouchard aneurysm. These are generally multiple small aneurysms only a few millimetres in diameter present on small arteries within the cerebral hemispheres. They occur in older, hypertensive individuals and are a common cause of intracerebral haemorrhage, a form of 'stroke'.

Atherosclerotic aneurysms are commonest in the abdominal portion of the aorta and they may present with massive haemorrhage or as a pulsatile mass in the abdomen, which may compress structures such as the ureters. Often they become complicated by thrombosis, with the risk of shedding emboli into lower limb vessels. These aneurysms occur in individuals with risk factors for atheroma and they develop due to thinning of the media exacerbated by hypertension. It is not known how atheroma, an intimal disease, produces medial damage. The aneurysms are generally fusiform in shape and often extend for several centimetres along the aorta. Aneurysms greater than 6 cm in diameter are likely to rupture so it is recommended that these are replaced by prosthetic grafts, as replacement after rupture carries a high mortality.

Cystic medial necrosis is a descriptive term for necrosis of the media associated with the formation of mucoid cystic lakes. The cause of cystic medial necrosis is unknown but it is associated with hypertension and may involve production of abnormal collagen, elastin and proteoglycans in the media, as occurs in Marfan's syndrome. It is important as a possible aetiological factor in aortic dissection, in which blood tracks down through the media.

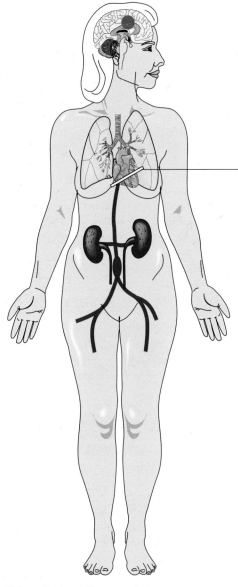

Brain
Microaneurysms and intracerebral haemorrhage

Lungs
Pulmonary oedema due to left ventricular failure

Heart
Left ventricular hypertrophy and failure; myocardial infarction

Kidneys
Ischaemic cortical damage

Blood vessels
Atherosclerosis and aneurysm formation

Figure 7.15 Complications of hypertension

Unfortunately, aortic dissection is often referred to as an aortic dissecting aneurysm, despite the vessel not being dilated.

Aortic dissection usually occurs in the 40- to 60-year-old group and affects men more commonly than women, although it does occur in pregnant women, possibly because of generalized hormonal actions that soften connective tissue. Patients complain of sudden severe pain in the centre of the chest, similar to that felt in myocardial infarction, but this often radiates to the back and moves as the dissection progresses. The first event in aortic dissection is a tear in the intima, so that blood enters the media and tracks down between the middle and outer thirds of the media. The tear often occurs in the ascending aorta and is thought to be due to shearing forces on the intima because of turbulent blood flow. Any hypertension will exacerbate both the turbulence and the forces splitting the media. Once the blood begins to track along the

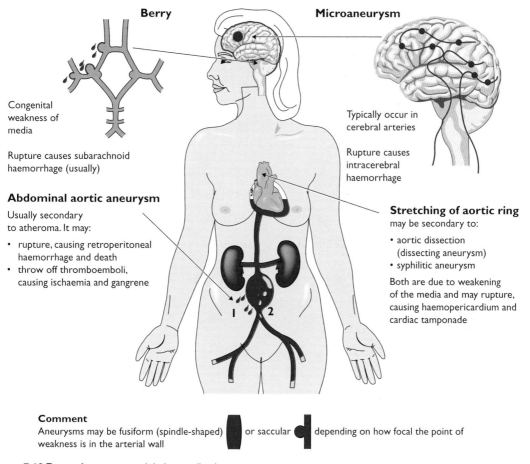

Berry

Congenital weakness of media

Rupture causes subarachnoid haemorrhage (usually)

Abdominal aortic aneurysm

Usually secondary to atheroma. It may:

- rupture, causing retroperitoneal haemorrhage and death
- throw off thromboemboli, causing ischaemia and gangrene

Microaneurysm

Typically occur in cerebral arteries

Rupture causes intracerebral haemorrhage

Stretching of aortic ring may be secondary to:

- aortic dissection (dissecting aneurysm)
- syphilitic aneurysm

Both are due to weakening of the media and may rupture, causing haemopericardium and cardiac tamponade

Comment

Aneurysms may be fusiform (spindle-shaped) or saccular depending on how focal the point of weakness is in the arterial wall

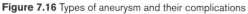

Figure 7.16 Types of aneurysm and their complications

media, it can travel in either direction and it can rupture back into the aorta or out into the peritoneal cavity, pericardial sac or pleural cavity. Rupture outwards is catastrophic and common, whereas rupture into the aorta is rare but has a good prognosis and will produce a double-barrelled aorta. Extension of the dissection will occlude the mouths of any tributaries which become involved and this commonly affects the coronary, renal, mesenteric, iliac or cerebral vessels. More recently, dissection of the vertebro-basilar vessels has been described.

Aneurysms secondary to inflammation include those due to syphilis, arteritis and infection. Syphilitic aneurysms tend to occur in the ascending aorta and arch of the aorta, where they are ideally situated to cause mischief. Those that arise close to the aortic valve ring lead to dilatation of the ring

and hence to aortic incompetence, the result of which is overload of the left ventricle and cardiac failure. Aneurysms may rupture into the trachea or oesophagus to produce haemoptysis (coughing up blood), haematemesis (vomiting blood) or death. Any cause of aortic expansion within the chest can produce difficulty in breathing or swallowing due to compression, persistent cough due to irritation of the recurrent laryngeal nerves, or problems of bone erosion. Fortunately, syphilis is now an uncommon disease in the Western world and these complications are rare.

Aneurysms secondary to vasculitis, such as polyarteritis nodosa, tend to occur in the renal and mesenteric vessels where they lead to local ischaemia. Patients may therefore present with renal failure or with intestinal infarction and peritonitis, all of which have a significant mortality.

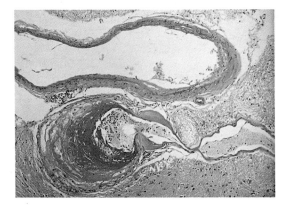

Figure 7.17 Photomicrograph showing microaneurysm with a thrombus

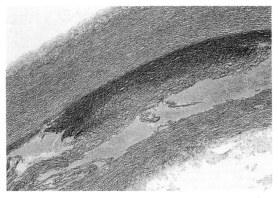

Figure 7.18 Elastin stain of aorta showing dissection of the wall by blood (stained yellow) (Courtesy of Dr S. Edwards, SGHMS)

Aneurysms secondary to infection are called mycotic aneurysms. Such aneurysms tend to be 'saccular', i.e. the wall is weakened in a particular focus which 'blows out' to form a sac. Most of the other conditions we have mentioned cause more diffuse weakening of the arterial wall, which dilates to form a 'fusiform' or spindle-shaped aneurysm.

SHOCK

Shock is a wonderful word! It means such different things to medical and lay people. How often we hear news reports that someone has been taken to hospital suffering from shock after witnessing some tragic event. No doubt that person is surprised and possibly emotionally disturbed but they are not in a state of circulatory collapse, which is what a doctor regards as shock.

The 'shocked' patient is desperately ill and requires intensive treatment both to correct the condition that has produced the circulatory collapse and also to cope with the widespread ischaemic damage resulting from shock. By definition, the patient will have hypoperfusion of many tissues. The blood pressure may be low but need not be, as the body may either have compensated by increasing peripheral vasoconstriction to keep the pressure normal or the patient may have had a high blood pressure which has now dropped. There may be pallor, cold extremities, sweating and a tachycardia; the first two signs due to poor perfusion and the other two resulting from the attempt to compensate, which includes the release of adrenaline.

What has happened to precipitate this disastrous state? Logically, there will be a sudden generalized poor perfusion if the pump fails or if there is insufficient blood, so-called cardiogenic and hypovolaemic shock. Abrupt heart failure may result from myocardial infarction, arrhythmias and cardiac tamponade while hypovolaemic shock follows fluid loss due to haemorrhage, severe burns, diarrhoea or vomiting. Shock following pulmonary embolism mimics cardiogenic shock but the heart is normal and the reduced output occurs because the left atrial filling has dropped. A rather special but clinically very important form of shock is 'septic shock' due to overwhelming infection, especially those caused by Gram-negative bacteria that have

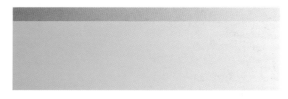

Key facts

Important mediators of vascular dilatation and increased permeability in septic shock

- Histamine
- Thromboxane
- Serotonin
- Prostaglandins
- Leukotrienes
- TNFα
- IL-1α
- C3a and C5a

endotoxic lipopolysaccharides (page 32). Here the pathogenesis is complicated because of the varied effects of the bacterial products on endothelial cells, platelets and leukocytes, which leads to a veritable web of interactions resulting in DIC and reduced blood volume because of vasodilatation and increased vascular permeability. Similar mechanisms probably operate in anaphylactic shock and neurogenic shock.

Let us concentrate first on cardiogenic shock as this follows naturally from the previous chapter on atherosclerosis and hypertension.

MYOCARDIAL INFARCTION

A typical clinical scenario may be as follows: A 63-year-old man presents to the Accident and Emergency department complaining of chest pain. He

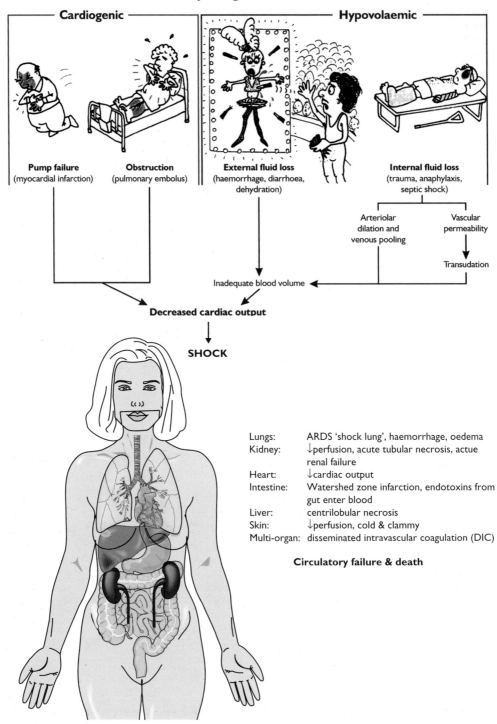

Figure 8.1 The pathogenesis and clinical effects of shock. Shock may be due to pump failure (cardiogenic shock) or loss of blood volume (hypovolaemic shock) but, if treatment is unsuccessful, the clinical outcome is much the same. ARDS, adult respiratory distress syndrome, see Fig. 8.15. For DIC see Fig. 6.14

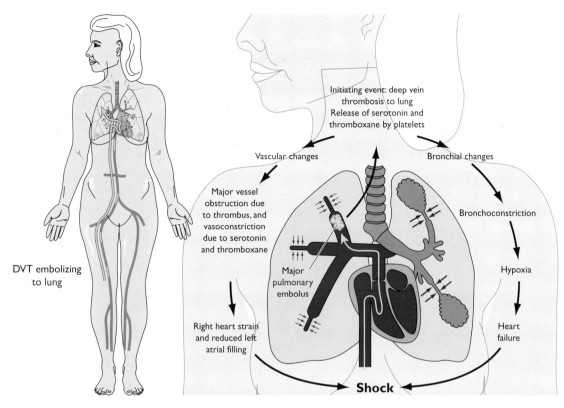

Figure 8.2 The pathogenesis of shock in pulmonary embolism

has had central chest pain for 6–8 hours and the pain radiates down the left arm and into his neck. He is feeling nauseated and also complains of shortness of breath. He has had a history of hypertension for the last 5 years and has been receiving treatment. He also smokes 25 cigarettes per day and is obese. He has a family history of hypertension: his father died at the age of 55 of a 'heart attack'. His brother is also hypertensive.

On examination he is found to have a pulse rate of 40 beats/min, blood pressure of 110/80 and is in cardiac failure. An electrocardiogram (ECG) confirms an inferior myocardial infarction and he is found to be in complete heart block. He receives treatment for his pain, a temporary pacing wire is inserted and he is transferred to the intensive care unit for observation.

As house physicians and residents, you will encounter this sort of situation with alarming regularity. So what is the pathological sequence of events that leads to a myocardial infarction and what are the complications that may arise as a consequence?

What mechanisms lead to myocardial infarction?

In myocardial infarction the cardiac muscle cells die because of a lack of nutrients, most importantly oxygen. Generally, this results from poor blood flow to the myocardium because of narrowing or total occlusion of one or more coronary arteries. The extent of the infarction will depend on the amount of collateral flow, the metabolic requirements of the cells and the duration of the insult. Atheroma of the coronary vessels accounts for the majority of cases, but rarer causes include vascular spasm, emboli, arteritis and anaemia.

We have learnt in Chapter 7 that plaques can be stable or unstable. Stable plaques narrow the coronary arteries so that blood flow is insufficient for even a moderate increase in cardiac work, such as walking upstairs, and the patient will complain of chest pain on exercise which is relieved on resting. This is called **angina** and occurs because the myocardial cells become ischaemic but the damage is reversible. Unstable plaques may not produce any clinical problems until an 'acute' event occurs when the fibrous cap of the plaque splits and blood from the lumen can reach the soft necrotic centre. This can distort and enlarge the plaque but, most significantly, the plaque contents activate the thrombotic cascade. Platelets and fibrin will aggregate to block the lumen and the platelet constituents (thromboxane A_2, histamine and serotonin) may worsen the situation by promoting spasm in the vessel wall. It is not known why the plaque fissures but it may be influenced by macrophage activity in the soft atheromatous centre, by vasospasm in the wall, by bending and twisting of the vessel as the heart contracts or by altered distribution of stresses on the wall. It is often stated that coronary artery stenosis is not likely to produce clinical symptoms unless the cross-sectional area is reduced by 75 per cent. This is true for long-standing fibrosed areas of atheroma, but the majority of plaques which fissure to produce occlusion are fairly small and have an abundance of soft lipid. You will recall

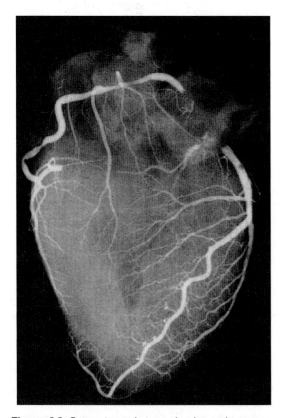

Figure 8.3 Coronary arteriogram showing main coronary arteries and numerous collateral vessels

that soft plaques are more likely to fissure than hard, fibrous plaques.

Vasospasm is an elusive mechanism for a pathologist to identify because there will be nothing to see at autopsy. However, it may be seen on angiography in some patients with angina or infarction and principally occurs in areas damaged by atheroma. It is potentially of great therapeutic importance because it may be influenced by drugs. Nitric oxide (NO) (originally called endothelin-derived relaxing factor) may be important in vasospasm either through reduced local production, reduced responsiveness of the smooth muscle cells or early neutralization.

PATTERNS OF INFARCTION

Occlusion of a single vessel, as described above, will produce a regional infarct, occupying the segment of myocardium that is normally supplied by a particular coronary artery. The infarct may involve a variable thickness of the myocardial wall, but when it involves the full thickness of the wall, it is referred to as a transmural infarction. Ninety per cent of transmural infarctions result from thrombosis complicating atheroma. Myocardial infarction is much commoner in the left ventricle and interventricular septum, but approximately 25 per cent of posterior infarctions will extend into the adjacent right ventricle or even into the atria. Occasionally, the infarcted region does not correlate with the thrombosed vessel and this is termed 'infarction at a distance'. It occurs because the patient has had previous coronary artery problems and has developed a collateral circulation so that, for example, long-standing poor flow through the left anterior descending coronary artery may make the anterior wall of the left ventricle dependent on collateral flow from the right coronary artery. Thus sudden occlusion of the right coronary artery may result in infarction of the region normally associated with the left anterior descending artery.

The other important pattern of myocardial damage is the subendocardial infarction. The pathogenesis of this type of infarction is different from that of regional infarction as there is generally widespread atherosclerosis in all coronary vessels but no specific occlusion. The subendocardial region is the most vulnerable part of the myocardium for two reasons: first, any collateral supply that is developed tends to supply the subepicardial part of the myocardium, and secondly, the subendocardium is under the greatest tension from the compressive

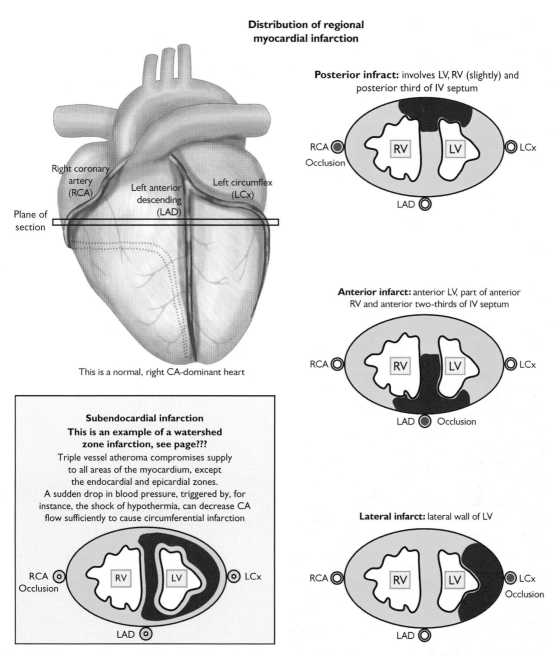

Distribution of regional myocardial infarction

This is a normal, right CA-dominant heart

Posterior infract: involves LV, RV (slightly) and posterior third of IV septum

Anterior infarct: anterior LV, part of anterior RV and anterior two-thirds of IV septum

Subendocardial infarction
This is an example of a watershed zone infarction, see page???
Triple vessel atheroma compromises supply to all areas of the myocardium, except the endocardial and epicardial zones. A sudden drop in blood pressure, triggered by, for instance, the shock of hypothermia, can decrease CA flow sufficiently to cause circumferential infarction

Lateral infarct: lateral wall of LV

Figure 8.4 Patterns of myocardial infarction. The region of myocardium affected by coronary artery (CA) thrombosis is reasonably predictable, generally following the patterns illustrated here. The patterns may vary however: some people are 'right CA dominant' when much of the left CA territory is supplied by the right CA. Other modifying factors include the presence of a collateral circulation (see Fig. 6.11)

forces of the myocardium and, hence, most likely to be ischaemic.

Normally, blood will flow into the myocardium when the aortic root pressure exceeds the left ventricular cavity pressure as occurs during diastole. Generalized reduction in myocardial perfusion results from any combination of coronary stenosis, reduction in aortic root pressure, increase in left ventricular cavity pressure, myocardial thickening and shortening of diastole.

Subendocardial infarction is much less common than transmural infarction. It is confined to the inner half of the myocardium and may be regional or circumferential. A very thin layer of subendo-cardial muscle remains viable because it receives nutrients and oxygen from the ventricular luminal blood. It should be noted, however, that even a transmural, regional infarct probably begins in the subendocardial region and then spreads to the rest of the wall.

IS MYOCARDIAL INFARCTION PREVENTABLE?

You will realize from the preceding sections that any dietary or therapeutic factors that influence atherogenesis or thrombosis will alter the risk of myocardial infarction. If a patient has widespread severe atherosclerotic coronary heart disease, they may have their diseased vessels bypassed by a graft from their leg veins or by synthetic vessels. Alternatively, the internal mammary artery can be 'plumbed' into the coronary arteries to bypass the stenotic areas. If they have only a localized lesion, they may have this 'stretched' by inflating an intravenous balloon catheter in the affected area and the vessel may be stented to try to avoid restenosis. Low-dose aspirin may be used to reduce any thrombotic tendency by acting on platelets.

Once a coronary artery has become occluded, urgent action is required in the first 2 hours while ischaemic damage is in the reversible phase. An intravenous catheter may be used to attempt to dislodge the clot, lytic agents may help to dissolve it and the use of antithrombotic drugs will aim to prevent any extension of the thrombus.

What are the appearances of infarction?

Let us consider the clinical example described earlier in which the patient's ECG showed him to have had an inferior infarction. If he had died within a few hours, autopsy would have revealed a thrombus within the right coronary artery. This artery supplies the posterior wall of the left ventricle and the posterior third of the interventricular septum. Ischaemia of the septum would explain his complete heart block as this would damage the conduction pathway. No macroscopical abnormality would be seen in the myocardium, as the infarction would be only 6 hours old, but the area of infarction could be highlighted using histochemical techniques. Normal heart muscle contains dehydrogenases, which leak out of fibres that have been damaged by ischaemia. If a 1-cm slice of myocardium is dipped

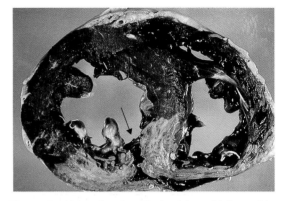

Figure 8.5 Heart slice through the right and left ventricles stained with NBTZ to demonstrate infarction in the area supplied by the left anterior descending artery. The left ventricular wall has ruptured (arrow), allowing blood into the pericardial space. (Slice viewed from below; right ventricle at the right of photograph)

into a solution of the yellow dye nitrobluetetra-zolium (NBTZ), the normal myocardium will appear blue because of the reduction of the dye by the dehydrogenase enzymes, while the ischaemic myocardium will be pale and unstained.

If the patient had died at 24 hours, the infarcted area would either appear pale or be red-blue due to the trapped blood. Later the dead myocardium becomes pale yellow, softened and better defined with a rim of hyperaemic tissue at the periphery. Over the next few weeks, the necrotic muscle is replaced by fibrous scar tissue and this is usually complete by 6 weeks. The exact time course depends on the size of the infarct and any complications that may occur.

Under the light or electron microscope, the cardiac muscle will show the typical changes of reversible and irreversible ischaemic damage (page 12).

What complications may occur?

Our 63-year-old man was in cardiac failure and complete heart block, two of the commonest complications of myocardial infarction. First, we will consider arrhythmia. This may be a type of heart block, ventricular tachycardia or bradycardia, ventricular fibrillation or asystole. Arrhythmias are responsible for many cases of sudden death following myocardial infarction and their prompt diagnosis is of crucial importance in the management of these patients. Arrhythmias occur either because of

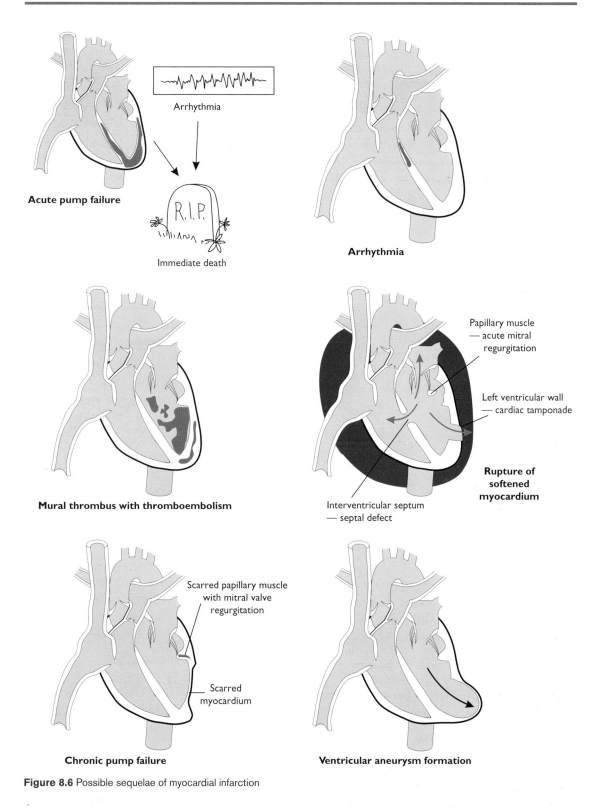

Acute pump failure

Arrhythmia

Immediate death

Arrhythmia

Mural thrombus with thromboembolism

Papillary muscle
— acute mitral
regurgitation

Left ventricular wall
— cardiac tamponade

**Rupture of
softened
myocardium**

Interventricular septum
— septal defect

Scarred papillary muscle
with mitral valve
regurgitation

Scarred
myocardium

Chronic pump failure

Ventricular aneurysm formation

Figure 8.6 Possible sequelae of myocardial infarction

ischaemia or death of the specialized conducting tissue of the heart or as a result of interruption of the conduction of impulses within the damaged myocardium. A damaged atrioventricular node, for instance, may lead to complete heart block, while damage to the conducting fibres within the ventricles will produce left or right bundle branch block. Damaged myocardial fibres may also be 'arrhythmogenic' and so initiate abnormal impulses, which may terminate in ventricular fibrillation. It is interesting that many of the drugs used to treat arrhythmias, which act by altering the action potential, are also capable of inducing them. Potentially fatal ventricular arrhythmias without specific myocardial damage can also occur as a result of an acute thrombosis linked to plaque fissuring, and probably represents the extreme end of the spectrum of unstable angina.

The second complication mentioned was cardiac failure. His cardiac failure could be due to complete heart block, so restoring normal sinus rhythm will be important in his treatment. Cardiac failure may also occur because of extensive death of muscle cells in the left ventricular wall or because they have been 'stunned' by a short period of ischaemia and are temporarily unable to contract, in which case they may recover over a few days. If a papillary muscle is damaged then mitral valve incompetence will produce cardiac failure. Initially, the papillary muscle is likely to be intact but incapable of contraction. After 4–5 days, the infarction has softened and the muscle may rupture, allowing the valve leaflet to prolapse, i.e. to float upwards into the left atrium. Similar softening occurs in infarcted tissue in the left ventricular wall so that it may rupture. This occurs in transmural infarction (i.e. full thickness) but not in subendocardial infarction. Within 24–48 hours of transmural infarction, the damaged ventricular muscle stretches, i.e. it becomes thinner, and is liable to aneurysm formation or rupture. This is often referred to as 'infarct expansion', but it should be appreciated that the amount of tissue damage is not increasing, it is merely a stretching of the damaged area.

Rupture may take place in the interventricular septum, which creates a ventricular septal defect (VSD), or through the ventricular wall so that the blood leaks into the pericardial cavity, producing a haemopericardium, which inhibits the normal action of the heart – so-called cardiac tamponade. Either of these complications is generally fatal and is most likely to occur 5–7 days after a myocardial infarction.

The body's immune system responds to the infarction so that the pericardial surface overlying the infarcted area usually becomes inflamed (pericarditis) by the second or third day. In most cases, this is self-limiting, but the friction between the pericardial surfaces produces a pericardial rub, which may be heard through a stethoscope. Similar changes occur on the endocardial surface of the infarct, which, in combination with stasis, predispose it to mural thrombosis. Whenever there is thrombosis, there is a risk of embolism. In this case, these would be systemic emboli affecting organs such as the brain or kidneys.

Finally, the healed and fibrotic wall may balloon out to produce a cardiac aneurysm, which itself can be a site of thrombus because of stasis.

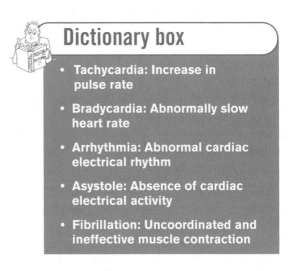

Dictionary box

- **Tachycardia: Increase in pulse rate**

- **Bradycardia: Abnormally slow heart rate**

- **Arrhythmia: Abnormal cardiac electrical rhythm**

- **Asystole: Absence of cardiac electrical activity**

- **Fibrillation: Uncoordinated and ineffective muscle contraction**

Extreme circulatory failure, as in shock, is a consequence of decreased cardiac output due to pump failure or blood volume loss. Lesser degrees of poor tissue perfusion can occur through any combination of pump failure, blood abnormalities and peripheral vascular disease. We have discussed heart and vessels quite extensively and should now turn our attention to the blood.

ANAEMIA

It is beyond the scope of this book to describe the whole of haematology, but we can provide a framework for thinking about blood disorders and help you to appreciate that abnormalities in the blood can manifest as symptoms and signs in almost any organ, i.e. it is a common mechanism of disease.

The key components of blood (excluding platelets and clotting factors) are the fluid, the red cells with their haemoglobin for oxygen transport, and the white cells with their defence functions. What can go wrong with each of these? The simple answer is too much, too little or the wrong sort. Abnormalities of white cells are discussed in Chapters 4 and 10. Derangements of fluid balance are best looked up in a physiology or renal book. This leaves us to consider the red cells, but first a brief overview may help.

What is anaemia?

> The modern haematologist, instead of describing in English what he can see, prefers to describe in Greek what he can't.
> *Richard Asher* (Lancet 1959)

A few key words or parts of words will help us through the maze of blood disorders. Any word ending in '... aemia' relates to the blood (e.g. poly-cythaemia, hypoalbuminaemia) just as words ending in '... uria' relate to the urine (e.g. haematuria – blood in the urine, anuria – not passing urine). A prefix of 'hypo' indicates too little, 'micro' means too small, 'hyper' is too much and 'macro' is too big. Leukaemia literally means white blood but has become synonymous with a malignancy of blood cells. Anaemia strictly means a lack of blood, which is not really correct because there is a reduction in red blood cells rather than an absence. The term is now used to indicate a reduction in haemo-globin concentration in the blood. What are the possible causes?

The red blood cells contain haemoglobin, which is important in the transport of oxygen. The haemoglobin level may drop because the number of red cells is low (reduced red cell mass) or the content of haemoglobin is reduced. Red cell numbers may be reduced because of impaired produc-tion, acute or chronic blood loss through bleeding or a reduced lifespan for a variety of reasons.

Anaemia can be classified according to its cause (Table 8.1) or according to the appearance of the blood (Table 8.3). It is important to know both because the first investigation of a pale patient is to perform a full blood count, which will detail the haemoglobin level in the blood, the number of

Dictionary box

- **Anaemia: Reduction in haemoglobin in blood**
- **Pancytopenia: Reduction in all blood cell types**
- **Neutropenia: Reduction in neutrophils**
- **Thrombocytopenia: Reduction in platelets**
- **Polycythaemia: Increase in red cells**
- **Thrombocythaemia: Increase in platelets**
- **Leukocytosis: Increase in white cells**
- **Leukaemia: Malignant haematopoietic cells in blood**
- **Aplastic marrow: No haematopoiesis in marrow**
- **Hypoplastic marrow: Reduced haematopoiesis in marrow**
- **Hyperplastic marrow: Increased haematopoiesis in marrow**
- **Leukoerythroblastic: Red and white cell precursors in peripheral blood may indicate marrow replacement by fibrosis, tumour, abscesses**

Red cell changes

- **Normocytic: Normal cell size**
- **Macrocytic: Increased mean corpuscular volume (MCV)**
- **Microcytic: Decreased MCV**
- **Normochromic: Normal haemoglobin (Hb) concentration**
- **Hypochromic: Decreased mean corpuscular haemoglobin concentration (MCHC)**
- **Poikilocytosis: Variation in shape**
- **Anisocytosis: Variation in size**
- **Howell–Jolly bodies: Nuclear remnants in delayed maturation**

Table 8.1 Causes of anaemia

Decreased red cell production

Defective haemoglobin production
    Iron deficiency
    Anaemia of chronic disease
    Sideroblastic anaemia
Defective DNA synthesis (megaloblastic anaemia)
    Vitamin B12 deficiency
    Folic acid deficiency
Stem cell failure, e.g. aplastic anaemia
Bone marrow replacement, e.g. infiltration by
    malignant disease
Inadequate erythropoietin stimulation,
    e.g. chronic renal failure
Other nutritional and toxic factors
    Scurvy
    Protein malnutrition
    Chronic liver disease
    Hypothyroidism

Increased red cell destruction, i.e. haemolytic anaemias

Intrinsic defect of erythrocytes
Congenital
    Haemoglobinopathies, e.g. sickle cell anaemia and
    thalassaemias
    Membrane defects, e.g. hereditary spherocytosis
    Enzyme deficiency, e.g. glucose 6-phosphate
    dehydrogenase deficiency (G6PD)
Acquired, e.g. paroxysmal nocturnal haemoglobinuria

Extrinsic cause for haemolysis
Immune-mediated
    Autoimmune haemolytic anaemia
    Haemolytic disease of the newborn
    Blood transfusion-related haemolysis
    Drug-induced immune haemolytic anaemia
Direct acting
    Infections, e.g. malaria
    Snake venom
    Physical trauma, e.g. microangiopathy
    Hypersplenism

Blood loss

red blood cells, the size of the red cells (mean corpuscular volume, MCV) and the average concentration of haemoglobin in a red cell (mean corpuscular haemoglobin concentration, MCHC). If the haemoglobin level indicates that the patient is anaemic, then you can use the MCV and MCHC to classify the anaemia on cell size and haemoglobin concentration and also look up the possible causes in Table 8.1. Let us try it for an imaginary patient. Remember that '...cytic' refers to the cell and '...chromic' refers to the haemoglobin concentration.

A 21-year-old woman goes to see her general practitioner for a prenatal health check as she is wanting to become pregnant for the first time. The doctor advises her about the risks of smoking and alcohol on the fetus and performs a physical examination and finds no abnormalities. Her blood pressure is normal and he takes a blood sample for further analysis. The results are shown in Table 8.2 along with normal levels.

Table 8.2 Normal peripheral blood values and an anaemic patient's results

	Normal values	Patient's values
Haemoglobin (g/dL)	14–18 (male), 12–16 (female)	8.2
Erythrocytes ($\times 10^{12}$ per L)	4.6–6 (male), 4.2–5.4 (female)	4.7
Haematocrit (PCV) (per cent)	42–50 (male), 37–47 (female)	31
MCV (fL)	80–95	69
MCHC (per cent)	32–35	24.5
Reticulocytes ($\times 10^9$ per L)	20–70	96

PCV = packed cell volume, MCV = mean corpuscular volume, MCHC = mean corpuscular haemoglobin concentration.

When she returns to the surgery the following week, the doctor explains that she has a minor problem because she is anaemic and probably has iron deficiency. How do you classify her anaemia?

Hopefully you have concluded that our patient has small red cells with a reduced haemoglobin concentration, i.e. a microcytic hypochromic anaemia. To search further for a cause, you need more information. The commonest causes of anaemia can be identified through a combination of:

- reticulocyte count
- morphological appearance of the cells in the peripheral blood
- haemoglobin electrophoresis
- serum iron
- bone marrow examination

Table 8.3 Morphological classification of anaemia

Type	MCV	MCHC	Common causes
Normocytic/normochromic	Normal	Normal	Anaemia of chronic disease Chronic renal failure
Microcytic/hypochromic (Fig. 8.11)	↓	↓	Iron deficiency β-Thalassaemia trait Anaemia of chronic disease (severe)
Macrocytic (megaloblastic) (Fig. 8.12)	↑	Normal	Folic acid deficiency Vitamin B12 deficiency
Macrocytic (non-megaloblastic)	↑	Normal	Liver disease, alcohol ingestion Hypothyroidism
Leukoerythroblastic anaemia (Fig. 8.7)	Normal	Normal	Replacement or infiltration of marrow

MCV = mean corpuscular volume, MCHC = mean corpuscular haemoglobin concentration.
Megaloblastic refers to abnormal maturation of erythroid cells detectable on examination of the marrow.

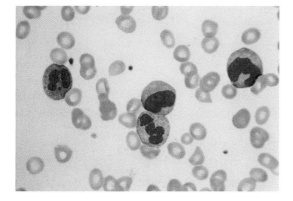

(a)

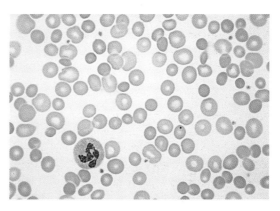

Figure 8.8 Peripheral blood in a patient with spherocytosis

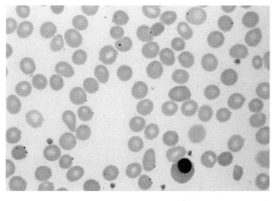

(b)

Figure 8.7 Two areas from the peripheral blood from a patient with leukoerythroblastic anaemia. Photograph (a) shows myelocytes, while (b) shows an erythroblast (nucleated red cell)

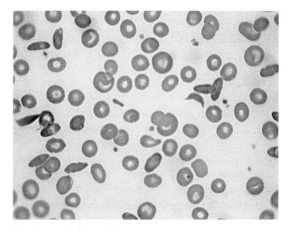

Figure 8.9 Sickle cell disease

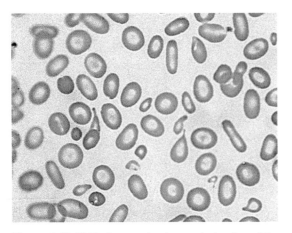

Figure 8.10 HbH disease showing marked anisopoikilocytosis

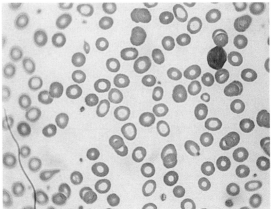

Figure 8.11 Microcytosis and hypochromia in a case of iron-deficiency anaemia

- serum ferritin (serum iron and iron binding capacity were originally used)
- serum vitamin B12 and folate levels
- Schilling test
- Antibody screens (e.g. parietal cell and intrinsic factor antibodies).

Reticulocytes are newly released red cells that are slightly larger than mature red cells and have a more basophilic (blue) cytoplasm on routine Giemsa staining. Approximately 1 per cent is the normal level and an increased number indicates increased red cell turnover. Normally the reticulocytes become mature red cells in the marrow and it is only when demand for red blood cells exceeds supply that these immature forms are released in significant numbers. Our patient has a normal reticulocyte count, so the most likely diagnosis is iron-deficiency anaemia, which is a common finding in premenopausal and pregnant women and easily treated with iron tablets. The doctor is not likely to investigate any further in this case unless the patient has other problems, but we shall digress to discuss the causes of iron deficiency and iron overload.

Iron deficiency is important to understand because it is common. Iron overload is worth remembering as an example where homeostasis cannot be achieved through increased excretion. Think about it! You drink too much water and the kidney responds. Take too much salt or vitamin C and you excrete what you do not need. However, there is no controllable excretion method for iron. Is this a unique situation? No, just consider calorie intake!

Iron-deficiency anaemia

Iron is an important element with well-known roles in haemoglobin, myoglobin, cytochromes and various enzyme systems in the cells. Approximately 80 per cent of the body's iron is in one of these functional forms while the remaining 20 per cent is stored as ferritin or haemosiderin. Iron is absorbed in the upper small intestine and transported in the blood bound to the glycoprotein transferrin. There is no control over the excretion of iron, and iron loss from the body is through loss in secretions, exfoliated cells and menstrual blood. There is some control over the absorption of iron, with between 10 per cent and 20 per cent of dietary iron being absorbed. This does not leave much of a safety margin so iron deficiency is the commonest cause of anaemia and occurs because of an imbalance between absorption and loss. In developed countries, an average diet contains about 15 mg of iron and the daily requirement for *absorbed* iron is 0.5–1.0 mg for men and 0.7–2.0 mg for women. This means that any reduction in dietary iron, problem with absorption or increased requirement for iron will lead to deficiency (Table 8.4). Iron balance is particularly precarious in premenopausal women because of menstrual blood loss. Fifty millilitres of whole blood contains about 25 mg of iron, which would require an extra 250 mg of iron in the diet to be back in balance.

There are no immediate problems for the person developing iron deficiency because red cell production continues, but the iron stores in the

Table 8.4 Causes of iron-deficiency anaemia

Inadequate intake

Deficient diet

Malabsorption

   Generalized malabsorption,
   e.g. coeliac disease

   Postgastrectomy (rapid
   gastrojejunal transit)

Increased iron loss

Reproductive tract

   Heavy menstruation

   Pregnancies and miscarriages

Gastrointestinal tract

   Oesophageal varices

   Peptic ulcer disease

   Chronic aspirin ingestion

   Hookworm infestation

   Haemorrhoids

   Tumours

Miscellaneous

   Epistaxis

   Haematuria

   Haemoptysis

Increased demand for iron

Early childhood

Pregnancy and lactation

marrow become depleted. Once the iron stores are inadequate, red cells are still produced but they are small (microcytic) with too little haemoglobin (hypochromic) and the patient will become tired and lethargic, breathless on exertion and appear pale. They may also have problems due to the effects of iron deficiency on epithelial cells if they do not receive treatment but remain chronically iron deficient. This complication, however, is rare in most countries. The mucous membranes of the mouth, tongue, pharynx, oesophagus and stomach become thin (atrophic) which may cause difficulty in swallowing (dysphagia) and produce mucosal webs in the upper oesophagus. Finger nails become spoon-shaped (koilonychia) and split easily and the thinned stomach wall does not produce a normal amount of acid. This combination of problems in severe iron deficiency is called the Plummer–Vinson syndrome and is cured by giving iron.

Small Print

The Paterson–Kelly–Plummer–Vinson syndrome

This syndrome was first described in 1909 by Donald R Patterson (ear, nose and throat (ENT) surgeon in Cardiff) and Adam B Kelly (ENT surgeon in Glasgow). It was also described by Henry S Plummer (Physician, Mayo Clinic, USA) and Porter P Vinson (Physician in Virginia, USA). In medical textbooks, you may come across a variety of combinations of these names.

Megaloblastic anaemia

The next woman in our prenatal clinic has Crohn's disease, which is an inflammatory disease that can affect any area of the gastrointestinal tract. The terminal ileum is commonly involved and this can result in anaemia due to vitamin B12 deficiency. Her blood results are as follows:

Haemoglobin (g/dL)	5.0
Erythrocytes ($\times 10^{12}$ per L)	1.7
Haematocrit (PCV) (per cent)	21
MCV (fL)	128
MCHC (per cent)	35
Reticulocytes ($\times 10^{9}$ per L)	40

The MCV is increased and the MCHC is normal, consistent with a macrocytic anaemia. We are going to concentrate on the subset of macrocytic anaemias that have abnormal erythroid maturation in the bone marrow, resulting in large precursors

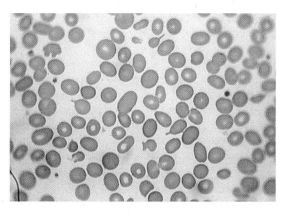

Figure 8.12 Oval macrocytes in a case of pernicious anaemia

Table 8.5 Causes of megaloblastic anaemia

Vitamin B12 deficiency

Inadequate diet
    Strict vegans excluding milk, eggs and cheese
Absorption problem
    Intrinsic factor deficiency, e.g. pernicious anaemia,
    total and subtotal gastrectomy
    Terminal ileal disease, e.g. Crohn's disease, surgical
    removal
Competition by microorganisms
    Bacterial overgrowth in blind loops
    Fish tapeworm infection

Folic acid deficiency

Inadequate diet
    Malnutrition
    Chronic alcoholism
Absorption problem
    Generalized malabsorption
    Tropical sprue
    Gluten-induced enteropathy (coeliac)
Increased demand
    Early childhood
    Pregnancy
    Erythroid hyperplasia in severe haemolytic anaemias
Use of folic acid antagonists
    Anticonvulsants, e.g. phenytoin
    Anticancer drugs, e.g. methotrexate

and called 'megaloblastic'. Megaloblastic anaemia is most commonly caused by vitamin B12 or folate deficiency (Table 8.5). Both are co-factors for the conversion of deoxyuridine to deoxythymidine, an essential step in the synthesis of DNA.

Working down our list of investigations, we first ask for a reticulocyte count and a peripheral blood film. The laboratory tells us that there are few or no reticulocytes but the red cells contain Howell–Jolly bodies, which are nuclear remnants due to delayed maturation, the red cells are large (macrocytic) and of variable shape (poikilocytosis) and the neutrophils are hypersegmented (most normal neutrophils have three or four lobes, whereas hypersegmented cells have more). These are all features of megaloblastic anaemia. The next step is to measure the serum vitamin B12 level and serum and red cell folate levels. If the folate level is low, we have a diagnosis of folate deficiency whose cause should be identified by taking a good history. If the vitamin B12 is low,

we can investigate further and need to understand a little more about B12 absorption.

Vitamin B12 is absorbed in the terminal ileum as a complex bound to intrinsic factor. Intrinsic factor (IF) is produced by the parietal cells in the stomach. This means that you need an adequate diet and a normal stomach and terminal ileum to avoid B12 deficiency. We assume that our lady with Crohn's disease will fail to absorb the B12/intrinsic factor complex because she has a diseased terminal ileum, but how could we prove this? We could demonstrate that her bone marrow is vitamin B12 deficient by injecting some vitamin B12 and observing an almost immediate increase in reticulocytes. In people with a normal terminal ileum but a damaged stomach, the parietal cells are unable to produce intrinsic factor and so no absorption occurs. This can be detected by performing a Schilling test, in which radiolabelled vitamin B12 is given orally and the amount of radioactivity absorbed into the blood and excreted in the urine is measured. If lack of intrinsic factor is a problem, then absorption will be low unless intrinsic factor is also given orally. If absorption is low when vitamin B12 and intrinsic factor are given together, then the terminal ileum is likely to be damaged or there is something else blocking absorption of the B12/IF complex.

The commonest cause of B12 deficiency in the UK is pernicious anaemia. This is aptly named because patients with megaloblastic anaemia can have a very severe anaemia and may even die without treatment. In pernicious anaemia or Addison's anaemia the vitamin B12 deficiency results from autoimmune damage to the stomach, leading to chronic atrophic gastritis, in which an inflamed and thinned stomach mucosa fails to produce adequate intrinsic factor or acid. This disease occurs predominantly after the age of 50 years and is more common in females. As well as severe anaemia, the sufferers may have neurological problems, such as subacute combined degeneration of the cord and segmental demyelination of peripheral nerves. These are due to the lack of vitamin B12 and do not occur in folate deficiency. They are also at an increased risk of stomach carcinoma.

What would have happened to our patients if their anaemia had not been discovered at prenatal testing? Let us discuss the effects of anaemia first. The anaemic patient has too little haemoglobin and hence a potential problem with the transport of oxygen to the tissues. The demand from the tissues will depend on the person's level of activity so that an anaemic person may be asymptomatic when

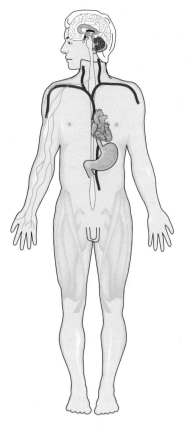

Clinical features of pernicious anaemia
Severe megaloblastic, macrocytic anaemia
Peripheral neuropathy
Subacute combined degeneration of the cord
  • demyelination of posterior and lateral columns
  • paraesthesia
  • loss of position and vibration sense
  • ataxia
  • weakness
  • spasticity
Increased risk of gastric carcinoma

Figure 8.13 Clinical features of pernicious anaemia

Key facts

Clinical features of pernicious anaemia

- Severe megaloblastic, macrocytic anaemia

- Peripheral neuropathy

- Subacute combined degeneration of the cord
  - Demyelination of posterior and lateral columns
  - Paraesthesia
  - Loss of position and vibration sense
  - Ataxia
  - Weakness
  - Spasticity

- Increased risk of gastric carcinoma

sitting at a desk but would have problems running a marathon; pregnancy can be regarded as a nine-month marathon (with a sprint finish!). An anaemic person can often compensate for the reduced amount of haemoglobin in the blood by pushing the blood round faster, i.e. increasing the cardiac output. However, in a normal pregnancy, cardiac output needs to increase by around 30 per cent so compensation for anaemia may not be possible. So who will suffer? The mother will suffer with breathlessness, tiredness, weakness and possibly dizziness or fainting. The baby will suffer because nutrition through the placenta may be inadequate, leading to a 'small for dates' baby lacking the normal stores of nutrients transferred between mother and baby in the last trimester.

ORGAN DAMAGE DUE TO POOR PERFUSION

Whatever the cause of poor perfusion, the effect at tissue level is similar, with a reduced delivery of

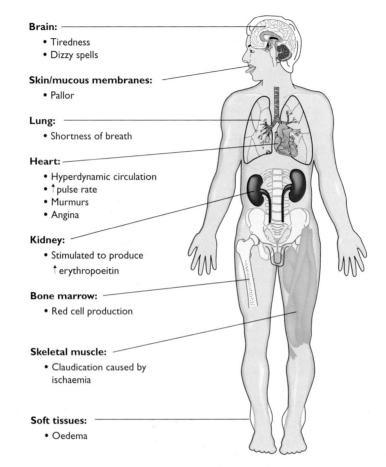

Brain:
- Tiredness
- Dizzy spells

Skin/mucous membranes:
- Pallor

Lung:
- Shortness of breath

Heart:
- Hyperdynamic circulation
- ↑ pulse rate
- Murmurs
- Angina

Kidney:
- Stimulated to produce
  ↑ erythropoeitin

Bone marrow:
- Red cell production

Skeletal muscle:
- Claudication caused by
  ischaemia

Soft tissues:
- Oedema

Figure 8.14 Presenting symptoms and systemic effects of anaemia

oxygen and nutrients so that cells' normal functions are disturbed. The details of reversible and irreversible cell injury have been discussed earlier (Chapter 1), so here we will concentrate on the clinical effects. The most important organs for immediate survival are the heart and brain, so the body has mechanisms for shunting blood from other tissues to protect these two organs. Frequently the kidneys and lungs will be underperfused and sufficiently damaged to be the immediate cause of death.

Adult respiratory distress syndrome

The lungs are fairly resistant to short periods of ischaemia but, if prolonged, the patient may develop 'shock lung' or 'adult respiratory distress syndrome' (ARDS) which can be life-threatening, as it is difficult to maintain adequate ventilation, even

with a mechanical ventilator. For oxygen to reach the alveolar blood, air must move in and out of the lungs and be able to diffuse across the alveolar septa. In 'shock lung' there is severe oedema affecting peribronchial connective tissue and alveolar septa and spaces. This both reduces the lung compliance and impairs alveolar diffusion, resulting in double trouble and a mortality rate of around 50 per cent.

The probable sequence of events (Fig. 8.15) is that the 'shock' causes the release of mediators, such as activated complement (C5a), leukotriene B_4 and platelet-activating factor, which promote leukocyte aggregation and activation in the lung. The neutrophils produce arachidonic acid metabolites, such as thromboxane, which cause pulmonary vasoconstriction, oxygen-derived free radicals, which injure the endothelial and epithelial cells, and lysosomal enzymes, which digest local structural proteins.

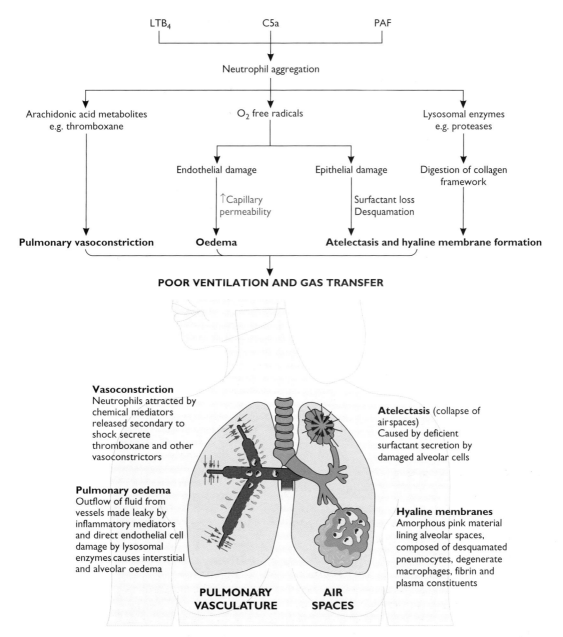

LTB$_4$ C5a   PAF

Neutrophil aggregation

Arachidonic acid metabolites
e.g. thromboxane

O$_2$ free radicals

Lysosomal enzymes
e.g. proteases

Endothelial damage   Epithelial damage   Digestion of collagen framework

↑Capillary permeability   Surfactant loss Desquamation

Pulmonary vasoconstriction   **Oedema**   **Atelectasis and hyaline membrane formation**

POOR VENTILATION AND GAS TRANSFER

Vasoconstriction
Neutrophils attracted by chemical mediators released secondary to shock secrete thromboxane and other vasoconstrictors

Atelectasis (collapse of air spaces)
Caused by deficient surfactant secretion by damaged alveolar cells

Pulmonary oedema
Outflow of fluid from vessels made leaky by inflammatory mediators and direct endothelial cell damage by lysosomal enzymes causes interstitial and alveolar oedema

Hyaline membranes
Amorphous pink material lining alveolar spaces, composed of desquamated pneumocytes, degenerate macrophages, fibrin and plasma constituents

PULMONARY VASCULATURE   **AIR SPACES**

Figure 8.15 Pathogenesis of adult respiratory distress syndrome (ARDS). An initiating event causes shock (see Fig. 8.1). Acute inflammatory mediators damage vascular endothelium, the alveolar walls and lining epithelium and cause pulmonary vasoconstriction, oedema, collapse and the formation of membranes over the alveolar surface

The damaged alveolar capillary endothelial cells are leaky, which leads to interstitial alveolar oedema and fibrin exudation. The damaged alveolar epithelial cells, particularly the type I pneumocytes, desquamate to form the characteristic hyaline membranes in combination with surfactant and protein-rich oedema fluid (Fig. 8.16). These are the same as the hyaline membranes in neonatal hyaline membrane disease and in both situations indicate severe epithelial injury with lack of surfactant. The lack of surfactant leads to collapse of alveolar air spaces (atelectasis) and so further reduces compliance and gas transfer.

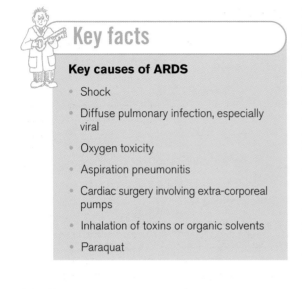

Key facts

Key causes of ARDS

- Shock
- Diffuse pulmonary infection, especially viral
- Oxygen toxicity
- Aspiration pneumonitis
- Cardiac surgery involving extra-corporeal pumps
- Inhalation of toxins or organic solvents
- Paraquat

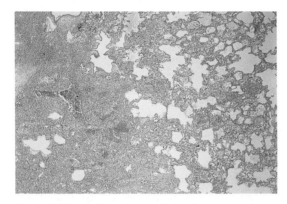

Figure 8.16 Lung photomicrograph showing adult respiratory distress syndrome. There is irregular ventilation due to the presence of hyaline membranes, exudate and cell debris within the alveolar spaces

Renal damage

Impaired renal blood flow results in acute tubular necrosis, a major cause of acute renal failure. This is not apparent immediately in a 'shocked' patient but will become evident once the 'shocked' state is under control and there is no circulatory reason for poor urine output. Then the patient will be noted to have oliguria (urine output of 40–400 mL/day, normal – 1500 mL/day), salt and water overload, a high plasma potassium and urea, and a metabolic acidosis. At this stage a renal biopsy would show numerous foci of tubular epithelial cell loss, affecting any area of the nephron, and epithelial 'casts', i.e. dead epithelial cells, present in the tubular

lumens. The important clinical point is that the patient can make a complete recovery if appropriately managed, e.g. by dialysis, and the cause of the shock rectified. After a few days, the tubular epithelium will regenerate and the urine volume will increase, often to above normal values because the tubules are unable to concentrate the urine, and there may be excessive loss of water, sodium and potassium: the so-called diuretic phase. Slowly the tubular epithelium returns to normal and reasonable renal function is restored.

Brain and cardiac damage

Despite the body's best efforts to protect the heart and brain, these organs may become underperfused. Damage to the brain may be mild or devastating. The neurons are most vulnerable to ischaemia, particularly the large Purkinje cells of the cerebellum and the pyramidal cells in the hippocampus. A short episode of hypoperfusion may not cause any irreversible neuronal damage, or the number of neurons damaged may be too few to produce any clinical effect beyond temporary confusion. However, prolonged ischaemia will result in infarction which most commonly affects the 'watershed' areas at the junctional zones between

Key facts

Organs damaged in a patient with shock

Kidney	Acute tubular necrosis
Lung	Adult respiratory distress syndrome (ARDS)
Heart	Ischaemic damage
Brain	Watershed infarcts
Liver	Fatty change/necrosis
Adrenal	Focal haemorrhagic necrosis
Pancreas	Pancreatitis
Stomach	Erosive gastritis
Duodenum	Ulceration
Small and large bowel	Haemorrhagic gastroenteropathy/ infarction

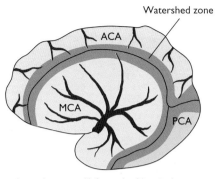

Lateral aspect of left cerebral hemisphere

Key:

MCA	Middle cerebral artery
ACA	Anterior cerebral artery
PCA	Posterior cerebral artery

Medial aspect of right cerebral hemisphere

Figure 8.17 Watershed zones. The brain, heart and colon are particularly at risk of ischaemic damage as they receive oxygenated blood from the most peripheral branches of supplying arteries with no territorial overlap. This supply can be compromised by hypotension, often due to shock. The regions affected in the brain are shown here. In the heart, subendocardial infarction may occur at the boundary between the peripheral myocardial blood supply from the coronary arteries and direct diffusion from the endocardial side (see Fig. 8.4). In the colon, the splenic flexure lies at the boundary between the inferior mesenteric and superior rectal arteries

the main arterial territories (Fig. 8.17). This may result in severe permanent cerebral damage or coma and death. It is important to remember that the 'watershed' effect operates in many organs if there is poor perfusion. In the heart, this is the subendothelial zone because the endocardium is nourished by direct diffusion from the blood in the cardiac chambers and the outer myocardium is supplied by arterioles penetrating from the outside. In the gut, areas such as the splenic flexure of the colon are at the boundary between arterial supplies and vulnerable to poor perfusion.

STROKES

As we reach the end of the section on cardiovascular disorders, it is a good moment to discuss 'strokes'. To understand 'strokes', you need to pull together the topics we have covered in these three sections: namely, thrombosis, embolism, atherosclerosis, hypertension, aneurysms and circulatory failure. So what is the clinical picture? 'Very variable' is the answer, because different areas of the brain perform very distinct functions and a patient's symptoms and signs will depend on the location of the damage.

First, a definition. A stroke is a sudden loss of some cerebral function due to a vascular lesion. It is usual to exclude haemorrhage caused by trauma (subdural and extradural haemorrhage) and to exclude global loss of function as might occur with generalized hypoxia or hypoperfusion (e.g. brain damage secondary to a cardiac arrest). If the loss of function lasts for less than 24 hours, it is called a transient ischaemic attack (TIA).

Second; are strokes a significant cause of death and disability? Approximately 10 per cent of deaths are due to stroke, which puts it in the top five causes of death. In the USA, there are approximately half a million cases of stroke each year. Roughly half will die and, of the remainder, half will have permanent significant disability. Around a third of strokes occur in people under 65 years of age. Thus, any intervention that can reduce the incidence or severity of strokes can have a major impact.

Third; what is the commonest type of stroke? Strokes occur when cerebral tissue is deprived of its blood supply. This is most commonly ischaemic in nature (80 per cent or more) due to blockage of an artery by thrombus (50 per cent or more) or embolus (30 per cent or more). You already know about the causes of thrombosis and the importance of unstable atheromatous plaques (page 172 and Fig. 7.4) and the types and sources of emboli (page 161). Most other strokes are due to haemorrhage, which can be intracerebral (about 10 per cent) or subarachnoid (about 5 per cent) and are associated with aneurysms (Fig. 8.18). Around 80 per cent of intracerebral haemorrhages occur in the presence of hypertension.

Cerebral blood supply and strokes

The clinical effect of a disease process will depend on how well the body can respond to the insult. With vascular problems affecting the brain,

The circle of Willis is an anastomosing complex of arteries at the base of the brain, derived from the right and left internal carotid and vertebral arteries, linked by the anterior and posterior communicating arteries. Three major branches, the anterior and middle and posterior cerebral arteries, supply each side of the brain. Despite the anastomoses proximally, the distal branches have no alternative route for blood flow and obstruction of small vessels by thromboembolus leads to infarction (75% of strokes). Patients with hypertension are at risk of haemorrhagic stroke, often following the development of a microaneurysm. These are different from berry aneurysms, which form at sites of congenital weakness at the branches of the circle of Willis and its immediate branches, which tend to cause subarachnoid, rather than intracerebral, haemorrhage should they rupture

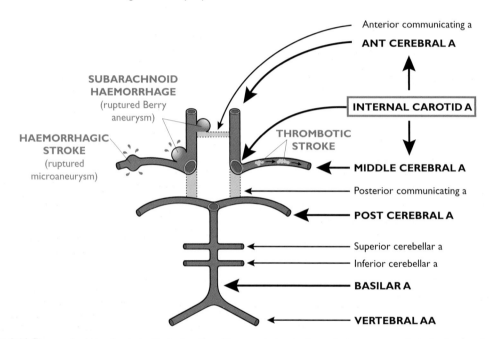

Figure 8.18 The cerebral blood supply, illustrating the difference between the main two causes of stroke, haemorrhagic and thrombotic, and typical sites of Berry aneurysm

this is influenced by the vascular anatomy and so it is time to revise some basic facts. You will recall that some vessels are endarteries and blockage will lead to infarction of a clearly defined tissue segment (see Fig. 1.13, page 18 for kidney and Fig. 8.4, page 189 for heart). In the brain, the small cerebral vessels are endarteries but the others are not and, to a greater or lesser extent, may compensate for blockage through being part of a collateral circulation.

The brain receives blood through two internal carotid arteries and two vertebral arteries. The two vertebral arteries join to become the basilar artery which, with the two internal carotid arteries, feeds the circle of Willis at the base of the brain. If the circle of Willis is anatomically normal and free from significant atheroma, it can be an effective collateral route, such that one internal carotid artery can be totally blocked without causing damage. Blockage

of the vertebrobasilar system, however, is less easy to compensate for.

The blood supply to the brain has two other unusual features. One is the effect of brain swelling (cerebral oedema) and the other is the ability to respond to and protect the brain from the effects of high or low blood pressure (autoregulation). The brain is encased in a hard, non-elastic structure (the bony skull) which has some fibrous internal dividing walls (tentorium cerebelli and falx cerebri) and one significant opening (foramen magnum). If a part of the brain increases in size, a so-called space-occupying lesion, then it presses on adjacent structures and may interrupt the blood supply directly or by herniation. For example, tentorial herniation can stop flow in the posterior cerebral or superior cerebellar arteries. The swelling that accompanies infarction can cause this (Fig. 8.19).

Autoregulation refers to changes in the resistance of cerbral arterioles in response to changes in blood pressure. This is believed to be able to compensate for systolic blood pressures as low as 50 mmHg (as in 'shock') or as high as 160 mmHg in normal individuals and is an example of effective homeostasis. However, this mechanism is disturbed after strokes, head injury or anaesthesia.

Dictionary box

Hernia: protrusion of part of an organ through an aperture

Transient ischaemic attacks have similar causes to ischaemic strokes and indicate an increased likelihood of having a stroke of anything from 10 to 50 per cent. The main mechanisms are poor perfusion as a result of sudden cardiac problems or thromboembolism. Their recognition is particularly important now that preventative treatment is becoming more effective (see below).

Who is most likely to have a stroke and how can it be prevented?

You have already worked through the risk factors and preventative measures for coronary artery disease (Fig. 7.1, page 166) and you should not be surprised to learn that they are similar for cerebrovascular disease. That is the advantage of understanding the key mechanisms of disease; once the principles are appreciated they can be applied to other situations. Combining the factors for thromboembolism, hypertension and atherosclerosis will give you the main pointers for stroke. For example, there is correlation between non-haemorrhagic stroke and raised serum total cholesterol, LDL cholesterol and triglycerides and lowered HDL cholesterol (i.e. as for myocardial infarction).

However, human autopsy examination has shown that atherosclerotic changes in cerebral arteries appear about 20 years later than in the coronary vessels and are more common in black individuals. Also, young patients with homozygous familial hypercholesterolaemia and severe involvement of coronary arteries may have no significant involvement of their cerebral vessels.

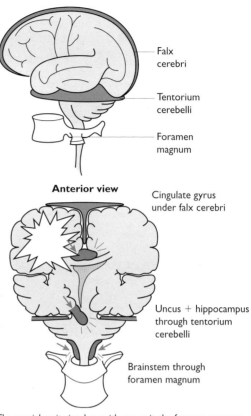

The cranial cavity is a box with one exit, the foramen magnum, and three interconnecting compartments divided by firm sheets of dura mater, the falx cerebri and the tentorium cerebelli. Increased pressure in one compartment causes brain tissue to be herniated under or through these structures. Death is caused by compression of, or secondary haemorrhage into, the brainstem and damage to the vital control centres, such as that governing respiration.

Figure 8.19 Sites of herniation in the brain

Prevention of stroke is improving, with the most important factor being the strict control of hypertension. Recently, an angiotensin-converting enzyme inhibitor (Ramipril) has been shown to decrease the risk of stroke and TIA in high-risk patients independently of any effect on blood pressure. As well as aiming to reduce the incidence of stroke, it is also important to limit the severity and permanent disability that may result and this appears improved by the combination of controlling hypertension and adding ACE inhibitors.

That brings us to the end of this section on circulatory disorders. We started with the words of William Harvey, conveying his despair at trying to understand the physiology of the motions of the heart. Physiology and pathology are of fundamental importance in clinical medicine and the words of Sir William Osler, perhaps the greatest physician of recent times, provide an appropriate ending:

A man cannot become a competent surgeon without the full knowledge of human anatomy and physiology, and the physician without physiology and chemistry flounders along in an aimless fashion, never able to gain any accurate conception of disease, practising a sort of popgun pharmacy, hitting now the malady and again the patient, he himself not knowing which.

Sir William Osler (1849–1919)

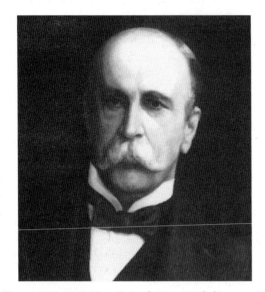

Figure 8.20 Sir William Osler (1849–1919) (Courtesy of Wellcome Institute for the History of Medicine)

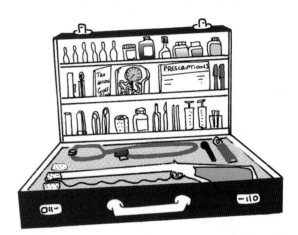

'Popgun pharmacy, hitting now the malady and again the patient. Sir William Osler'

Clinicopathological case study – circulatory failure

Clinical

A 65-year-old man complains of transient loss of vision in his right eye. He had two episodes in the previous month, each lasting for approximately 7–10 minutes. Two months ago, he also had transient slurring of his speech.

Examination:
Blood pressure 180/110.
Displaced apex beat and ejection systolic murmur.

Carotid bruits present.

No peripheral pulses palpable below the femorals.

Chest X-ray confirmed cardiomegaly but with no evidence of pulmonary oedema.

An ECG showed atrial fibrillation and features of an old anterior infarction.

An echocardiogram demonstrated thrombus within the left atrium.

Carotid doppler studies indicated moderate carotid artery stenosis.

Urine analysis: no glucose detected

Blood tests: Serial cardiac enzymes: normal

Urea and creatinine: slightly raised

Management and progress:
It was decided that he should be treated with antihypertensive agents to reduce his blood pressure and anticoagulants to reduce the risk of further thrombosis/embolism. However, within 24 hours he developed a right-sided weakness with hemiplegia and a right extensor plantar response. He died without regaining consciousness.

Pathological

Transient loss of vision or speech with full recovery is called a transient ischaemic attack. Generally it results from an embolus lodging in a small cerebral vessel and then being displaced or lysed. The commonest sites of origin are the heart or the carotid vessels.

He is hypertensive with an enlarged heart; i.e. left ventricular hypertrophy in response to increased workload.

The bruits indicate turbulent flow which is a result of stenosis and/or irregularities of the vessel wall due to atheroma.

Absent peripheral pulses indicate widespread arteriosclerotic disease.

The presence of pulmonary oedema would have indicated cardiac failure.

In atrial fibrillation, atria do not contract.

The resultant stagnation of blood predisposes to thrombus formation. Thrombus within the left atrium can be thrown into the systemic circulation. These can pass through the carotids to lodge in the cerebral vessels.

Dopplers detect turbulent flow. It is the electronic equivalent of the bruit.

A simple test for diabetes. Diabetics are at high risk of atheroma and may also suffer from sudden temporary loss of consciousness.

Test for myocardial infarction.

Mild renal impairment probably due to hypertension and atheroma.

The signs are of upper motor neuron damage involving the motor and sensory pathways with loss of consciousness. He has sustained a large left-sided cerebrovascular accident. The neural pathways cross, hence left-sided lesions give right-sided signs.

Postmortem findings:
Cardiovascular system – Left ventricular hypertrophy. Atheroma in all three coronary arteries with an old anterior infarction. No evidence of recent infarct and no vegetations. A small amount of thrombus present in the left atrium. Extensive atheroma in aorta and carotids with narrowing of the mouth of the renal arteries.
Central nervous system – A large haematoma in the region of the left internal capsule. Extensive atheroma in the cerebral vessels.
Genito-urinary tract – Small scarred kidneys showing ischaemic damage.
Clinically the stoke could have been due to an embolus but, in his case, it was a result of rupture of a microaneurysm on the lenticulostriate branch of the middle cerebral artery, due to hypertension. These are called Charcot–Bouchard aneurysms.

QUESTIONS

What are the causes and effects of vascular occlusion?

- Describe the clinical scenarios (i.e. type of patient most commonly affected and their symptoms and signs) for deep vein thrombosis, pulmonary embolism, heart attack and ischaemic stroke (pages 146 and 157; Figs 6.6, 6.7, 7.1 and 7.3).
- Explain the factors influencing thrombus formation, different types of emboli and stable and unstable atheromatous plaques (page 146; Fig. 7.4; page 161).

How are bleeding and clotting mechanisms kept in balance?

- Describe the vessel wall elements and blood constituents involved in producing and dissolving thrombus (Figs 6.2–4).
- Explain how these are altered in diseases (e.g. haemophilia) or by drugs (page 152).
- Mention disseminated intravascular coagulation (DIC) as a disease due to a loss of this homeostasis (Fig. 6.14).

Which atheromatous plaques are most likely to cause clinical problems?

- Describe the structure of an atheromatous plaque and the changes which increase the risk of plaque rupture (pages 167 and 168; Figs 7.4 and 7.7).
- Mention the influence of diet and drugs on lipid composition (pages 171–2; Figs 7.9 and 7.10).
- Discuss the impact of local arterial anatomy (e.g. endarteries and collateral system), regional MI, circle of Willis, etc. (Figs 6.11, 6.12, 8.4 and 8.17).

What are the causes, signs and symptoms of anaemia?

- Describe the causes under the headings of reduced red cell production, increased red cell destruction, abnormal haemoglobin and bleeding (page 193; Tables 8.1, 8.3–5).
- Signs and symptoms are listed on page 203 (see Figs 8.13 and 8.14).

What mechanisms operate in hypertension and what are the most significant complications?

- Describe primary and secondary hypertension, the mediators influencing vascular tone and the therapeutic options for treating hypertension (pages 178 and 179; Table 7.2; Fig. 7.11).
- The most significant complications are aneurysms, atherosclerosis and left ventricular failure (page 181; Figs 7.12, 7.15, 7.16).

FURTHER READING

Blann, A.D., Landray, M.J. and Lip, G.Y.H. (2002) Clinical review – ABC of antithrombotic therapy – An overview of antithrombotic therapy. *British Medical Journal* **325**, 762–5.

Pocock, S.J., McCormack, V., Gueyffier, F. *et al.* (2001) A score for predicting risk of death from cardiovascular disease in adults with raised blood pressure, based on individual patient data from randomised controlled trials. *British Medical Journal* **323**, 75–81.

Turpie, A.G.G., Chin, B.S.P. and Lip, G.Y.H. (2002) Clinical review – ABC of antithrombotic therapy – Venous thromboembolism: pathophysiology, clinical features, and prevention. *British Medical Journal* **325**, 887–90.

Underwood, J.C.E. (2000) *General and Systematic Pathology*, 3rd edition. Churchill Livingstone, London.

Weissberg, P.L. (2000) Atherogenesis: current understanding of the causes of atheroma. *Heart* **83**, 247–52.

Woolf, N. (1998a) Cardiovascular system. In: *Pathology: Basic and Systemic*, ch. 32, pp. 327–55. W.B. Saunders, Philadelphia.

Woolf, N. (1998b) Disorders of blood flow. In: *Pathology: Basic and Systemic*, ch. 18, pp. 198–217. W.B. Saunders, Philadelphia.

PART 4
Disorders of Cell Growth

Introduction

Does early death come
As a punishment?
Or
Does it come too late,
For those who are tortured
By incurable pain?
Is death really cruel?
Or
Is it merciful?
Gitanjali (1961–1977)

Gitanjali, as beautiful as the famous poem by Rabindranath Tagore (page 275), died at the age of 16 of cancer. To many people, cancer is a disease that appears suddenly, takes a tight grip, progresses relentlessly and causes a slow and painful death.

In 1731, Lorenz Heister, a German surgeon wrote, 'The name *Scirrhus* is given to a painless tumour that occurs in all parts of the body, but especially in the glands, and is due to stagnation and drying of the blood in the hardened part. … When a schirrus is not reabsorbed, cannot be arrested, or is not removed by time, it either spontaneously or from maltreatment becomes malignant, that is, painful and inflamed, and then we begin to call it *cancer* or *carcinoma*; at the same time the veins swell up and distend like the feet of a crab (but this does not happen in all cases), whence the disease gets its name; it is in fact, one of the worst, most horrible, and most painful of diseases.'

Is this pessimism really justified?

There are two facts that we all tend to forget. Everything that comes to life dies – death is an integral part of life. Secondly, we have created a world that is fearful of death and the word 'pain' is seldom far from the word 'death'. Yet here are some facts – about 20 per cent of people will die of cancer, which is less than the number dying from cardiovascular disease (approximately 30 per cent), but heart disease does not usually generate such intense dread.

Interesting? Could it be that death from cancer is 'unfair' and therefore painful but death from a heart attack is self-induced by overeating and smoking and therefore 'deserved'?

A BRIEF HISTORY OF CANCER

Johannes Müller, a German microscopist, established that tumours were made of cells (1883). This laid the foundation for his pupil, Rudolf Virchow, who divided tumours into 'homologous' and 'heterologous'. The homologous group resulted from proliferation of cells already present and were generally benign, while the heterologous group showed a change in the character of the cell and were generally malignant. Virchow, however, failed to recognize the mechanism of metastasis which was later described by Billroth (1856) and von Recklinhausen (1883). Many investigators have looked for causes of cancer. One of the most famous was Percival Pott who, in 1775, identified that scrotal cancer in chimney sweeps was related to chronic contact with soot. Occupational exposure to industrial tar and paraffin was recognized by von Volkmann in 1875 as causing cancers and many such associations have since been described.

Recently, advances in molecular and cell biology techniques have facilitated the investigation of these associations at the level of genetic material. We are now in a position to attempt to answer some of the fundamental questions relating to the control of normal growth and differentiation and how these mechanisms go wrong in the process of neoplasia.

In this section, we consider the benign disorders of cell growth and the premalignant changes that are clues of early cancer and are important in screening programmes. We will go on to look at the symptoms that occur in cancer, how it is diagnosed and which features are important for prognosis and treatment. Then we will turn to the aetiology (causes of cancer) and the pathogenesis (natural history) of tumours, and finally, how they behave and what treatments are available. Perhaps at the end, you will be able to ask yourself again whether our views about cancer, about death and about pain are justified.

CHAPTER 9
Benign growth disorders

Cells have to adapt to any changes in nutrient supply or workload in order to survive and continue performing their cellular function (i.e. to maintain homoeostasis). These adaptations take place at both the cellular and subcellular levels. We will discuss these adaptations with an emphasis on the changes that are important in pathology, and we will consider the clinical situations in which they are encountered. The changes that we will discuss are: hyperplasia, hypertrophy, atrophy, metaplasia and dysplasia and benign neoplasms.

CLINICAL CASE – PROSTATIC HYPERPLASIA

A 70-year-old man visited the urology clinic complaining of difficulty with micturition. He passed urine 15–20 times per day and several times during the night (nocturia). The stream of urine was poor and he found that on some occasions it dribbled. The urologist detected an enlarged prostate on rectal examination and the patient had part of his prostate removed to improve the flow.

Some of you may be wondering why an enlarged prostate obstructing urine flow through the urethra should result in increased urinary frequency. The reason (as indicated in Fig. 9.1) is that the enlarged median lobe protrudes into the bladder to produce a dam behind which some urine stagnates. This means that after micturition there is still urine in the bladder and the patient feels the urge to pass urine again. The stagnant urine is also prone to infection or stone formation. The poor urine flow is due to narrowing of the prostatic urethra and the 'ball valve' effect of the median lobe pressing forward on the urethral orifice.

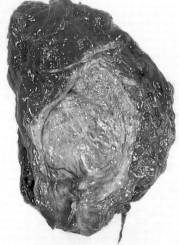

Figure 9.1 Macroscopic specimen with prostatic hyperplasia and bladder showing numerous trabeculae due to urinary obstruction by a nodular enlarged prostate

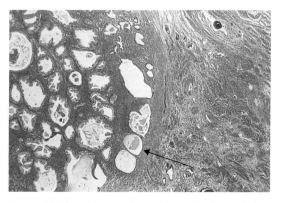

Figure 9.2 Photomicrograph showing nodular hyperplasia of the prostate

HYPERPLASIA AND HYPERTROPHY

Hyperplasia is defined as an increase in the **number** of cells in an organ or tissue, while hypertrophy is an increase in cell size. Often the two coexist in a tissue because some cell types are incapable of division and so must increase their size (hypertrophy) to cope with any extra work, while other cells can proliferate to share their additional work (hyperplasia). In Chapter 4 (page 114), we noted that cardiac and skeletal muscle and nerve cells are unable to replicate, whereas epithelial cells and fibroblasts can. Smooth muscle cells can respond by a combination of hyperplasia and hypertrophy. This means that in the prostate the glandular epithelium and the fibroblastic stroma will show hyperplasia and the smooth muscle is hypertrophic and hyperplastic. Why should the prostate enlarge with age, since its workload does not increase? Presumably there is an overreaction to years of androgen stimulation, but nobody really knows.

When the hypertrophy or hyperplasia is useful, i.e. it allows the organ to cope with extra work, it is called **physiological**. If the enlargement does not appear to serve a purpose, then it is termed **pathological**. Thus the prostatic changes would be pathological. **Physiological hyperplasia and hypertrophy** may be mediated through hormonal changes or growth factors. Pregnancy is an example of hormone- induced hyperplasia and hypertrophy that allows an organ the size of a pear to enlarge to accommodate a full-term baby and prepares the breasts for lactation. The smooth muscle cells of the uterus enlarge (hypertrophy and hyperplasia) ready for the work of pushing the baby into the world (aptly named 'labour') and the number of glandular milk-producing cells in the breast increases (hyperplasia).

A fascinating example of physiological hyperplasia that occurs in the body is the regeneration of the liver following partial hepatectomy (Fig. 9.3), as illustrated in the Greek myth about the fate that

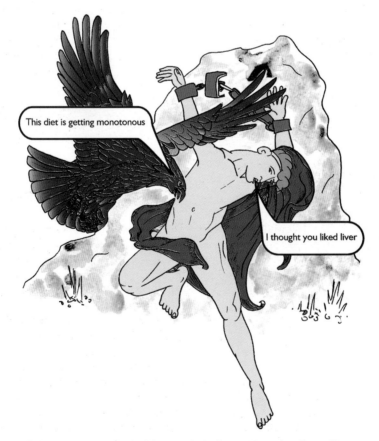

Figure 9.3 The Ancient Greeks appreciated the body's capacity for liver regeneration. Prometheus was punished by Zeus for bringing fire to humanity. Every night for years his liver was torn at by a vulture

befell Prometheus. The mighty Zeus, enraged that he had stolen fire from the Gods, had Prometheus chained naked to a pillar in the Caucasian mountains, where a vulture tore at his liver all day, year in, year out. Of course there was no end to his pain because the liver grew back each night! It is not recommended that you try this experiment on your colleagues.

The evidence suggests that when the liver is damaged, the remaining liver cells produce a growth factor called transforming growth factor alpha, which causes an increase in mitotic activity and hence an increase in the cell number. What is remarkable is that it knows when to stop! It is believed that a growth inhibitor, transforming growth factor beta, is involved in this process. The ancient Greeks had remarkable insights into the body's capacity to regenerate.

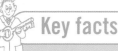

Key facts

Examples of hyperplasia and hypertrophy and their causative factors

- Hypertrophy of myocardium due to hypertension

- Skeletal muscular hypertrophy due to exercise

- Red cell hyperplasia in bone marrow secondary to low atmospheric oxygen (living at high altitude)

- Uterine hyperplasia/hypertrophy secondary to hormonal changes of pregnancy

- Hyperplasia of epidermis and connective tissue due to release of growth factors to aid wound healing

ATROPHY

Atrophy is defined as a decrease in cell size and/or cell number. Surplus cells are lost through the process of apoptosis described in Chapter 1. Strictly speaking, the reduction in cell numbers is called involution. Since this is part of normal development, it is termed physiological atrophy and the classic example is the involution of the thymus gland during development. It is distinguished from pathological atrophy, which results from an abnormal state. An example of pathological atrophy is the severe muscle wasting that may follow an episode of poliomyelitis or the muscle wasting that is commonly observed in limbs immobilized in plaster following a fracture.

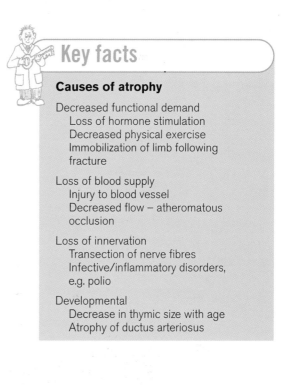

Key facts

Causes of atrophy

Decreased functional demand
　Loss of hormone stimulation
　Decreased physical exercise
　Immobilization of limb following
　fracture

Loss of blood supply
　Injury to blood vessel
　Decreased flow – atheromatous
　occlusion

Loss of innervation
　Transection of nerve fibres
　Infective/inflammatory disorders,
　e.g. polio

Developmental
　Decrease in thymic size with age
　Atrophy of ductus arteriosus

METAPLASIA AND DYSPLASIA

The uterine cervix serves as a useful model for this discussion of metaplasia and dysplasia. The changes in the cervix are now well documented because of the national programme designed to screen women of reproductive age to detect early changes associated with cancer. Screening involves scraping some cells from the junctional zone of the cervix using a spatula. These are spread onto a glass slide, fixed and stained by the Papanicolaou technique.

The cervix has a transitional zone between the squamous epithelium of the ectocervix and the columnar epithelium of the endocervix. If there is chronic inflammation of the cervix, the columnar epithelium may be replaced by squamous epithelium – so-called squamous metaplasia. Metaplasia is the conversion of one type of differentiated tissue

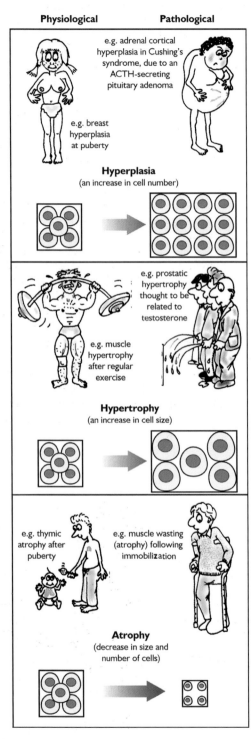

Figure 9.4 Hyperplasia, hypertrophy and atrophy may represent physiological responses to normal development or a pathological change in response to a disease process

into another type of differentiated tissue. This is most common in epithelial tissue although it can occur in other types of tissues such as mesenchymal tissues. In general, metaplasia is a response to chronic irritation and is a form of adaptation which involves, for example, replacing a specialized glandular or respiratory epithelium with a more hardy squamous epithelium.

Metaplasia is benign and reversible but its importance lies in the fact that the stimulants and irritants causing it may persist and play a role in carcinogenesis.

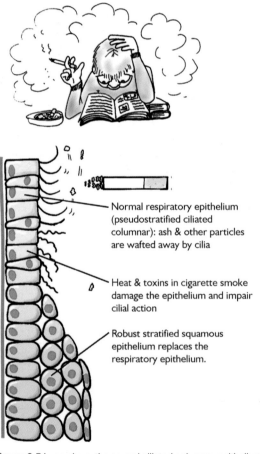

Figure 9.5 In smokers, the normal ciliated columnar epithelium lining the bronchus undergoes metaplasia to stratified squamous epithelium. This confers greater protection against heat damage. Metaplasia is reversible if the stimulus is removed. Metaplasia is not a premalignant condition, but areas in which metaplasia occurs are at increased risk of developing dysplasia, which *is* premalignant. In this example, carcinogens in the cigarette smoke may induce mutations in the exposed, rapidly dividing epithelial cells

The exfoliated cervical cells may show dysplasia, which is more worrying because it is a step on the road to an invasive tumour. The term dysplasia was originally used to mean an abnormality of development. Unfortunately, it is a term that is used too loosely and this causes confusion. In pathology reports concerning the microscopy of tissues, dysplasia refers to a combination of abnormal cytological appearances and abnormal tissue architecture. Its importance lies in its precancerous association. However, the term is still used to describe some gross abnormalities of development encountered in neonatal pathology, such as renal dysplasia and broncho-pulmonary dysplasia, which have no pre-cancerous association.

Dysplasia in the cervical squamous epithelium involves an increased cell size, nuclear pleomorphism (variation in size and shape), hyperchromatism (increased blueness due to abnormal chromatin), loss of orientation of the cells so that they are arranged rather haphazardly and abnormally sited mitotic activity (Fig. 9.8). These appearances are the same as those described in malignant change but they differ in *extent*. When the full thickness of the epithelium is involved, it can be called 'carcinoma *in situ*' while involvement of only the lower third is 'mild dysplasia'. Many pathologists and clinicians felt that it was inappropriate to have different names for the various stages and so the term 'cervical intraepithelial neoplasia' (CIN) was introduced. CIN I is the equivalent of mild dysplasia and describes abnormalities affecting the lower third of the epithelium, CIN II (replacing moderate dysplasia) is used for changes reaching the middle third, and CIN III (replacing severe dysplasia or carcinoma *in situ*) refers to full-thickness involvement.

Similar terminology can be used for changes in the squamous epithelium of the vulva (VIN) and larynx (LIN), although glandular epithelial changes (e.g. stomach or large bowel) are usually subdivided into mild, moderate or severe dysplasia.

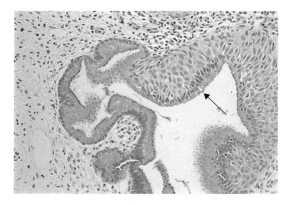

Figure 9.6 Photomicrograph showing squamous metaplasia of endocervical glands

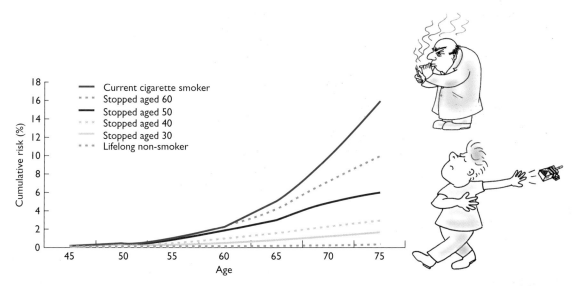

Figure 9.7 Effects of stopping smoking at various ages on the cumulative risk (%) of death from lung cancer by age 75 (© Cancer Research Campaign 2001)

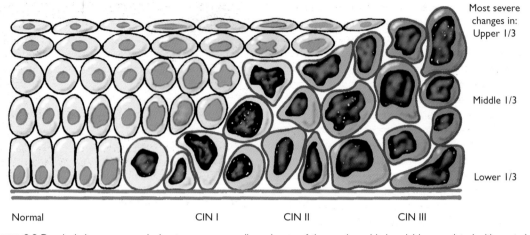

Most severe changes in:
Upper 1/3

Middle 1/3

Lower 1/3

Normal   CIN I   CIN II   CIN III

Figure 9.8 Dysplasia is a precursor lesion to squamous cell carcinoma of the cervix and is invariably associated with wart virus (human papillomavirus) infection. Warty change is called 'koilocytosis' and is visible microscopically as a halo effect around the nucleus, which appears spiky. Dysplasia is classified as CIN I, II or III (cervical intraepithelial neoplasia), depending on the degree of nuclear atypia seen. Nuclear atypical changes predominate in the lower one-third of the epithelium in CIN I and throughout all layers in CIN III. CIN III carries a very much higher risk of progression to cancer than CIN I or II

A potential problem with the terminology is that it implies a biological continuum from low-grade (CIN I) to high-grade lesions (CIN III), which may not be true. In some organ systems such as breast, it is clear that in most cases, high-grade *in situ* carcinoma does not develop from low-grade *in situ* carcinoma.

It should not be assumed that dysplasia is irreversible. It is believed that early stages of dysplasia may revert to normal if the stimulus is removed. However, severe dysplasia will often progress to cancer if left untreated and, for this reason, it is sometimes referred to as carcinoma *in situ*. If severe dysplasia is cancer confined to the epithelium, what are moderate and mild dysplasia? This is a good question and without a 'correct' answer. In practice, severe dysplasia is treated as a favourable type of cancer, while milder degrees of dysplasia can be managed slightly less aggressively but followed to ensure that they do not progress to more severe disease.

The concept of dysplasia fits with our current multistep theory of neoplasia (page 256) in that it represents a stage between benign hyperplastic proliferation and overt cancer. The concept of dysplasia as a cancer in its early stages has also led to the institution of screening programmes for cervical and breast carcinoma. The logic behind this is that if

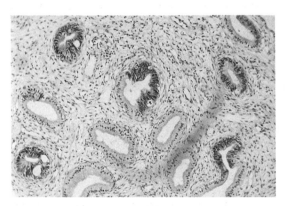

Figure 9.9 Dysplasia involving endocervical glands

dysplastic changes precede carcinoma by several months or years and patients with dysplasia can be identified and treated, we can reduce the death toll from that cancer. Obviously, deaths from that cancer must be fairly common to make this worthwhile and we must be confident that the 'at risk' group are being screened sufficiently often to detect the early changes. For example, if the progression from CIN II to invasive tumour took only 1 year, then it would be of limited value to screen patients every 3 years.

Much of the interest in genetic and immunocytochemical markers of malignancy lies in the hope that we will be able to detect ever earlier precancerous changes to increase the potential benefits of such screening programmes. Whether these screening programmes really save lives is a moot point. There is little doubt that they have had a modest effect on mortality and also have led to an improvement in the quality of radiological, pathological and clinical services. It is still a matter of hot debate as to whether the money spent is cost-effective. You must bear in mind that finding a lesion in its earliest stage when it may not progress for 30 or more years is not necessarily doing the patient a favour. This is an important health issue and worth thinking about and discussing with your colleagues. What would you do if you were the Minister of Health?

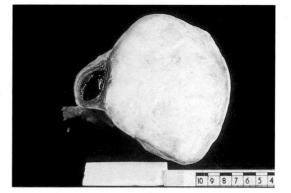

Figure 9.10 Benign leiomyoma

BENIGN NEOPLASMS

A neoplasm is defined as a new and abnormal growth, and particularly one in which the cell division is uncontrolled and progressive. Neoplasms may be benign or malignant. We will deal with malignant neoplasms in the next chapter. A benign neoplasm, such as an adenoma in the colon, is an uncontrolled focal proliferation of well-differentiated cells, which does not invade or metastasize. Unfortunately, the term is sometimes used inaccurately and some tumours do not quite fulfil these criteria, but it will serve as a working definition. Although benign, these tumours can cause many clinical problems as discussed in the section on the local effects of tumours (page 264). One of the most common benign tumours necessitating removal is the leiomyoma (fibroid) of the uterine myometrium (Fig. 9.10), which may contribute to heavy and painful menstruation. Benign melanocytic tumours of the skin are removed for cosmetic reasons or for fear of malignant change (Fig. 9.11). Endocrine tumours are generally benign but can cause dramatic systemic problems through excessive production of hormones (Fig. 9.12) and some 'benign' intracranial tumours like meningiomas can kill the patient because the skull cannot stretch to accommodate the 'benign' expansion. Remember that something which is 'benign' to the pathologist may appear 'malignant' to the patient!

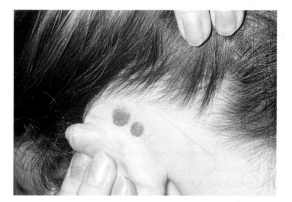

Figure 9.11 Benign naevi

Key facts

Hyperplasia and hypertrophy versus benign neoplasms

The difference between a benign neoplasm and hypertrophy/hyperplasia is that the neoplasm, by definition, exhibits uncontrolled cell proliferation. This is unlike hyperplasia and hypertrophy, in which the growth, either due to increase in cell numbers or cell size, is a response to a stimulus, and removal of this stimulus results in regression.

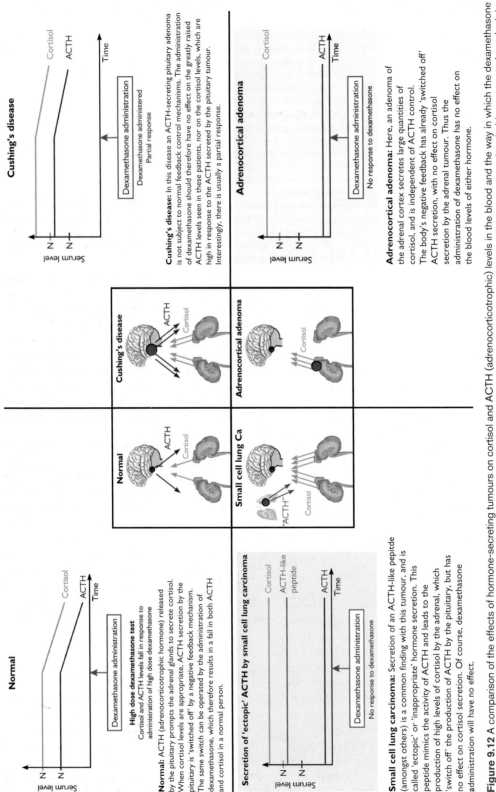

Normal

High dose dexamethasone test

Cortisol and ACTH levels fall in response to administration of high dose dexamethasone

Normal: ACTH (adrenocorticotrophic hormone) released by the pituitary prompts the adrenal glands to secrete cortisol. When cortisol levels are appropriate, ACTH secretion by the pituitary is 'switched off' by a negative feedback mechanism. The same switch can be operated by the administration of dexamethasone, which therefore results in a fall in both ACTH and cortisol in a normal person.

Cushing's disease

Dexamethasone administration

Dexamethasone administered

Partial response

Cushing's disease: In this disease an ACTH-secreting pituitary adenoma is not subject to normal feedback control mechanisms. The administration of dexamethasone should therefore have no effect on the greatly raised ACTH levels seen in these patients, nor on the cortisol levels, which are high in response to the ACTH secreted by the pituitary tumour. Interestingly, there is usually a partial response.

Secretion of 'ectopic' ACTH by small cell lung carcinoma

Dexamethasone administration

No response to dexamethasone

Small cell lung carcinoma: Secretion of an ACTH-like peptide (amongst others) is a common finding with this tumour, and is called 'ectopic' or 'inappropriate' hormone secretion. This peptide mimics the activity of ACTH and leads to the production of high levels of cortisol by the adrenal, which 'switch off' the production of ACTH by the pituitary, but has no effect on cortisol secretion. Of course, dexamethasone administration will have no effect.

Adrenocortical adenoma

Dexamethasone administration

No response to dexamethasone

Adrenocortical adenoma: Here, an adenoma of the adrenal cortex secretes large quantities of cortisol, and is independent of ACTH control. The body's negative feedback has already 'switched off' ACTH secretion, with no effect on cortisol secretion by the adrenal tumour. Thus the administration of dexamethasone has no effect on the blood levels of either hormone.

Figure 9.12 A comparison of the effects of hormone-secreting tumours on cortisol and ACTH (adrenocorticotrophic) levels in the blood and the way in which the dexamethasone test can help to distinguish between the causative lesions. Adenoma, benign glandular tumour; small cell lung carcinoma, malignant tumour of probable neuroectodermal origin

CHAPTER 10

Malignant neoplasms

CLINICAL CASE – BREAST LUMP

A 50-year-old woman presented to her family doctor with a lump in her left breast. She had noticed a recent enlargement in its size but the mass was not painful. She had no other medical problems but she had a positive family history, her mother having died of breast cancer 5 years previously. She had two daughters aged 27 and 25 years, who were both well.

The doctor could feel a 2-cm-diameter mass below the nipple in her left breast. This was hard, poorly defined and caused dimpling of the overlying skin. It was also fixed to the underlying tissues. The nipple and areola on that side had an eczematous appearance but the right breast and nipple were normal. No enlarged lymph nodes could be found in either axilla or supraclavicular fossa and there were no abnormalities in the rest of the body. The doctor suspected that this was a malignant tumour and so referred her to hospital for further investigation.

But why did the family doctor consider that this mass was malignant?

CLINICAL FEATURES OF MALIGNANT TUMOURS

It should be stressed that it was not a single criterion but a combination of factors that allowed the doctor to draw such a conclusion. In this case the lump was ill-defined, hard and involved adjacent tissues and skin. A characteristic feature of malignant tumours is that tongues of cancer cells infiltrate surrounding tissues, whereas benign tumours tend to grow with a smooth pushing edge. Thus while benign lumps are generally mobile, malignant tumours are often fixed relative to the surrounding structures. Many malignant tumours induce a proliferation of benign fibroblasts which produce dense collagenous connective tissue. This reaction is termed desmoplasia and gives the tumour its hard texture.

The lesion was bigger than most benign lesions, although size is a variable feature. More importantly, there was a recent rapid increase in size, which often indicates malignant growth. In this example, there was one other important clue for the doctor which is a peculiarity of some breast cancers. The 'eczema' that was noted over the nipple is referred to as Paget's disease of the nipple. This is caused by carcinoma cells growing along the breast ducts towards the nipple and then into the epidermis of the skin.

Two other factors, had they been present, would have influenced the doctor: these are pain and the presence of metastasis. Many tumours, both benign and malignant, are painless, but the presence of unremitting pain is suggestive of malignancy. The presence of metastatic disease is the definitive evidence that a tumour is malignant and it is important to understand possible routes of spread in order that the most likely sites for metastasis can be examined carefully. In this patient's case, there was no pain or evidence of metastatic tumour spread, so the doctor suspected that it was a localized malignant growth.

Evaluation in hospital

The patient was referred to hospital, where a series of tests were performed to make a more precise diagnosis and to assess the extent of her disease. Tests included haematological and biochemical blood tests to look for anaemia and changes in liver function which might suggest metastases to bone marrow and liver, mammography (X-ray of

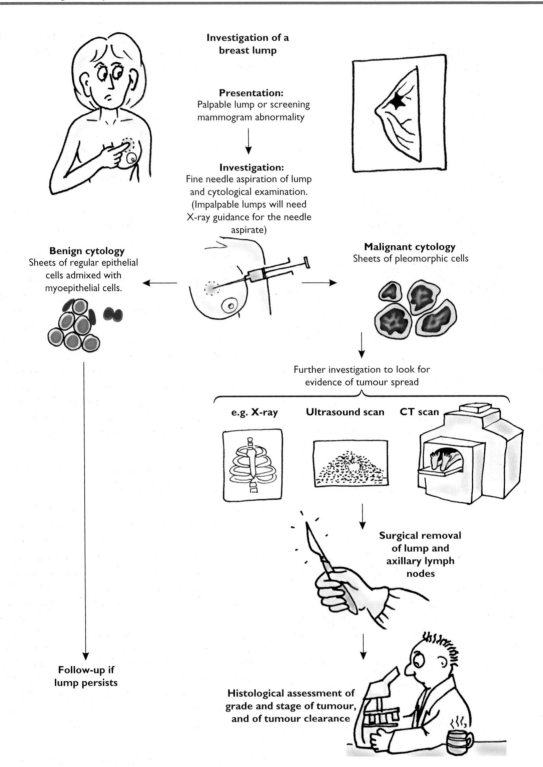

Figure 10.1 Investigation of a patient with a breast lump

In a case such as this the surgeon must make a definite diagnosis by obtaining some tissue from the breast lump. Various options are available:

- Fine needle aspiration (FNA) cytology – a needle is inserted attached to a syringe to suck out some cells for examination
- Trucut biopsy – a special biopsy needle is used to ream out a core of tumour about 3 mm wide and 10–15 mm long
- Excision biopsy – the patient is anaesthetized and part of the lump removed
- Wide local excision or mastectomy – the patient is anaesthetized and the whole lump removed.

In this particular case the surgeon opted for FNA cytology, which showed malignant cells.

Many centres use this type of 'triple approach' of clinical evaluation, radiology (mammography) and FNA cytology in the initial evaluation of patients. Since all three investigations were positive, the surgeon went on to excise the lump and sample the axillary lymph nodes. In due course, the surgeon received the pathologist's report on these tissues and used that information to guide the management of the patient. The report is reproduced below and we shall discuss its relevance for patient management and some points it raises about the biology of tumours.

What are the macroscopical features that distinguish malignant tumours?

Let us consider this report in more detail. First, there is the gross appearance that records points similar to the criteria used clinically by the family practitioner and surgeon for distinguishing malignant from benign lumps. This includes the size, the infiltrating margin and the consistency of the tumour. Other features include the presence or absence of necrosis and haemorrhage. Most importantly, there is an assessment of excision margins, since incomplete excision will result in rapid recurrence and increased opportunity for spread. The report of the microscopical appearances records the pathologist's conclusion, i.e. that it is a primary malignant tumour of breast tissue. Let us consider how this conclusion has been reached.

What are the microscopical features that distinguish malignant tumours?

Malignant tissues differ from benign tissues in that individual cells have an abnormal appearance and

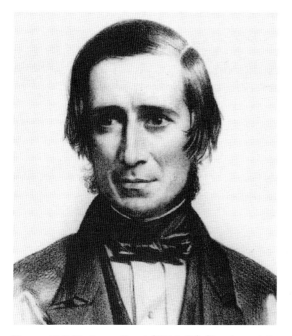

Figure 10.2 Sir James Paget (1814–99) (Courtesy of the Wellcome Institute for the History of Medicine) James Paget was born in Yarmouth, Norfolk. He was apprenticed to a surgeon at the local hospital at the age of 16 and enrolled as a medical student at St Bartholomew's Hospital, London at the age of 20 years. In 1837, a year after obtaining his MRCS, he was appointed Curator of the museum at the hospital. Paget was an excellent clinical observer and an eloquent lecturer. He is best remembered for his descriptions of Paget's disease of bone (osteitis deformans) and Paget's disease of the nipple. He was elected FRS (1851) and Surgeon Extraordinary to Queen Victoria (1858). He was created a Baronet in 1871

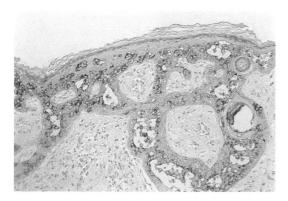

Figure 10.3 Photomicrograph of nipple stained with epithelial membrane antigen (EMA) showing tumour cells (red) within the epidermis

the breast), a chest X-ray and bone scan to look for tumour spread. The mammography showed a 2-cm spiculated mass with linear calcification. The rest of her investigations were unremarkable.

Pathology report

Name: Ida Hopps
Age: 50 years
Ward: Thompson
Consultant: I M Surgeon
Specimen: Wide local excision and axillary dissection
Date of operation: 12.11.02

Macroscopical appearance:
A wide local excision specimen, weighing 80 g. It consists of skin, including nipple, which measures 50 × 10 mm and covers fatty tissue with maximum dimension of 80 mm. In the tissue beneath the nipple, there is a pale, firm, gritty mass measuring 25 × 20 × 20 mm, which has an irregular, poorly defined margin. The closest excision margin (deep) is 5 mm from the mass. There is an area of erythema around the nipple. The axillary dissection measures 80 × 50 × 50 mm and 13 lymph nodes have been identified.

Microscopical appearance:
Sections show high-nuclear grade ductal carcinoma *in situ* of comedo type with coarse microcalcification. There is also an invasive adenocarcinoma of ductal type, Grade II, exhibiting a moderate amount of tubule formation, moderate nuclear pleomorphism and 5 mitoses/10 hpf. The maximum tumour dimension is 22 mm. There is no evidence of lymphatic or vascular permeation and both the *in situ* and invasive carcinoma are completely excised by 5 mm (deep margin). The sections of the nipple confirm the presence of Paget's disease. None of the 13 axillary lymph nodes contains tumour.

Both oestrogen and progesterone receptor status is positive (ER⁺, PR⁺) and Her-2 staining is negative.

Conclusion:
Left breast: *in situ* and invasive ductal carcinoma grade II, 22 mm (T2)
complete excision
ER⁺, PR⁺, Her-2⁻

Reported by Dr S P Ecimen

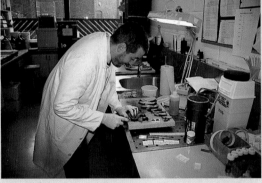

Figure 10.4 Gross examination of mastectomy specimen

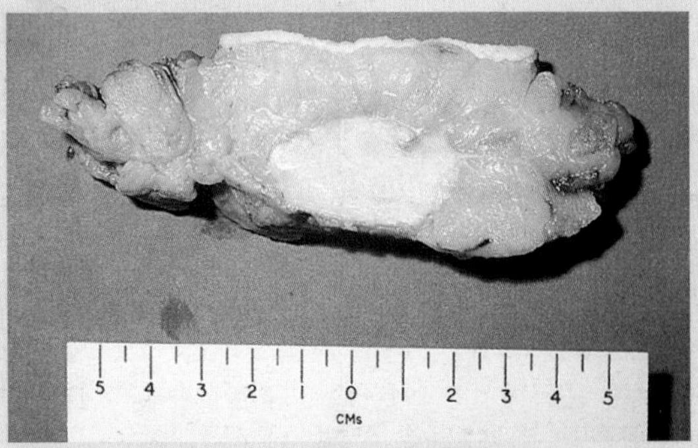

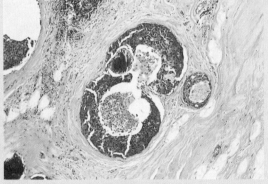

Figure 10.6 *In situ* ductal carcinoma with central necrosis and microcalcification

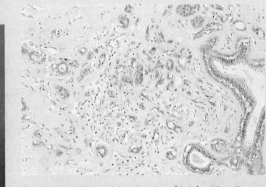

Figure 10.7 Normal breast duct (right) with adjacent tissue showing infiltration by moderately differentiated ductal carcinoma

Figure 10.5 Slice of lumpectomy specimen showing spiculated tumour close to the deep margin

their arrangement is deranged. The disordered growth pattern is easy to appreciate provided that you know the normal histological appearance of that tissue. Within the breast, the normal duct–lobular system is composed of an inner epithelial and an outer myoepithelial layer surrounded by basement membrane, which contrasts with the carcinoma shown in Fig. 10.11. A crucial factor, which is often

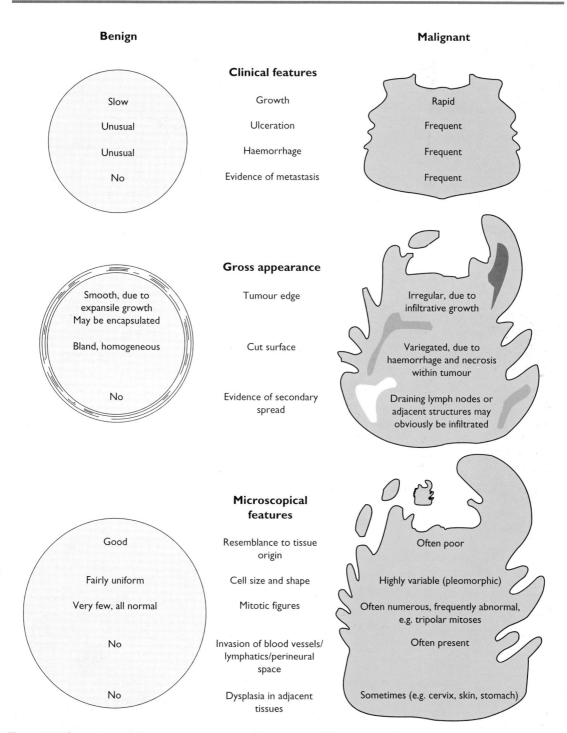

Benign   **Malignant**

Clinical features

Slow	Growth	Rapid
Unusual	Ulceration	Frequent
Unusual	Haemorrhage	Frequent
No	Evidence of metastasis	Frequent

Gross appearance

Smooth, due to expansile growth May be encapsulated | Tumour edge | Irregular, due to infiltrative growth

Bland, homogeneous | Cut surface | Variegated, due to haemorrhage and necrosis within tumour

No | Evidence of secondary spread | Draining lymph nodes or adjacent structures may obviously be infiltrated

Microscopical features

Good | Resemblance to tissue origin | Often poor

Fairly uniform | Cell size and shape | Highly variable (pleomorphic)

Very few, all normal | Mitotic figures | Often numerous, frequently abnormal, e.g. tripolar mitoses

No | Invasion of blood vessels/lymphatics/perineural space | Often present

No | Dysplasia in adjacent tissues | Sometimes (e.g. cervix, skin, stomach)

Figure 10.8 Comparison of clinical, gross and microscopical features of benign and malignant tumours

essential for diagnosing carcinoma, is that cells should have breached the basement membrane, which marks the boundary between epithelial and subepithelial tissues. Within the breast, it is possible to identify disordered growth that is still confined within the ducts – an *in situ* carcinoma.

An atypical appearance of individual cells (cytological atypia) is a rather more subtle change. The

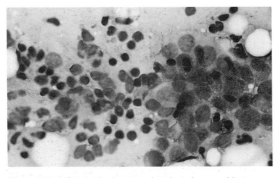

Figure 10.9 Cytological smear showing pleomorphic tumour cells admixed with smaller lymphoid cells

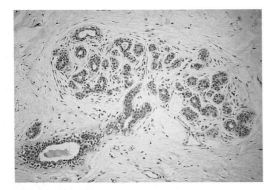

Figure 10.10 Normal terminal duct and lobule of breast

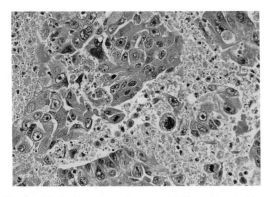

Figure 10.11 Breast carcinoma exhibiting pleomorphism, necrosis and mitotic activity

malignant cells do not only differ from normal cells but also from each other – this is called pleomorphism. Pleomorphism may involve both nucleus and cytoplasm. In practice, it often refers to the nucleus, which may be many times the size of a normal nucleus and may show marked variability in size and shape (nuclear pleomorphism). It may also have an altered distribution of chromatin and is a darker colour in stained sections (hyperchromatism). These alterations reflect the increased amount and abnormalities of nuclear chromatin, which is common in tumours as they are frequently aneuploid.

Dictionary box

Aneuploid: An abnormal number of chromosomes that is not an exact multiple of the haploid (23) number.

Most normal cells have a small single nucleolus. In malignant cells, there may be many nucleoli of varying sizes or, alternatively, a large single nucleolus. The position of the nucleus within the cell is often abnormal, i.e. it exhibits a loss of polarity. Thus, the nucleus of, for example, a normal colonic cell is situated at the cell's base with mucus in the cytoplasm nearer the surface, whereas the nucleus is more central in a malignant cell. There is also an increase in mitotic activity due to the increase in cell proliferation and abnormal mitotic figures may also be identified. The general appearance of the cells is altered as there is an increase in nuclear–cytoplasmic ratio, either because the amount of cytoplasm is less or the nucleus is larger or a combination of the two.

The cytoplasmic changes vary depending on the tissue but generally involve a loss of specialized features, for example, absence or reduction in mucin content in a colonic adenocarcinoma.

Ultimately, however, all of these features are only guidelines and the real test is whether the tumour behaves in a malignant fashion. Of course we cannot leave patients untreated just to see how the tumour behaves. Pathologists have learnt much about the behaviour of tumours from autopsy studies and, fortunately, tumours of similar appearance usually show similar behaviour in different patients.

Note that many of the features discussed here are same as those used for the assessment of dysplasia (page 218) and the distinction between grades of dysplasia and frank malignancy is based on both degree and extent of the changes.

WHAT FACTORS INFLUENCE PROGNOSIS?

Here we are concerned with factors that influence prognosis and that can be assessed routinely by histopathologists. The important aspects are:

- the type of tumour
- the grade of tumour
- the stage of the disease
- tumour markers.

First, it is essential to decide whether the tumour has arisen locally or whether it is a metastasis. Two points help make this distinction and these are whether there are precancerous changes or *in situ* carcinoma present and whether the lesion resembles tumours known to occur at that site.

In situ carcinoma is an alteration in the cytological appearance that is similar to that seen in malignant tumours but does not show any invasion through the basement membrane. If this tumour had been entirely *in situ* then it would have had an extremely good prognosis because the lack of local invasion would mean that the tumour had no ability to extend into lymphatic or blood vessels and no possibility of metastasis.

Precancerous lesions are harder to define but are changes (e.g. atypical hyperplasia) that have been shown in large studies to be associated with the subsequent development of cancer and are believed to represent an early, but possibly reversible, stage of malignancy.

To return to our patient; she has an adenocarcinoma which has *in situ* and invasive components. The *in situ* carcinoma tells us that it is locally arising. Therefore, this is a primary tumour of the breast. Within the breast, there are a large number of different subtypes and it is worth remembering that not only is cancer many diseases, but individual organs also have many different types of cancer. Our patient has a ductal carcinoma, which has a poorer prognosis than a mucinous carcinoma (Figs 10.12 and 10.13).

Although she has an invasive carcinoma, the tumour was not seen in lymphatic or blood vessels. The most important prognostic feature is the *type* of tumour but after that the prognosis is influenced by the grade and stage. The grade of a tumour depends on its histological appearance, while the stage of a tumour depends on its size and extent of spread. The histological grade is a crude measure of how much the tumour resembles normal tissue, combined with an estimate of its mitotic activity. There is a well-defined scoring system for breast tumours (Table 10.1), based on tubule formation, nuclear pleomorphism and the mitotic count. A tumour is given a score of 1 to 3 based on assessment

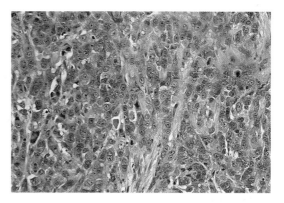

Figure 10.12 High-grade invasive ductal carcinoma

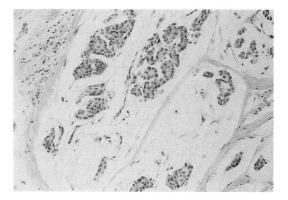

Figure 10.13 Invasive mucinous carcinoma of the breast

Table 10.1 Grading of breast cancer

	Score
Tubule formation	
Majority of tumour >75 per cent	1
Moderate amount 10–75 per cent	2
Little or none <10 per cent	3
Nuclear pleomorphism	
Mild	1
Moderate	2
Severe	3
Mitotic count – count per 10 high-powered fields – varies with type of lens	
0–5	1
6–10	2
>11	3
Total score	**Grade**
3–5	1
6–7	2
8–9	3

of each criterion and the scores are combined to determine the grade. Grade 1 tumours have a better prognosis than grade 3 tumours. Many sites have no formal grading system and so the pathologist will merely record whether the tumour is well-differentiated, moderately differentiated or poorly differentiated, by assessing similar features but in a less objective way.

The stage of a tumour is a measure of the extent of disease and depends on pathological, radiological and clinical information. A TNM staging system is often used for breast carcinoma, where T stands for size of primary tumour, N codes for regional node involvement and M for metastatic disease. Figure 10.14 illustrates the different pathological staging systems and its links with the TNM classification. This provides an easy shorthand for indicating the disease stage, which is helpful for deciding treatment and comparing the outcome of patients treated with new therapeutic regimens. Obviously, assessment of a new treatment regimen must take account of the stage of a patient's disease to avoid spurious results.

The pathology report on our patient states that none of the lymph nodes contained tumour and the clinical investigation did not show metastases. Therefore, she would be categorized as T2 (size 2.2 cm), N0, M0, which translates as stage II disease. This short coded message tells the doctor that she is in a relatively good prognostic group.

Immunohistochemical markers for tumour-associated gene(s) and gene products are sometimes carried out to help predict behaviour and decide on treatment options. Since the breast is an endocrine responsive organ and proliferates due to stimulation by oestrogen, breast cancers may express the oestrogen and progesterone receptors. Approximately 60–70 per cent of breast cancers will be ER and PR positive, and this not only gives a better prognostic index but also predicts for response to anti-oestrogenic treatment (e.g. tamoxifen). Her-2 is an oncogene (page 242) that is overexpressed in a quarter of breast cancers and is usually seen in high-grade cancers and predicts for a poorer prognosis. Recently, a monoclonal antibody (Herceptin) developed against the Her-2 receptor has shown promise in the treatment of advanced breast cancer.

When the doctor talks to the patient about these results, she may well ask a variety of questions about her prognosis, but before we attempt to answer those questions, we should digress to discuss the classification of tumours.

CLASSIFICATION OF TUMOURS

The pathological classification of tumours is illustrated in Fig. 10.15. You will recall that a knowledge of the normal structures at a particular site can be of great help in predicting the commonest tumours. In most organs, there is one particular type of malignant tumour that is more common than any other and this generally corresponds with the type of tissue proliferating at that site. The stomach and colon have active glandular epithelium, so the commonest malignant tumour at both sites is an adenocarcinoma, which is composed of malignant glandular epithelium. The bladder is lined by transitional epithelium, which gives rise to transitional cell carcinoma, and the skin has squamous epithelium and squamous carcinomas.

Since the tumour resembles part of the parent tissue, the classification is based on the assumed histogenesis. For example, because a transitional cell carcinoma has some similarities with transitional epithelium, it is assumed to arise from it.

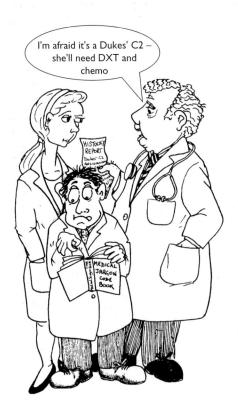

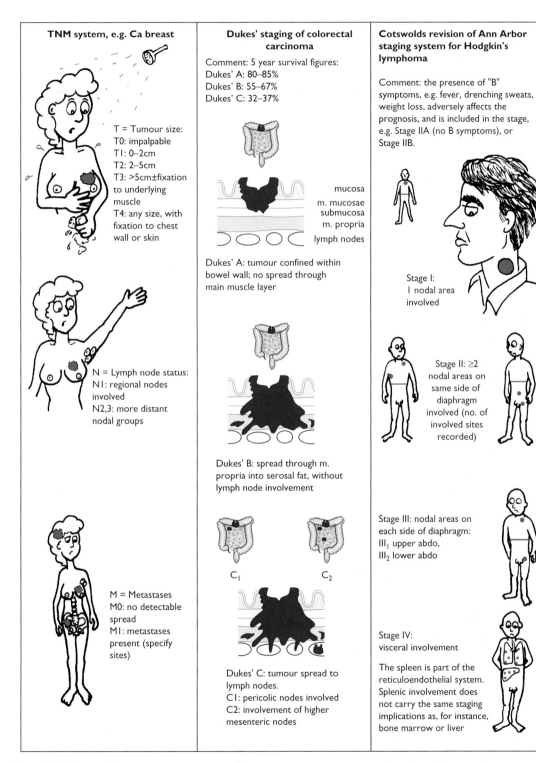

TNM system, e.g. Ca breast

T = Tumour size:
T0: impalpable
T1: 0–2cm
T2: 2–5cm
T3: >5cm±fixation to underlying muscle
T4: any size, with fixation to chest wall or skin

N = Lymph node status:
N1: regional nodes involved
N2,3: more distant nodal groups

M = Metastases
M0: no detectable spread
M1: metastases present (specify sites)

Dukes' staging of colorectal carcinoma

Comment: 5 year survival figures:
Dukes' A: 80–85%
Dukes' B: 55–67%
Dukes' C: 32–37%

mucosa
m. mucosae
submucosa
m. propria
lymph nodes

Dukes' A: tumour confined within bowel wall; no spread through main muscle layer

Dukes' B: spread through m. propria into serosal fat, without lymph node involvement

C_1　　C_2

Dukes' C: tumour spread to lymph nodes.
C1: pericolic nodes involved
C2: involvement of higher mesenteric nodes

Cotswolds revision of Ann Arbor staging system for Hodgkin's lymphoma

Comment: the presence of "B" symptoms, e.g. fever, drenching sweats, weight loss, adversely affects the prognosis, and is included in the stage, e.g. Stage IIA (no B symptoms), or Stage IIB.

Stage I:
1 nodal area involved

Stage II: ≥2 nodal areas on same side of diaphragm involved (no. of involved sites recorded)

Stage III: nodal areas on each side of diaphragm:
III_1 upper abdo,
III_2 lower abdo

Stage IV:
visceral involvement

The spleen is part of the reticuloendothelial system. Splenic involvement does not carry the same staging implications as, for instance, bone marrow or liver

Figure 10.14 Staging of tumours

TISSUE TYPE	BENIGN	MALIGNANT
Epithelium		**Carcinoma**
Squamous, e.g. skin	Squamous papilloma	**Squamous** carcinoma
Glandular, e.g. gastrointestinal tract	Adenoma	**Adeno**carcinoma
Transitional, e.g. urothelium	Transitional cell papilloma	**Transitional cell** carcinoma
Connective tissue		**Sarcoma**
Fat	Lipoma	**Lipo**sarcoma
Muscle: i. Smooth muscle, e.g. wall of gastrointestinal tract	Leiomyoma	**Leiomyo**sarcoma
Muscle: ii. Striated muscle, i.e. voluntary muscle	Rhabdomyoma	**Rhabdomyo**sarcoma
Fibrous tissue, e.g. tendon	Fibroma	**Fibro**sarcoma
Cartilage	Chondroma	**Chondro**sarcoma
Bone	Osteoma	**Osteo**sarcoma
Special categories	(non-systematic nomenclature retained mainly for historical reasons)	
Bone marrow-derived cells: Myeloid cells Lymphoid cells		Myeloid leukaemia Lymphocytic leukaemias Lymphomas
Plasma cells	Plasmacytoma	Myeloma
Central nervous system, e.g. glial cells		Gliomas
Melanocyte	Benign melanocytic naevus	Melanoma
Germ cells	Benign teratoma	Malignant teratoma Seminoma/Dysgerminoma
Placenta	Hydatidiform mole	Choriocarcinoma
Embryonal cells		Embryonal cell tumours (may show differentiation towards tissue types, e.g. neuroblastoma)

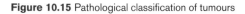

Figure 10.15 Pathological classification of tumours

The broad classification divides tumours into those arising from epithelia (carcinomas), from connective tissue (sarcomas), from lymphoid tissue (lymphomas) and 'the rest', which includes specialized tissues such as the brain. Included in this table are the benign counterparts arising from the same tissues.

At this point there needs to be a word of caution because, although this classification originated from ideas on histogenesis, it is now apparent that cells of one tissue type may 'differentiate' to resemble cells of another type (a process called metaplasia – see page 215). For example, bronchial glandular epithelium may become squamous due to the chronic irritation from smoking. A tumour arising in such a patient may hence appear squamous, although the original epithelium at this site was glandular. The histogenetic approach to classification is destroyed in such circumstances. Fortunately, we only have to claim that we will classify tumours according to their type of differentiation and we eliminate the problem! Thus a tumour resembling squamous cells is a squamous cell carcinoma regardless of the true origin. You will discover that, although rare, it is possible to get squamous carcinoma in the breast and adenocarcinoma in the bladder! Sometimes a tumour cell is very poorly differentiated so that, even

to the trained histopathologist's eye, it does not resemble a particular type of normal cell. In this situation, special stains to demonstrate cytoplasmic or surface molecules can be helpful. Thus the presence of intracellular mucins would suggest an adenocarcinoma, and immunohistochemical stains for different intermediate filaments or lymphoid antigens would help to distinguish between a wide variety of tumours. If it is not possible to demonstrate any differentiation, the tumour is referred to as anaplastic.

Some of these substances are also released into the blood, which is useful both for diagnosis and for following the patient's response to treatment. For example, prostatic-specific antigen (PSA) levels can be measured in the blood to help screen for prostatic adenocarcinoma, although levels are also raised in some non-malignant prostatic disorders because the antigen is present on both benign and malignant prostatic cells. The β subunit of human chorionic gonadotrophin (βHCG) and α fetoprotein (AFP) are also useful markers in patients with teratoma.

Now we must turn to the patient's questions. What causes cancer? How will it behave? What treatments are available? Will there be a lot of pain?

If we are not to be stumped by these questions, we have to understand a little more about the natural history of cancer.

CHAPTER 11

What causes cancer?

CANCER AS A DISEASE OF GENETIC MATERIAL

The view that cancer originates within a single cell due to abnormalities within its DNA is now generally accepted. The evidence comes from five main sources:

1 Some cancers have a heritable predisposition – examples include familial retinoblastoma and familial adenomatous polyposis.
2 Many tumours exhibit chromosomal abnormalities and karyotypic studies have even identified specific changes in some tumours (e.g. 8:14 translocation in Burkitt's lymphoma).
3 A number of rare inherited disorders involve an inability to repair damaged DNA. For example patients with xeroderma pigmentosa have an increased susceptibility to skin cancer following damage to DNA from ultraviolet light.
4 Many chemical carcinogens are also mutagens, i.e. they have been shown to cause genetic mutations.
5 DNA recombinant technology has demonstrated that DNA from tumour cells, when transferred into a normal cell, can convert them into tumour cells of the same type.

The isolation of genes with a direct role in tumour formation (oncogenes) has firmly established cancer as a disease of genetic material. We will now consider the many predisposing and aetiological factors that lead to tumour formation. Although it appears that these factors must alter either the DNA structure or function in some way, the details of many of these processes remain unclear.

One of the concerns that patients often ask about is what causes cancer and the risk factors that were important in his or her case.

AGE AS A RISK FACTOR FOR CANCER

The advent of antibiotics, improved sanitation and good nutrition has extended people's expected lifespan so that they can now achieve an age in which there is a high incidence of malignant tumours, particularly those of breast, colon, lung, prostate and bronchus. It is postulated that carcinogens may have a cumulative effect over time and that this may explain an increased incidence with age. The ability of carcinogens to induce genetic mutations is well known, and the large number of cell divisions with increasing age may contribute to the neoplastic process. Cell division itself is a risk, since each time the DNA is copied there is a potential to introduce mistakes within the genome. Although there are elaborate DNA-repair mechanisms in place to correct such errors, mutations in genes coding for proteins involved in DNA repair will allow such errors to pass on to the next generation of cells. All these factors, together with the age-related metabolic or hormonal changes, may combine to account for the increasing incidence of tumours with age.

Of course tumours are not just confined to the elderly, and some malignancies, such as leukaemias, are more common in children. In some childhood tumours (e.g. retinoblastoma) heredity plays a major part in the aetiology.

GENETIC FACTORS AND CANCER

In our case of breast carcinoma discussed in Chapter 10, the doctor discovered that the patient's mother had died of breast carcinoma. She also had two daughters who at the time were both well. This history of malignant disease within family members is of relevance as there are several tumour types in which the risk of cancer in close family members is increased. How much the risk is increased in individual cases and with different tumours is not easy to specify but, in general, it is about two to three times the general population. Obviously, tumour development is not inevitable and many other factors such as environmental and dietary influences may modify the risk.

In some tumours, the genetic susceptibility is better understood and in two autosomal dominant conditions, familial polyposis coli and retinoblastoma, it involves loss of a tumour suppressor gene or anti-oncogene (see later). Familial polyposis coli (familial adenomatous polyposis) is a disorder in which individuals develop hundreds of polyps in the gastrointestinal tract. These polyps show varying degrees of dysplasia (page 218) and although benign, should be regarded as premalignant because practically all of these patients will develop a colonic carcinoma if the colon is not removed by the age of 25 years. Retinoblastoma is a malignant tumour of the eye which is commonest in children. Between 25 and 30 per cent of cases of retinoblastoma are hereditary and the rest are sporadic. Both familial and sporadic cases arise due to two mutations in the retinoblastoma gene but the familial cases inherit one mutation through the germline cells (see later).

GEOGRAPHY AND RACIAL FACTORS IN CANCER

Geographical factors merge with environmental factors, as a geographical factor is only an environmental factor that affects the population of a particular area. This may be a sunny climate, radioactive rock formations or a carcinogen in the water supply.

Let us discuss, as an example, the increased incidence of stomach cancer in Japan compared with North America. The tumour is seven times commoner in Japanese people living in Japan than in Americans living in the United States. Is this a racial difference or an effect of some climatic, geological or dietary factor which operates in Japan? To answer this we need to know the incidence in Japanese people who move to America and raise families. They will keep their racial (genetic) factors and may import their dietary factors but not their geographical factors. We find that the incidence drops in these immigrants and is halved in

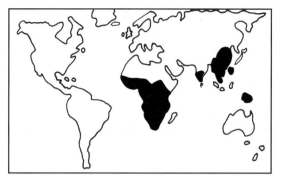

Hepatocellular carcinoma
Sub-Saharan black Africa
Far East

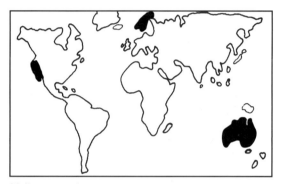

Malignant melanoma
Australia
Scandinavia
North America: Californian whites at highest risk

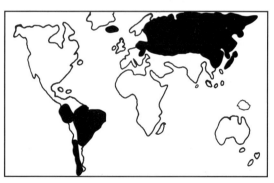

Gastric carcinoma
Japan, China
Brazil, Colombia, Chile
Iceland, Finland,
USSR, Poland, Hungary

Figure 11.1 Geographical variations in tumour incidence

their first-generation offspring but is still higher than that in non-immigrant Americans, so we haven't achieved a definite answer to our question. Some reports suggest that the incidence drops further in future generations until it equals the American rate. This would appear to rule out a racial (genetic) factor and may implicate a cultural dietary change.

A much easier example is the incidence of melanomas in white-skinned Australians. Here there is a racial predisposition, because they do not have sufficient skin pigmentation to protect them from ultraviolet light, and the geographical factor of a sunny climate. If the Australian emigrates at birth to a cold, grey country, then his risk of melanoma drops dramatically.

ENVIRONMENTAL AGENTS AND CANCER

Numerous environmental agents have been implicated in the causation of cancer. Everybody knows that there is a strong association between smoking and lung cancer. This problem may not only affect the smoker but also the 'innocent bystander' who inhales exhaled tobacco smoke (passive smoking).

Asbestos exposure increases the risk of developing lung carcinoma and malignant mesothelioma of the pleura and peritoneum. Exposure to beta-naphthylamine, which may occur in the rubber and dye industries, increases the risk of transitional cell tumours of the bladder. Exposure to vinyl chloride in the plastic industry enhances the development of liver angiosarcoma (malignant tumour of blood vessels).

One of the first examples of an environmental cancer was described in 1775 by Percival Pott, surgeon to St Bartholomew's Hospital in London. He had observed that chimney sweeps had a very high incidence of scrotal cancer, and correctly deduced that this was due to chronic contact with soot. In fact, Percival Pott achieved a double, describing an environmental carcinogen and an occupational cancer in one go! He is also remembered for his description of spinal tuberculosis, referred to as Pott's disease.

CARCINOGENIC AGENTS

So far we have discussed carcinogenesis under the broad headings of age, genetics, race, geography and environment. The next step is to consider what type of agent is operating (the aetiological agent) and to look at ideas on how the agent converts a normal cell to a malignant cell (pathogenesis).

It is worth remembering that, as in the case considered earlier of the woman with breast cancer, by the time a patient presents with a tumour, a large number of cellular events and many thousands of cell divisions have already taken place. Consequently, we are looking at a growth that has been in existence for quite some time. Identifying the responsible aetiological factors at this stage can be extremely difficult. There are three major groups of agents involved in carcinogenesis that we need to consider. These are:

- chemical carcinogens
- radiation
- viruses.

These groups should not be viewed in isolation. Chemicals may, for example, interact with ionizing radiation or with oncogenic viruses. Several different agents within any one group may also interact with each other. Further, all these extrinsic agents may interact with endogenous or constitutional factors in the host such as genetic susceptibility or hormonal status, emphasizing that the carcinogenic process is complex and multifactorial.

Chemical carcinogens

Figure 11.2 illustrates classical experiments of chemical carcinogenesis using mouse skin, which provide the basis for the multistep theory (page 256) and lead to the descriptions of the processes of initiation and promotion. We now know that tumour development in humans is much more complex than depicted in the figure.

Let us consider Fig. 11.2. If you apply a low dose of polycyclic aromatic hydrocarbon (initiator) to the shaved skin of the mouse and don't do any more, then no tumours will result. However, if you later apply another chemical, croton oil (promoter), to the same skin, local tumours will develop. The important points are that the initiator must be applied before the promoter and that the promoter must be applied repeatedly and at regular intervals. There may be a long time interval between initiation and promotion, which suggests that initiation provokes an irreversible change in the DNA that is fixed by cell division. In contrast, the promoter acts in a dose-related, initially reversible fashion and appears to modify the expression of altered genes. Some chemicals (complete carcinogens) can act as both initiator and promoter whereas others (incomplete carcinogens) only fulfil one action.

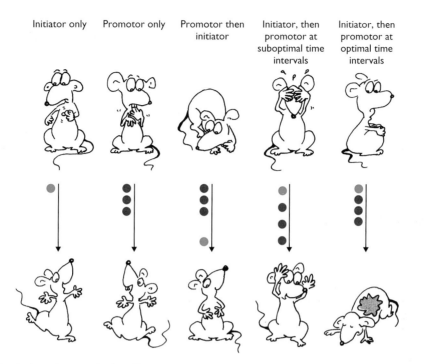

Figure 11.2 Chemical carcinogenesis: the effects of tumour promoters and initiators. Key: green dot − initiator; red dot − promoter

Evidence that certain chemicals are carcinogenic in humans is provided by epidemiological studies. Some chemical carcinogens occur naturally; for example, the potent hepatocarcinogen aflatoxin B_1 is a metabolite from the fungus *Aspergillus flavus*, a common contaminant of grain and other crops in the tropics. Several carcinogens occur as complex mixtures, as in tobacco smoke. Chemical carcinogens typically take 20 or more years to exert their effects, hence there is a long latent period between first encounter with the chemical and the appearance of a tumour.

The dose required to induce tumours also varies widely. Carcinogens act on a number of fairly specific target tissues, broadly determined by the initial routes of exposure and by subsequent patterns of absorption, distribution and metabolism. Beta-naphthylamine is an interesting example. It enters the body mainly via the respiratory system and is inactivated by conjugation with glucuronic acid. Following excretion in the urine, it is activated again due to the action of urinary glucuronidase, which splits the conjugate, releasing the active molecule. Its carcinogenic effects are therefore confined to the urinary tract where it causes transitional cell tumours.

Chemical carcinogenesis is complex and occurs in several steps, to which both genotoxic and non-genotoxic events contribute. Genotoxic carcinogens react with DNA. Various types of genetic damage will follow and, if the damage is not lethal to a cell, it will be transmitted to the daughter cells after cell division. The only protection the cell has is its array of DNA-repair enzymes, which must reconstitute the DNA before the next cell division or else the abnormality will be 'stamped' in by being transmitted to the daughter cells. Most genotoxic carcinogens undergo metabolic changes and are converted from inactive procarcinogens to activated ultimate carcinogens that bind to DNA. Some genotoxic chemicals react directly with DNA without previous metabolic activation. The conditions that determine whether a potential genotoxic chemical is activated or detoxified are very complex, but two main groups of enzymes are involved: the family of cytochrome P450-dependent monooxygenase isoenzymes, and various conjugating enzymes that catalyse the formation of water-soluble glucuronides.

The process by which activated genotoxic carcinogens bind to DNA is equally complex. Once an activated carcinogen is bound to DNA, a number

Table 11.1 Some chemical carcinogens and their associated tumour types

Carcinogen	Tumour type
Aromatic amines, e.g. β-naphthylamine	Transitional cell carcinoma of lower urinary tract (principally of the bladder)
Polycyclic aromatic hydrocarbons, e.g. benzo(a)pyrene	Skin cancer, lung cancer
Vinyl chloride and thorotrast	Angiosarcoma of liver
Arsenic	Skin cancers
Aflatoxin B_1	Liver cell carcinoma

of consequences follow, depending on the nature and extent of the DNA damage that has been sustained. If this damage is extensive and irreversible, the cell will die. If less severe, the damage can be restored by the process of error-free DNA repair. The third possibility, mentioned earlier, is that the cell will survive with damaged DNA which will then be passed on to the daughter cells following cell division.

Non-genotoxic carcinogens, by contrast, do not bind to DNA and do not directly damage it. They appear to act on cells in the target tissues mainly by directly stimulating cell division, or by causing cell damage and death (and thus indirectly stimulating cell division through the process of regeneration and repair). Other effects are less clearly understood, but the general mode of action of non-genotoxic chemicals can be thought of as causing disruption of normal cellular homeostasis. Some non-genotoxic chemicals, such as hormones, act through receptors on the surface of target cells.

One final point should be made. Some genotoxic chemicals exert both genotoxic and non-genotoxic effects in the target tissues. So although genotoxic and non-genotoxic effects are both required for tumour development, they do not necessarily depend on separate genotoxic and non-genotoxic agents.

Radiation

Ionizing radiation includes electromagnetic rays, such as ultraviolet light, X-rays and gamma rays, and particulate radiation, such as alpha particles, beta particles, neutrons and protons. All of these are carcinogenic.

As ionizing radiation passes through tissue, it interacts with atoms in its path to destabilize them. This disturbance in the electron shell of atoms may lead to chemical changes.

The precise mechanisms are still obscure. Radiation causes chromosomal breakage, translocations and mutations. Various protein molecules are also damaged and there are two principal theories to account for the observations. The direct theory states that ionizing radiation directly ionizes important molecules within the cell, while the indirect theory states that ionization first affects water within the cell, which leads to the production of oxygen free radicals, which cause the damage. Whichever mechanism operates, the end result is that DNA is altered, analogous to the initiator effect in chemical carcinogenesis.

The carcinogenic effect of radiation is related to its ability to produce mutations and it is known that this depends on the type and strength of the radiation and the duration of exposure. Some tissues, such as bone marrow and thyroid, are particularly sensitive to the effects of radiation and children are more susceptible than adults.

Ultraviolet light is particularly important, as sun exposure causes vast numbers of melanomas, squamous cell carcinomas and basal cell carcinomas of the skin. Fortunately, squamous cell carcinomas and basal cell carcinomas generally can be cured by complete local excision, but melanomas metastasize early and kill. Many of the pioneers who studied radioactive materials and X-rays developed skin cancers, and miners of radioactive elements have a high incidence of lung cancers. The radiation from the atomic bombs dropped on Hiroshima and Nagasaki resulted in increased incidence of leukaemia, especially acute and chronic myeloid leukaemia, breast, lung and colonic cancers. In contrast, a dramatic increase in thyroid carcinomas has been described in children living in Ukraine and Belarus, who were exposed to fallout after the Chernobyl accident. Interestingly, no increase in the incidence of other types of childhood or adult solid cancers has been noted.

Viruses

A large number of viruses have been implicated in the causation of cancer (Table 11.2). In this

Table 11.2 Viruses and their associated cancers

Virus	Associated tumour
Oncovirus	
HTLV-1	Adult T cell leukaemia/ lymphoma
Hepadnavirus	
Hepatitis B	Liver cancer
Papovavirus	
Papillomavirus types:	
1, 2, 4, 7	Benign skin papillomas
6, 11	Genital warts
16, 18	Cervical cancer
10, 16	Laryngeal cancer
5	Skin cancer
Herpes virus	
Epstein–Barr (EBV)	Burkitt's lymphoma
	Nasopharyngeal Ca
	Hodgkin's lymphoma
	Immunoblastic lymphoma
Herpes simplex virus 8	Kaposi's sarcoma
	Body cavity B-cell lymphoma

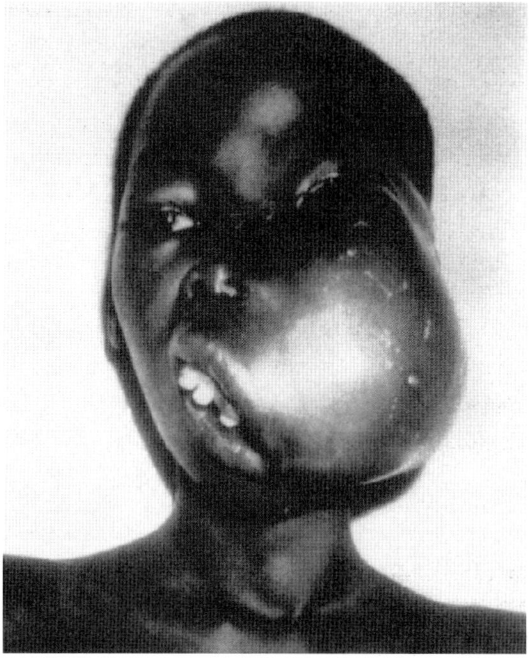

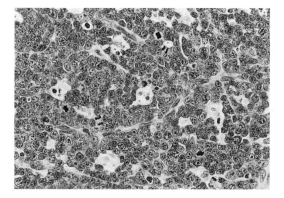

Figure 11.3 Young child with a large maxillary tumour distorting the face. This is a classical presentation of Burkitt's lymphoma

Figure 11.4 Photomicrograph showing classical 'starry sky' appearance of Burkitt's lymphoma

section we will discuss Epstein–Barr virus, human papillomavirus, hepatitis B virus, human T cell leukaemia virus I (HTLV-I) and Kaposi's sarcoma-associated herpesvirus (KSHV).

EPSTEIN–BARR VIRUS (EBV)

Epstein–Barr virus is a member of the herpesvirus family. It is implicated in two major types of cancers: Burkitt's lymphoma and nasopharyngeal carcinoma.

There is a very strong association between EBV and the African variety of Burkitt's lymphoma, since over 98 per cent of the African cases show EBV genome in the tumour cells and all the patients have a raised level of antibodies to EBV membrane antigens. However, EBV does not inevitably cause cancer, as EBV is a common infection in developed countries, where it causes a flu-like illness called infectious mononucleosis or glandular fever. Burkitt's lymphoma can occur without EBV and few non-African Burkitt's lymphomas (15–20 per cent) have the EBV genome. Therefore, EBV must be just one factor involved in the transformation of B lymphocytes to a B cell malignancy.

It is interesting that the African regions where Burkitt's lymphoma is common are also regions where malaria is endemic. It would appear that malaria causes a degree of immuno-incompetence that allows the EBV-infected B cells to proliferate and, hence gives them an increased risk of mutation. Burkitt's lymphoma exhibits a specific mutation resulting in 8:14 translocation, regardless of whether EBV is involved. This translocation moves the c-*myc* gene from its position on chromosome 8

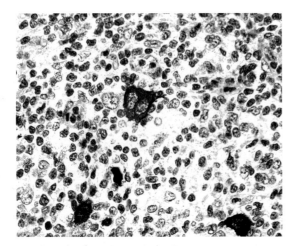

Figure 11.5 Reed–Sternberg cell in Hodgkin's disease, staining positively for Epstein–Barr virus

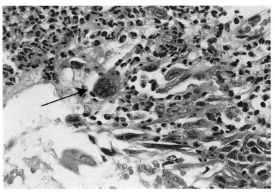

Figure 11.6 Inflamed cervical epithelium with multinucleate giant cell due to HPV infection

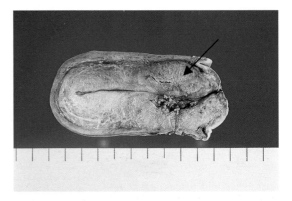

Figure 11.7 Macroscopical picture showing invasive cervical carcinoma

to be adjacent to the immunoglobulin heavy chain gene on chromosome 14. c-*myc* codes for proteins that control cell proliferation and the effect of this translocation is to increase its transcription, possibly because that zone of chromosome 14 is an area of frequent transcriptional activity.

HUMAN PAPILLOMAVIRUS (HPV)

Human papillomavirus is a papovavirus which has long been known to be associated with skin papillomas (warts). Its role in causing cancer was recognized during the study of a very rare disease called epidermodysplasia verruciformis, in which patients have defective cell-mediated immunity and numerous skin papillomas. These papillomas may transform into squamous cell carcinomas, which frequently contain the genome of HPV 5, 8 or 14. HPV is not a single virus but a group of around 85 genetically distinct viruses. Interestingly, some types appear to produce benign tumours while others predispose to malignancy. Thus HPV 16 and 18 (the most common amongst many others) are implicated in squamous cell carcinoma of the uterine cervix, while HPV 6 and 11 are common in benign cervical lesions.

HPV can be transmitted by sexual intercourse and it is noted that there is a high incidence of carcinoma of the cervix in those who begin sexual activity at an early age and in those who are promiscuous. The question is: why doesn't our immune system eradicate the virus? Many people have skin warts on their hands and feet (verrucae)

as children but appear to develop immunity so that the warts are less common in later life. HPV genome comprises a number of genes, two of which are believed to be important in malignancy. The protein products of the E6 and E7 genes bind to p53 and retinoblastoma protein respectively, inactivating their function in regulating the cell cycle (page 251).

Now that we know the viral types involved in some cancers, it opens the door for developing vaccines. Unfortunately, immunization against cervical cancer is not yet available, but immunization for the prevention of hepatitis B and its associated hepatocellular carcinoma is already in progress.

HEPATITIS B VIRUS (HBV)

Hepatitis B virus is associated with the production of a chronic hepatitis, cirrhosis and carcinoma of the liver.

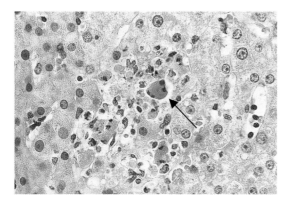

Figure 11.8 Photomicrograph of liver showing inflammation and necrosis due to viral hepatitis

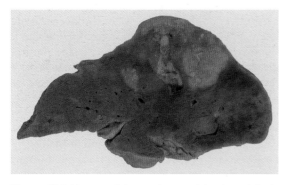

Figure 11.9 Hepatocellular carcinoma arising in a cirrhotic liver

In subSaharan Africa and South-East Asia, where infection with HBV is endemic, the infection is transmitted vertically from mother to child during pregnancy or at childbirth. These children, therefore, have chronic HBV infection and a high incidence of hepatocellular carcinoma at a relatively young age (20–40 years).

The importance of HBV in hepatocellular carcinoma (HCC) is apparent from this sort of epidemiological work and also from molecular biological investigation looking for integrated HBV DNA sequences. These have been identified in the hepatocytes of some patients with chronic HBV infection and some HCC tumour cells. It appears that integration of the viral genome precedes malignant transformation by several years but, to date, no known oncogenic sequences have been identified. The HBV genome does contain a transactivating gene, termed X, which codes for a product that alters the level of transcription of other genes, including the genes in the hepatocytes. An additional mechanism that has been postulated is that HBV infection also leads to liver cell injury and regeneration due to the effect of cytotoxic T cells. It is possible that both the direct (DNA effect due to X) and indirect mechanism (proliferation in response to immune-mediated injury) are important in the aetiology of HCC.

Liver cell carcinomas are also associated with alcoholic liver disease, androgenic steroids and aflatoxins. Aflatoxins are toxic metabolites of a fungus, *Aspergillus flavus*, which can contaminate food in the tropics. Aflatoxin B is thought to contribute to the high incidence of liver cancer in parts of South-East Asia and Africa. Possibly these agents act by causing damage that leads to regenerative activity and, hence, the production of proliferative nodules that are susceptible to further cellular alterations by HBV.

HUMAN T CELL LEUKAEMIA VIRUS I (HTLV-I)

HTLV-I is important because it is the only example (so far!) of a retrovirus causing a human cancer. It is implicated in adult T cell leukaemia/lymphoma (ATLL), which is a rare tumour of the lymphoid system. HTLV-I infection is most common in southern Japan, South America and parts of Africa and precedes the development of malignancy by decades. It has a transactivating gene, *tat*, that increases IL-2 receptor expression in infected T cells, promoting their growth. The study of retroviruses has advanced our knowledge of the role of genes in tumour biology by allowing the identification of specific transforming genes (discussed in greater detail in Chapter 2). However, to date, they have not been shown to be important in common human tumours.

KAPOSI'S SARCOMA-ASSOCIATED HERPESVIRUS (KSHV), HHV-8

Kaposi's sarcoma is an important vascular neoplasm which has come to prominence in HIV-infected patients. Since the early 1980s it has been frequently associated with patients who have AIDS. It is an endemic lesion in central Africa, predominantly in healthy men but also in women and children. Evidence is accumulating that this odd vascular tumour is due to a novel herpesvirus, which has been termed Kaposi's sarcoma-associated herpesvirus (KSHV) or human herpesvirus 8 (HHV-8). There is strong evidence that this virus is linked to several other neoplasms, such as body

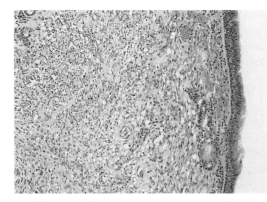

Figure 11.10 Kaposi's sarcoma with slit-like channels within the trachea

cavity B cell lymphoma, multiple myeloma, benign lymphoproliferative disease, angiosarcoma of the face, angiolymphoid hyperplasia with eosinophilia, and multicentric Castleman disease. Although the data are unclear, there is a suggestion that HHV-8 may play a role in some enigmatic inflammatory diseases, such as sarcoidosis. The study of HHV-8 has thrown light on several aspects of carcinogenesis. The genome of this virus encodes proteins that take part in molecular mimicry of cell cycle regulatory and signalling proteins (see Chapter 12).

The study of viruses has helped enormously in unravelling the relevance of genes in human cancer. Of particular use are the retroviruses, which normally contain just three genes; two coding for structural proteins (*gag* and *env*) and one (*pol*) for the enzyme, reverse transcriptase, that produces DNA from RNA. The addition of a fourth gene can often give the virus acute transforming properties; that is, infection with the altered virus can produce tumours under experimental conditions, so-called transfection experiments. These viruses have acted as tools to enable scientists to identify the genetic sequences that can transform cell lines. Many of the viral oncogene sequences were recognized as variants of cellular genes that the retrovirus had acquired from the human genome. This focused attention on the human cells' proto-oncogenes and led to an understanding of the mutations and translocations that can lead to their activation.

ONCOGENIC RNA VIRUSES

Oncogenic RNA viruses are all retroviruses (i.e. they contain reverse transcriptase) and they can be divided into acute transforming viruses, slow

transforming viruses and transactivating viruses. The acute transforming viruses produce tumours within a few weeks in infected animals and often are capable of transforming cell cultures. The slow transforming viruses take months to produce tumours, which are frequently forms of chronic leukaemia.

These two groups of viruses alter the infected cell in different ways. The acute transforming viruses are usually incapable of normal replication because they have lost some genes related to replication but gained genes which confer their transforming capabilities. These additional genes are variants of their host's genes, genes that are called proto-oncogenes when in the host and viral oncogenes when in the virus. The proto-oncogene is a normal cell gene that is normally involved in growth or differentiation. The viral oncogene is not identical to the proto-oncogene, although there is quite extensive sequence homology. The viral oncogene is structurally altered, which, in some way, deregulates cell growth. Alternatively, at the time of inclusion into the viral genome, the proto-oncogene may be inserted near a potent viral promoter, resulting in increased expression. In some cases, acute transforming viruses and normal retroviruses co-infect cells so that the non-transforming retrovirus can provide the replication information that the transforming virus lacks.

Slow transforming retroviruses do not contain oncogenes, have the normal three gene structure to their genome and are capable of replication. They alter the host cell's behaviour by inserting near to a cellular proto-oncogene, so that they either cause increased activity of the cellular gene or, possibly, induce a structural change in the gene. This is called insertional mutagenesis.

Transactivating viruses do not contain oncogenes but, in addition to the *gag*, *pol* and *env* genes, they have a fourth region, which confers transforming properties. The human T cell leukaemia virus is in this group and its extra genes (*tat*) code for a variety of proteins, one of which activates the host's IL-2 and IL-2 receptor genes, resulting in uncontrolled cell proliferation.

ONCOGENIC DNA VIRUSES

Oncogenic DNA viruses contain genes that act early in infected cells to increase expression of a wide variety of genes. The purpose of this is to activate later viral genes concerned with replication and assembly. However, it can also have the effect of inducing excessive expression of host cell genes responsible for growth regulation. For example, the 'early genes' of the virus can produce proteins (e.g. T proteins of polyoma and SV40 viruses) that localize in the nucleus and alter the regulation of DNA synthesis. In some cases, this is through binding to the p53 protein so that its half-life is increased and DNA synthesis remains activated. Some 'growth enhancing' actions may actually result from inhibiting normal 'growth inhibiting' proteins.

There is an old wives' saying that 'where God puts disease, he also puts a cure'. Viruses undoubtedly cause infectious disease and can be one step on the road to cancer. However, they may also provide a possible cure for disease as they may be the ideal vehicle for altering the genetic code within human cells. Ultimately, it would be best if patients with single-gene disorders could have their defective gene replaced by the correct gene. In theory, this is possible by using retroviruses to introduce the gene, but in practice there are many problems to conquer. The most useful practical application of our rapidly expanding knowledge of the genes is in the manufacture of specific proteins.

SUMMARY

Although we started the chapter with the statement that cancer is a disease of genetic material, it should be evident that it is also a multifactorial disorder. This might appear initially as a paradox, but remember that in any given person, the combination of a genetic make-up, the environment in which the person lives and the factors to which he or she is exposed, the longevity of the person and 'chance' will combine to produce the genetic changes (mutations) that may ultimately lead to cancer. One could argue that at least in some circumstances, the cancer is a direct payback for an evolutionary advantage of the past. It is not difficult to envisage a genetic make-up that gives such an advantage; a good example could be decreased pigmentation in races living in the cloudy and colder northern regions of the world, which would help in obtaining adequate amounts of vitamin D from sunshine. This advantage from the genetic make-up becomes a distinct disadvantage if put into the context of chance mutations, increased exposure to sunlight due to sunbathing on numerous holidays to the tropics and a long enough life for the mutations to result in a cancer – a melanoma.

Key facts

Major aetiological factors involved in tumour formation

- Age
- Genetic factors
- Geographical and racial factors
- Environmental agents
- Carcinogens: chemicals, radiation, viruses

CHAPTER 12

Molecular genetics of cancer

It is now well over a hundred years since Gregor Mendel first carried out his experiments with peas and almost exactly a century since Mendel's laws were 're-discovered'. It is also exactly a century since Theodore Boveri proposed that alterations in the chromosomes were the basis of cancer formation. Remarkably, it was half a century later that the Philadelphia chromosome (discussed below) was identified.

There is little doubt that Theodore Boveri is one of the giants of twentieth century cancer genetics. His classic experiments on the fertilization of sea urchin eggs with two sperms demonstrated the phenomenon of abnormal chromosomal segregation, and he was quick to realize that this abnormal chromosomal number may account for the unrestricted growth of tumours. In fact, he made a number of pertinent remarks relating to regulation of the cell cycle, the presence of oncogenes and tumour suppressor genes and genetic instability in tumours. To put it into context, Boveri made his observations between 1902 and 1904, the Philadelphia chromosome was identified in the 1960s, Knudson's 'two-hit' hypothesis and the identification of the first dominant oncogene in the 1970s, the cloning of the first tumour suppressor gene, retinoblastoma gene (*RB*) in the 1980s, discovery of mismatch repair defects in tumours and cloning of *BRCA1/2* in the 1990s and the publication of the first draft of the human genome in 2000. What an incredible century!

CYTOGENETICS

Not surprisingly, following Boveri's publications, some of the earliest indications for genetic alterations came from classical karyotypic analysis. This type of study reveals gross abnormalities at the chromosomal level. Classical examples of tumours showing such gross chromosomal abnormalities include chronic myeloid leukaemia and Burkitt's lymphoma. We have already considered Burkitt's lymphoma in the section on viruses (page 236). We will briefly consider chronic myeloid leukaemia here.

The Philadelphia (Ph1) chromosome is present in 90 per cent of cases of chronic myeloid leukaemia and can be used as a diagnostic marker. It is produced by a reciprocal and balanced translocation between chromosomes 22 and 9. The breakpoint on chromosome 9 occurs at the locus of the *abl* proto-oncogene and the breakpoint on chromosome 22 is in the region termed the breakpoint cluster region (*bcr*). Some recent work suggests that the *bcr* genes code for a protein kinase that could have oncogenic potential. The *abl* proto-oncogene has sequence homology with the tyrosine kinase family of oncogenes but it is only after translocation to chromosome 22 that it produces a mutant protein with tyrosine kinase activity. This particular tyrosine kinase activity is located in the nucleus, where it is believed to influence transcription of DNA. Further examples of tumours and cytogenetic abnormalities are listed in Table 12.1.

CANCER-PRODUCING GENES – ONCOGENES

The term 'oncogene' refers to any mutated gene that contributes to neoplastic transformation in the cell. Two major types of oncogenes have been identified; dominant oncogenes and tumour suppressor genes (anti-oncogenes).

Some oncogenes involved in carcinogenesis are mutated versions of normal cellular genes (called

Table 12.1 Chromosomal alterations in human tumours

Tumour type	Chromosomal aberration	Possible action	Gene(s)
Haematopoietic tumours – translocation			
Chronic myeloid leukaemia	t(9;22)(q34;q11)	Alteration of nuclear tyrosine kinase	BCR-ABL
Burkitt's lymphoma	t(8;14)(q24;q32)	Cell cycle regulation	c-myc-IgH
	t(2;8)(p12;q24)		Igk, Igλ,
	t(8;22)(q24;q11)		c-myc
Acute myeloid leukaemia	t(8;21)(q22;q22)		ETO
Mantle cell lymphoma	t(11;14)(q13;q32)		Bcl-1-IgH
Follicular lymphoma	t(14;18)(q32;q21)		IgH-bcl-2
Solid tumours – translocation			
Ewing's sarcoma/PNET	t(11;22)(q24;q12)		EWS-FL1
	t(21;22)(q22;q12)		EWS-ERG
	t(11;22)(q13;q12)		EWS-WT1
Synovial sarcoma	T(X;18)		
	(p11.23,q11.2)		SYT-SSX1
	T(X;18)		
	(p11.21,q11.2)		SYT-SSX2
Malignant melanoma	t(1;19)(q12;p13)		?
	t(1;6)(q11;q11)		?
	t(1;14)(q21;q32)		?
Salivary adenoma	t(3,8)(p21;q12)		CTNNB1
Renal adenocarcinoma	t(X;1)(p11;q21)		TFE3
	t(9;15)(p11;q11)		?
Solid tumours – deletions			
Retinoblastoma	del13q14	Loss of oncosuppression	RB
Wilm's tumour	del11p13	Loss of oncosuppression	WT-1
	del11p15		?
	del17q12–21		FWT1
Bladder-transitional cell carcinoma	del11p13		?
Lung cancer-small cell type	del17p13	Loss of oncosuppression	TP53
Colorectal adenocarcinoma	del17p13	Loss of oncosuppression	TP53
	del 5q21	Loss of oncosuppression	APC
Breast cancer	del17p13	Loss of oncosuppression	TP53
	del17q21	Loss of oncosuppression	BRCA1
	del13q12–13	Loss of oncosuppression	BRCA2
	del16q22.1	Loss of oncosuppression	
Solid tumours – amplification			
Neuroblastoma		Cell cycle control	N_MYC
Breast cancer		Increased growth factor activity	CERBB2

proto-oncogenes). The function of these normal genes is enhanced by the mutations and hence they are referred to as 'activating' or 'gain-in-function' mutations. These genes are also known as 'dominant' oncogenes since mutation of one allele is sufficient to exert an effect, despite the presence of normal gene product from the remaining allele. It is over 25 years since such genes were discovered.

Dictionary box

Allele: Alternative form of the gene found at the same locus in homologous chromosomes.

In contrast, tumour suppressor genes are normal genes whose function is inactivated by mutations; hence these are known as 'inactivating' or 'loss-of-function' mutations. Tumour suppressor genes are also known as 'recessive' oncogenes since inactivation of both alleles is required to have an effect at the cellular level. Evidence for the existence of such genes has been largely circumstantial and was based on classical genetics, cytogenetics and molecular genetics. You should beware that the terms 'dominant' and 'recessive' refer to action at the genetic level; confusion sometimes occurs because the terminology has been borrowed from classical Mendelian genetic inheritance patterns.

Where do oncogenes come from? There are both exogenous and endogenous sources. The exogenous sources include viral oncogenes (v-*onc*), which may be introduced into cells by tumour viruses. Endogenous genes are called cellular oncogenes (c-*onc*) and these are genes that are normally present in the cell but have been altered to produce the oncogene. As mentioned above, the normal gene from which the oncogene is derived is called the proto-oncogene.

The viral or exogenous oncogenes can be divided into two types: those that show similarity to normal cellular genes and those that are completely different. This is important because viral oncogenes that resemble cellular genes are actually derived from the cell's genes. This is quite amazing when you think

about it. A virus infects a cell and incorporates some of the cellular genes into its own genome. These genes, finding themselves in a new piece of DNA or RNA, become altered in their properties and are then viral oncogenes. When the virus infects another cell, it can introduce the viral oncogene (a process called transduction), which leads to altered growth of the infected cell. Retroviruses, which consist of RNA that becomes incorporated into the host DNA through the action of the enzyme reverse transcriptase, can readily 'pick up' some host DNA and thus carry viral oncogenes derived from cellular oncogenes. Oncogenic DNA viruses generally possess gene sequences that are uniquely viral and have no homology with cellular oncogenes.

How can oncogenes promote cell growth?

There are a number of ways in which the function of oncogenes can be altered, including point mutations, amplification, gene rearrangement/translocation, deletion of part or whole of chromosome and altered expression. Since most of the mechanisms described apply to both types of oncogenes, they are considered here together; however, there are differences in the pattern of alterations between dominant oncogenes and tumour suppressor genes. In contrast to dominant oncogenes, which are mutated in a consistent manner either by point mutation (e.g. *ras*), translocation (e.g. *abl*) or gene amplification (e.g. N-*myc*), mutations in tumour suppressor genes tend to be diverse both in type and position within the gene (e.g. *TP53*).

POINT MUTATIONS

Point mutation results in the substitution of one base pair by another (e.g. substitution of G:C by A:T).

Table 12.2 Main differences between dominant oncogenes and tumour suppressor genes

	Dominant oncogenes	Tumour suppressor genes
No. of alleles in normal cells	Two	Two
No. of alleles mutated to exert effect	One	Two
Effect of mutation on the function of the protein product	Enhanced	Reduced
Germline (inherited) mutations identified, i.e. important in genetic predisposition	Rare-*RET, KIT*	Many-*TP53, RB* etc.
Adjectives to describe mutations	Activating, gain in function, dominant	Inactivating, loss of function, recessive

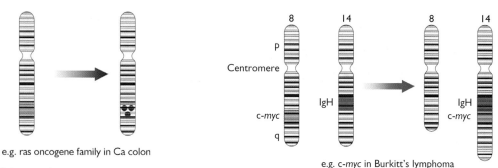

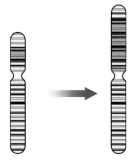

e.g. ras oncogene family in Ca colon

Figure 12.1 Point mutation

e.g. c-*myc* in Burkitt's lymphoma

Figure 12.2 Translocation

e.g. N-*myc* in neuroblastoma

Figure 12.3 Gene amplification

The effect of the point mutation depends on its position and includes alteration of the protein structure by change in the amino acid composition and insertion of a stop codon with premature termination of the protein. The clearest example of point mutations in human tumours are found in the *ras* family. Mutations at codons 12, 13 and 61 of H-, K- and N-*ras* contribute to oncogenesis in many of the main types of human tumours. Mutations in *ras* are encountered in both benign and malignant neoplasms. The *kit* gene encodes a transmembrane tyrosine kinase receptor that is consistently expressed in hematopoietic stem cells, mast cells, melanocytes, germ cells, and interstitial cells of Cajal (ICC). Activating germline mutations of *kit* gene are associated with ICC hyperplasia, familial gastrointestinal stromal tumours (GISTs), cutaneous mastocytosis, and cutaneous hyperpigmentation. Depending on the site where the mutation has occurred, patients present with a combination of all or some of the above lesions.

GENE REARRANGEMENTS/TRANSLOCATIONS

This refers to the production of a hybrid chromosome due to joining of part of one chromosome with another. The rearrangement of DNA sequences can lead to creation of an altered gene (and product) either as a result of structural change or due to change in the control of transcription. Examples include 8:14 (or 8:22, 2:8) translocation in Burkitt's lymphoma and the 9:22 translocation in chronic myeloid leukaemia (CML).

AMPLIFICATION

The normal genome contains two copies of each gene (the two alleles). In amplification, one copy is multiplied numerous times and may result in

increased mRNA and hence increased protein product. At the level of the chromosome, these areas of amplification are seen as double minutes (DM) or homogeneously staining regions (HSR). DMs are extrachromosomal chromatin bodies without centromeres that segregate randomly during mitosis. HSRs are expanded chromosomal regions that are linked to the centromere and therefore segregate in the normal way. Most classes of oncogenes have been shown to be amplified in human malignancy. Examples include N-*myc* in neuroblastoma and c-erbB-2 in breast cancer. Only some of these amplifications have been demonstrated to have pathological significance. N-*myc* amplification is correlated with advanced stage and recurrence of neuroblastoma and c-erbB-2 amplification in breast cancer correlates with poor prognosis. It should be noted, however, that in many tumours, overexpression of mRNA and protein are seen in the absence of gene amplification.

DELETIONS

Deletions range from the loss of a single base pair to the loss of an entire chromosome. Small intragenic

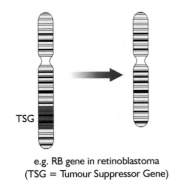

TSG

e.g. RB gene in retinoblastoma
(TSG = Tumour Suppressor Gene)

Figure 12.4 Deletion

deletions have similar effects (abnormal protein, stop codons) to point mutations. Larger deletions will, of course, inactivate many genes at a time.

ALTERED EXPRESSION

The inactivation of a gene via deletions or intragenic mutations is now a familiar story. It has recently become apparent that some putative tumour suppressor genes do not exhibit these common phenomena in certain tumours. Instead changes in the methylation patterns of the promoter region of the gene or even alterations in the chromatin pattern regulated by histone deacetylases lead to an altered expression in some genes (i.e. alteration in the transcription of the mRNA and translation of the protein). This occurs without any mutational event in the gene and if the gene was sequenced, no changes would be detected. Some good examples are the inactivation of *p16* gene on chromosome 9p21, the inactivation of *BRCA1* gene in sporadic breast carcinomas, and the inactivation of the second allele in some rare types of gastric carcinomas (isolated or signet ring cell gastric carcinoma). It is worth bearing in mind that in tumorigenesis, methylation and acetylation play roles in the downregulation of the expression of tumour suppressor genes.

Mode of action of dominant oncogenes

Normal cell growth is believed to be influenced by growth factors binding to receptors on the surface of the cell. This produces a stimulus through a 'signal transduction pathway(s)', which influences the cell's nucleus to produce instructions for proliferation. Within the nucleus itself there are also molecules that regulate transcription and those that regulate the cell cycle during cell division. Therefore, cell growth could be stimulated as a result of:

- increased growth factor production
- increase in growth factor receptors on the cell's surface
- abnormal growth factor receptors
- abnormal signalling through the cascade of signal transduction pathways in the cytoplasm
- abnormalities in the nuclear acting molecules
- alterations to the control of the cell cycle.

Oncogenes that act through each of these mechanisms have been identified.

GROWTH FACTORS AND GROWTH FACTOR RECEPTORS

Growth factors are polypeptides that act locally to stimulate proliferation and, sometimes, differentiation. If tumour cells produce substances that act as growth factors, then they will be continually self-stimulating (autocrine stimulation). Several classes of growth factors have been classified according to sequence homology and biological activity. The categories include epidermal growth factor family (EGF and TGFα), the fibroblast growth factor family (acidic and basic FGF, HST and INT-2), platelet-derived growth factor (PDGF), colony-stimulating factors (CSF), interleukins and the insulin-like growth factors (IGF).

Growth factors act by binding to a receptor residing in the plasma membrane. The binding leads to activation of the receptor and signal transduction to the interior of the cell.

When the normal cell surface receptors are activated by growth factors, the receptors usually dimerize, leading to phosphorylation of tyrosine residues and an increase in their tyrosine kinase activity. When the genes coding for these receptors are abnormal, there is persistent activity without receptor binding. The growth factor receptors can be activated in this way by a number of mechanisms, including gene amplification, rearrangement and overexpression. For example, the c-erbB-2 gene (also known as HER-2) is amplified in about 25 per cent of breast cancers and also in a variety of other cancers such as lung. Breast cancers that express the HER-2 receptor are more aggressive and have a poor prognosis. Recently, a humanized monoclonal antibody against HER-2 has been developed and is used to treat patients with breast cancer. In other situations, the receptor may not be

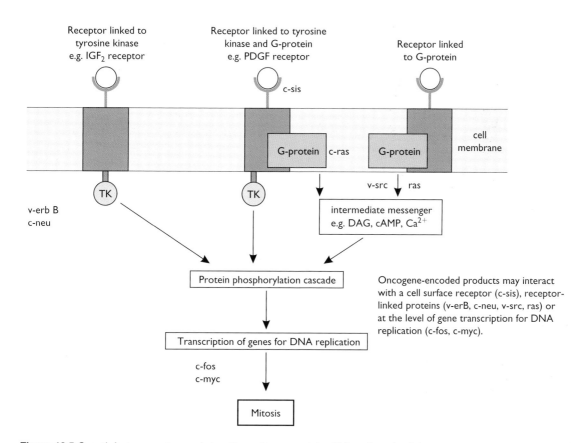

Figure 12.5 Growth factor receptors and signalling pathways: points of interaction of cellular oncogenes

overexpressed but may instead have altered kinase activity as with c-erbB-1. Some tyrosine kinases are not attached to a receptor but are anchored to the plasma membrane and participate in signalling. The c-src oncogene alters the activity of one of these non-receptor tyrosine kinases.

SIGNAL TRANSDUCTION PROTEINS: GTP-BINDING PROTEINS

Three mammalian ras genes – H-ras-1, K-ras-2 and N-ras – have been identified. They form one of the most important families of oncogenes identified to date. ras genes usually acquire transforming activity as a result of point mutation within their coding regions. These activating point mutations are restricted to certain sites, notably codons 12, 13 and 61. The p21 products of both ras proto-oncogene and transforming genes are located in the inner surface of the cell membrane. They bind guanosine nucleotides (GDP and GTP) and possess intrinsic GTPase activity. These biochemical properties resemble those of the G proteins, which are

associated with the cell membrane and are implicated in the modulation of signal transduction. It is becoming clear that ras proteins function as critical relay switches that regulate signalling pathways between the cell surface receptors and the nucleus.

Overall, point mutation in the ras gene is the commonest dominant oncogene abnormality in human tumours. It appears to play a major role in colon, pancreatic and thyroid cancers, as well as in myeloid leukaemia.

NUCLEAR ONCOPROTEINS

These oncoproteins share the features of nuclear localization and proven or suspected ability to bind to specific DNA sequences.

An important family of such genes involved in human malignancy is myc. This was originally identified as the oncogene carried by several acutely transforming retroviruses. The myc family consists of c-myc, N-myc, L-myc, R-myc, P-myc and B-myc. They have been isolated on the basis of homology to v-myc or one of the myc proto-oncogenes. c-myc

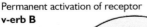

↑Growth factor
c-sis

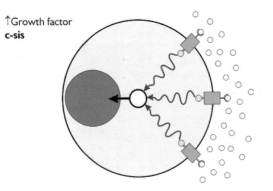

Permanent activation of receptor
v-erb B

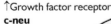

↑Growth factor receptor
c-neu

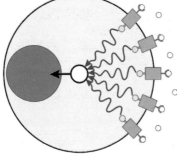

Abnormal signal transduction
c-K-ras

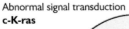

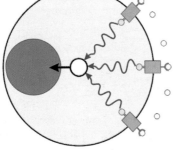

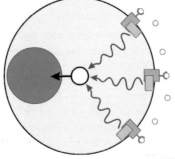

Figure 12.6 Mechanisms of oncogene activation

is expressed in many tissues and correlates with cell proliferation. Activation due to gene amplification occurs in breast cancer and small cell lung cancer (SCLC). In B and T cell lymphomas, translocation to an immunoglobulin (Ig) or T cell receptor locus is seen.

The end result of all the signalling pathways is the transition of the cell through the cell cycle. Here another important family of molecules is critical. These are the cyclins and cyclin-dependent kinases (CDKs). The cyclins activate the CDKs by phosphorylation and these activated kinases are critically important in allowing the various stages of the cell cycle to progress smoothly. The control of the cell cycle also involves the products of tumour suppressor genes such as retinoblastoma (see below).

Tumour suppressor genes/recessive oncogenes

Although 'activated' or 'dominant' oncogenes held centre stage 20 years ago, it is interesting that there was evidence for yet another type of gene long before that. The successful identification of genes whose proteins are physiological inhibitors of growth stemmed from two main types of studies: investigations of somatic cell hybrids and genetic studies of inherited cancer syndromes. Furthermore, cytogenetic studies had already shown that many tumours exhibit loss of DNA involving almost all chromosomal arms.

In somatic cell hybrids, the normal cell is fused with a transformed ('malignant') cell to form a

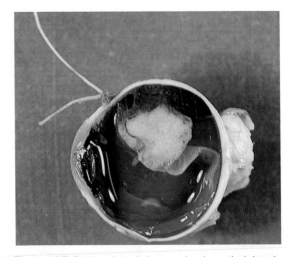

Figure 12.7 Section through the eye showing retinal detachment due to underlying tumour

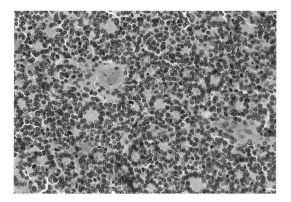

Figure 12.8 Photomicrograph showing characteristic rosettes of retinoblastoma

hybrid cell. The main action of fusion was to produce a non-transformed state. This phenomenon of tumour suppression suggested that the normal cell must replace a defective function in the cancer cell. The first tumour suppressor to be identified was found during the study of a rare familial disease called retinoblastoma.

Retinoblastoma, a tumour arising from the embryonal neural retina, has a world-wide incidence of 1:20 000. The tumour is of interest because it has both a sporadic form and a familial form, with approximately 25–30 per cent of the tumours being heritable. These cases tend to present earlier and develop bilateral disease. In contrast, the sporadic cases have unilateral tumours. Advancement in surgery and radiotherapy led to improved survival and it became clear that 50 per cent of the offspring of patients with bilateral tumours were themselves at risk of the disease. Evaluation of family pedigrees clearly shows the inherited form as Mendelian dominant.

In 1971, Alfred Knudson proposed his 'two hit' hypothesis (Fig. 12.9). He pointed out that if cancer arises as a result of a series of somatic events, then it is possible that sometimes, one of these changes is inherited in the germline and hence is present in every cell of the body. All the cells are therefore already one step along the pathway of carcinogenesis and this forms the basis for the dominantly inherited cancer susceptibility. In addition, a further mutation occurring somatically during life in the same gene would knock out the function of the gene. Hence, while the susceptibility is dominant, the action at the cell level is recessive. This therefore predicted for a class of genes that had to be inactivated or to have 'loss of function' in order

to provide the malignant phenotype. Knudson examined data relating to the age of first appearance of the tumour in both familial and sporadic cases and showed that it followed the expected statistical model based on this hypothesis.

Cytogenetic studies had revealed that a few of the familial tumours showed germline deletions of chromosome 13, and careful karyotyping revealed deletions of 13q14. The retinoblastoma gene (*RB1*) was cloned in 1986. It was the first tumour suppressor gene to be isolated. With the cloning of the gene, it could be confirmed that familial retinoblastoma is indeed caused by an inactivating mutation. Further evidence for oncosuppression comes from fusion experiments. Insertion of the 4.7 kb complementary DNA sequence (cDNA) into retinoblastoma and osteosarcoma cell lines led to reversion of the tumorigenic phenotype, and introduction of these cells into nude mice failed to produce tumours. Interestingly, mutations of the retinoblastoma gene and expression of the protein product have also been seen in almost every tissue despite the restricted oncogenic effects. Mutations are also found in other types of tumours such as breast carcinoma, although breast cancer does not form part of any syndrome in association with retinoblastoma.

THE MODE OF ACTION OF TUMOUR SUPPRESSOR GENES

Interestingly, although the mode of action of genes that are inhibitory for growth might follow the same pathways as those that promote growth, there is much less information on this topic than on dominant oncogenes.

Perhaps the best examples of molecules that act at the cell surface are the cadherins, which are cell-to-cell adhesion molecules. E-Cadherin (an epithelial cell–cell adhesion molecule) is abnormal in a special type of breast cancer called lobular carcinoma. Mutations in the E-cadherin gene are also responsible for predisposition to inherited gastric cancer of diffuse type in a small percentage of patients.

Another good example is the binding of transforming growth factor beta (TGFβ) to its receptor, which leads to the transcription of genes that inhibit growth. The TGFβ signalling pathway is abnormal in colonic and pancreatic cancers.

A good example of a protein that regulates cell signalling is the APC (adenomatosis polyposis coli) protein. The *APC* gene, which predisposes to familial adenomatous polyposis (FAP), is an important

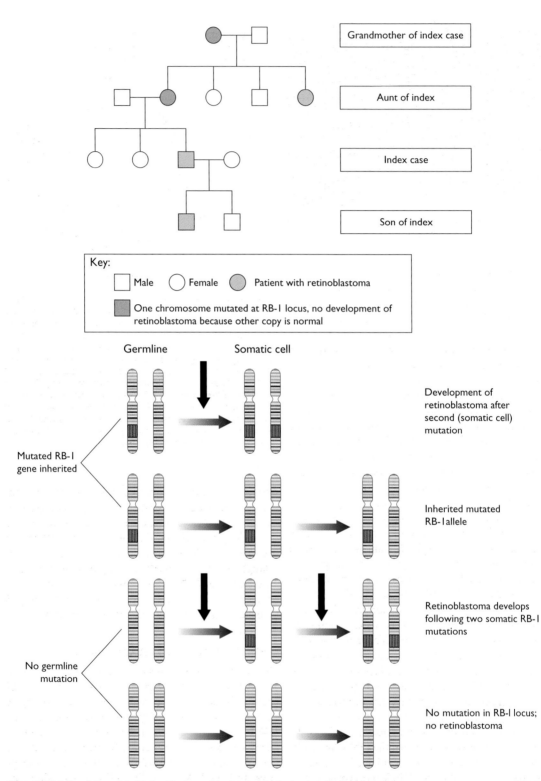

Figure 12.9 Two-hit model of retinoblastoma. Black arrow indicates inactivating mutation

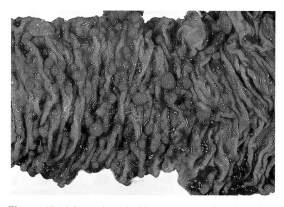

Figure 12.10 Large bowel with numerous polyps in patient with familial adenomatous polyposis

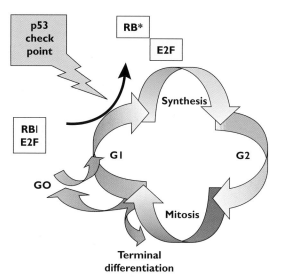

Figure 12.11 The cell cycle is largely governed by the actions of cyclins and cyclin-dependent kinases (cdk), some of which are manufactured during the cycle, others are recycled. Phosphorylation of the retinoblastoma protein (product of the RB-1 gene) enables the transition from G1 to the synthesis phase by releasing E2F protein, which activates DNA synthesis genes. p53 protein operates a quality control system at this checkpoint: if DNA damage or mutation is identified the defect is either repaired by DNA-repair enzymes or the cell is consigned to apoptosis. G2 is the pre-mitotic phase, during which preparation is made for mitosis. The resultant cells either re-enter the cycle, terminally differentiate and leave the cell cycle, or enter a resting phase, G0.

player in the development of colonic carcinoma. The APC protein plays an important role in the signalling pathway that involves a molecule called β-catenin. This protein acts in the nucleus to increase the activity of growth-promoting genes. APC causes degradation of β-catenin, hence removing the proliferative signal. It is easy to see then that mutations in the *APC* gene will lead to increased levels of β-catenin and hence increased proliferating signal.

Not surprisingly, most information relating to the function of tumour suppressor genes comes from the study of *RB* and *p53*. These molecules have an effect on nuclear transcription and the regulation of the cell cycle. The regulation of the cell cycle is complex and illustrated in Fig. 12.11.

Briefly, when the cells are in the resting or quiescent stage, the retinoblastoma protein is hypophosphorylated. In this state, RB is able to bind to a transcription factor called E2F and hence prevent the activation of genes that play a role in pushing the cell through division. Various growth factors, including the EGF family (discussed above), activate the proteins of the cyclin family. The cyclin D/CDK4, CDK6 and cyclin E/CDK2 complexes phosphorylate the RB protein, leading to release of the E2F molecule, which is then free to bind to DNA and activate transcription of genes involved in cell division. This process is balanced by signals that inhibit the process – p16 playing an important role.

Unlike RB, p53 protein does not play a role in maintaining a check on the normal cell cycle. However, if damage is caused to the DNA by irradiation or by chemicals, its actions kick in. Levels of p53 protein rise following DNA damage and this leads to two main effects: cell cycle arrest by the transcription of an inhibitor of CDK called p21

and, if the damage is too severe, cell death (apoptosis). The cell cycle arrest is necessary and important as it allows the cell time to repair the damage before completion of cell division. It is not too difficult to see that if cells undergo cell division to produce daughter cells without repairing the defect, they in essence consolidate that damage; this is one of the features of tumour cells. No surprise then that p53 has been called 'the guardian of the genome'.

OTHER TUMOUR SUPPRESSOR GENES

Many tumour suppressor genes have now been identified and although the exact mechanism of action is not clear in every case, the biology is slowly being unravelled. Examples include the *BRCA1/2* genes that predispose to hereditary breast and ovarian cancer. The proteins produced are thought to have a role in controlling transcription and in DNA repair. The *NF-2* gene predisposes to the development of neurofibromatosis type 2. The protein is believed to have a role in cell–matrix

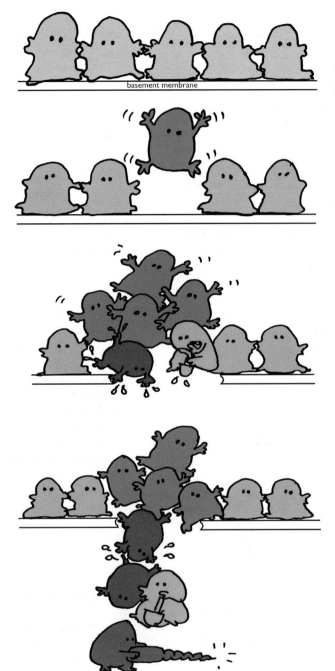

Normal epithelial cells, with cell–cell junctions and normal regulation of proliferation

Mutation in one cell confers freedom from normal growth control mechanisms. It proliferates without restraint

During proliferation, new mutations occur, some of which confer an increased growth advantage and an ability to spread through basement membrane

Further mutations occur. Thus, although the tumour has originated from a single mutated cell (i.e. it is clonal), it is clear that the final population is mixed, each new population evolving to the advantage of the tumour. This is clonal evolution

Figure 12.12 Clonal evolution

interaction, although the exact mechanism is unclear at present. Other examples include the *WT-1* gene involved in Wilm's tumour and the *PTEN* gene on chromosome 10, which predisposes to an autosomal dominant disorder characterized by benign and malignant thyroid disease, multiple hamartomas and breast cancer.

Some examples of tumour suppressor genes that have a familial predisposition are shown in Table 12.3.

Table 12.3 Tumours and familial predisposition

Syndrome	Principal tumour types	Genetic locus/gene
Familial polyposis coli	Colorectal carcinoma	5q21 (*APC*)
MEN I	Pituitary, parathyroid thyroid, adrenal cortex, islet cell tumour	11q13
MEN IIa	Medullary carcinoma of thyroid, phaeochromocytoma, parathyroid tumours	10q11 (*RET*)
MEN IIb	Medullary carcinoma of thyroid, phaeochromocytoma, mucosal neuromas	10q11 (*RET*)
Von Hipple–Lindau	Haemangioblastoma of cerebellum & retina, renal cell carcinoma, phaeochromocytoma	3p25 (*VHL*)
Tuberous sclerosis	Angiomyolipoma	9q34 (*TSC1*) 16p13.3 (*TSC2*)
Familial retinoblastoma	Bilateral retinoblastoma, osteosarcoma	13q14 (*RB*)
Neurofibromatosis type I	Neurofibromas, neurofibrosarcoma, glioma, meningioma, phaeochromocytoma	17q11 (*NF1*)
Neurofibromatosis type II	Bilateral acoustic schwannomas, multiple meningiomas	22q (*NF2*)
Li–Fraumeni	Breast cancer, sarcoma	17p13 (*TP53*)
Breast ovarian	Breast cancer, ovarian cancer	17q21 (*BRCA1*)
Breast	Breast cancer, ovarian cancer, prostate cancer	13q12–13 (*BRCA2*)
Hereditary non-polyposis colorectal cancer (HNPCC)		Colorectal carcinoma 2p (*MSH2*) 3p (*MLH1*) 7p (*PMS2*)
Familial gastrointestinal stromal tumours (GIST) cells of Cajal, mastocytosis, hyperpigmentation		Multiple GIST, hyperplasia of intestinal 4q12 (*c-Kit*)
Wilms' tumour (WAGR syndrome)	Wilms' tumour, aniridia, genitourinary abnormalities, mental retardation	11p13.3 (*WT1*)

MEN = multiple endocrine neoplasia.

DNA REPAIR

If the human genome is not to fall apart as a result of exogenous (environmental chemicals, radiation) and endogenous (DNA replication) damage, it has to have efficient DNA-repair mechanisms and the ability to execute programmed cell death. There are many different types of DNA-repair mechanisms within the cell and undoubtedly our knowledge will become more complicated and refined with time. Since some of the important genes involved in cancer are already being assigned to have a role in particular types of DNA-repair mechanisms, they will be listed here, but it is not the intention that you should be able to regurgitate the different mechanisms in detail.

The mechanisms include homologous recombinational repair (HRR), non-homologous end joining (NHEJ), nucleotide excisional repair (NER), base excisional repair (BER) and mismatch repair. HRR, as its name suggests, relies on the homologous chromosome to provide the template for repairing the defective strand. It is therefore an accurate and error-free way of dealing with damage. In contrast, NHEJ is prone to error, as no complementary strand is available to provide a template for accurate replication. The recently identified breast cancer predisposition genes, *BRCA1/2*,

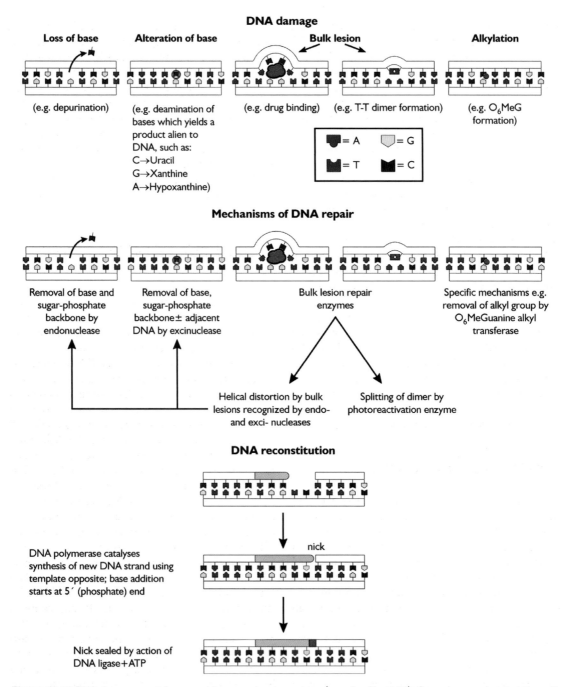

Figure 12.13 DNA damage can take several forms, some shown here (see also Fig. 2.26). Several enzymes patrol the cell's DNA to detect DNA distortion or mismatch and effect DNA repair. Once a cell has divided, any mutation will be perpetuated if the daughter cell is capable of further division. This may lead to tumour development

are involved in DNA repair through HRR. In their absence following mutations in the genes, DNA repair is still possible but it now occurs through the error-prone pathway of NHEJ, making the cell more susceptible to further genetic changes and hence cancer formation.

The other major pathway that has been identified to play a role in tumour formation is mis-match repair. Genomic instability plays an important role in the development of tumours in patients with hereditary non-polyposis colorectal cancer (HNPCC). Most HNPCC patients have mutations in the DNA mismatch repair genes *MLH-1* and *MSH-2*. Mutations in these genes leads to an inability to repair DNA mismatch (mistakes that happen during DNA replication) and hence contribute to neoplastic transformation by allowing mutations to be transmitted to daughter cells.

Microsatellites are repeat units generally found within the non-coding part of the genome. They are highly polymorphic (the two alleles differ in size) and hence they provide a useful tool for the investigation of mutations within the genome. Patients with HNPCC show widespread alterations in these microsatellites and are therefore said to exhibit microsatellite instability (or a mutator phenotype). If microsatellite instability is found then the implication is that the mismatch repair genes must be inactivated, otherwise the mismatch repair proteins would have corrected the mutations identified in the microsatellites. Analysis of microsatellite instability therefore provides indirect evidence for mismatch repair gene abnormality, and patients with high levels of instability can have direct genetic testing to look for the mutations in the mismatch repair genes.

APOPTOSIS AND CANCER

Following genetic damage, the cell may have an opportunity to repair the defect via the pathways described above. Occasionally the damage is so severe that the cell is unable to do this and a set of signals are initiated that lead to programmed cell death. This is an important protective mechanism as a cell with severe genetic damage is no threat if it is dead! It is only when it manages to go through the cell division cycle with its damage and pass the alterations onto the daughter cells that problems are likely to occur.

Apart from showing increased proliferation, cancer cells also fail to undergo apoptosis and hence have an increased lifespan compared with normal cells. The inability of cancer cells to commit suicide is an important contributory factor to tumour growth both at the primary site and at the sites of metastatic spread.

Many genes involved in the control of apoptosis have now been identified. The first to be identified was *bcl-2*. This gene is a member of a large family of genes, some of which are pro-apoptotic (*bax*, *bad*), while others are anti-apoptotic (*bcl-2*, *bcl-xL*). The mechanisms controlling apoptosis are complex. In response to DNA damage, a whole series of cascades are set up, the balance of which determines whether the cell is sent into a death programme. In the presence of an overall death outcome, the Bcl-2 family of proteins operate via the activation of a series of proteolytic enzymes called caspases, which chop up the DNA into fragments.

Two other genes that are also prominent in the apoptotic pathway are *p53* (discussed above) and c-*myc* oncogene.

TELOMERES, TELOMERASE AND CANCER

Telomeres consist of a series of short tandem nucleotide repeat sequences of six base pairs (TTAGGG) that are found at the ends of chromosomes. They cap the chromosomes and protect the ends from degradation during the DNA replication that occurs as part of cell growth and differentiation. They also work as a molecular counting mechanism (an intracellular clock), because with each round of DNA replication, the telomeres shorten until the cell reaches a 'crisis' (also known as the Hayflick limit). At this point the chromosomal ends become dysfunctional, end-to-end joining occurs and the cell is sent into apoptosis via a p53-mediated pathway.

An enzyme called telomerase plays a role in the maintenance of the telomeres by preventing the erosion of telomeres that occurs during replication. This enzyme is a ribonucleoprotein reverse transcriptase that is composed of two components, hTERC (the RNA subunit that acts as the template for addition of new telomeric repeats) and hTERT (the catalytic protein component). Its expression is tightly regulated during development and, after this period, in humans, it is expressed in quantities sufficient to prevent telomere erosion in male germ cells, lymphocytes and stem cell populations, including basal keratinocytes. The state when the cell cannot divide anymore is called 'cellular senescence'.

It is becoming clear that in order to create a cancer cell, two barriers must be overcome: cellular senescence and the crisis that limits replicative potential. This hypothesis seems to be valid for both benign and malignant tumours, at least in *in vitro* experiments. It is not difficult to postulate that cancer cells have learnt how to circumvent the erosion of telomeres. This is indeed the case and, unlike normal, non-germ cells, most cancer cells have detectable and increased telomerase activity or develop an alternative mechanism for telomere lengthening (ALT), which is thought to involve recombination mechanisms and results in abnormal telomeres.

Several lines of evidence have supported the major role of telomerase in oncogenesis. When normal cells reach the 'crisis' (complete erosion of telomeres), lack of telomerase leads to major chromosomal abnormalities (aneuploidy and chromosomal fusions). Other connections between telomerase and other oncogenes and tumour suppressor genes are currently under intense investigation and over the next 5 years, the progress in this field is likely to be fast and exciting.

MULTISTEP MODEL OF CARCINOGENESIS

In the course of examining malignant tissues, histopathologists frequently encounter lesions that show transitions with appearances half-way between normal morphology and frank malignancy. Occasionally such lesions are closely associated with an invasive cancer. This led to the suggestion that many of these lesions may be precursors of the invasive carcinoma. With the identification of dominant oncogenes and tumour suppressor genes, genes involved in DNA repair and apoptosis, it became possible to investigate tumours and putative precursor lesions using molecular techniques. The study of colorectal carcinoma with its well-defined pre-invasive lesion, the adenoma, has paved the way for this type of investigation (Fig. 12.14). The results demonstrate that both activating and inactivating events are involved and it is the co-ordinated involvement of many of these types of alterations that are important in colon tumour formation. Furthermore, it is not just the timing of the events but the sequential accumulation of genetic damage that is also important in tumour formation. This

idea that it is not one event but a sequence of genetic alterations that produces tumours is referred to as the multistep theory of neoplasia.

The idea of the multistep model has been extended to almost every tumour type and there is good evidence that cancers in general develop in this way. The idea behind this type of model has also been fundamental in recommending screening programmes for cancer, the argument being that if you pick up a 'tumour' either when it is very small or still in its early stages of development, you can cure it. While the idea is a good one, it has also opened up a whole lot of problems. The screening programmes are identifying lesions at a very early stage in development and the classification and natural history of many such lesions is at present unknown. Once a lesion has been removed, the patient inevitably wants to know what it is and what its implications are. Since this is not always possible to predict with accuracy, it can cause much distress, for the clinician as well as for the patient.

NEW MOLECULAR TECHNIQUES

There has been a hope that new molecular techniques will help us to understand the biology of cancer and in particular the early lesions. So what are these techniques and how are they helping with patient management?

Loss of heterozygosity (LOH)

Following on from Knudson's 'two-hit' hypothesis for the presence of tumour suppressor genes, it was recognized that the second mutation that leads to inactivation of the gene is usually in the form of a large deletion. This led to the development of the loss of heterozygosity (LOH) technique by Cavenee and colleagues. The technique relies on that observation that markers (microsatellites) that are heterozygous and near the tumour suppressor gene would become homo- or hemizygous in the tumour compared with normal tissue. This was confirmed in the case of retinoblastoma, where markers close to the gene were seen to exhibit LOH in both sporadic and familial cancers.

Since the introduction of the technique, there have been numerous studies looking at LOH in many cancer types. Although patterns of LOH have been reported in some series as being of prognostic

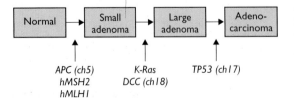

Figure 12.14 Multistep model for colorectal carcinoma

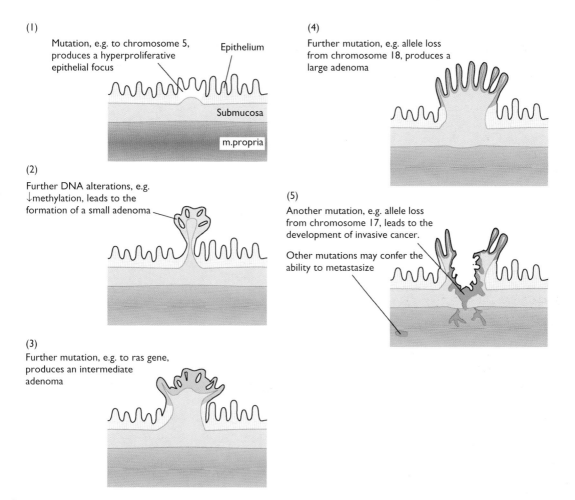

(1)

Mutation, e.g. to chromosome 5, produces a hyperproliferative epithelial focus

Epithelium

Submucosa

m.propria

(2)

Further DNA alterations, e.g. ↓methylation, leads to the formation of a small adenoma

(3)

Further mutation, e.g. to ras gene, produces an intermediate adenoma

(4)

Further mutation, e.g. allele loss from chromosome 18, produces a large adenoma

(5)

Another mutation, e.g. allele loss from chromosome 17, leads to the development of invasive cancer.

Other mutations may confer the ability to metastasize

Figure 12.15 The colonic adenoma–carcinoma sequence

significance, this information has not yet translated into routine practice. LOH has also been used extensively to investigate precancerous lesions in the hope that patterns of LOH would help to stratify lesions into 'benign' and 'malignant'. It has become apparent that many lesions traditionally thought of as 'benign' are monoclonal, and that there is considerable overlap in LOH between these lesions and those accepted as 'malignant' (e.g. ductal carcinoma *in situ*). At present there are no robust profiles using LOH that help to definitively distinguish such lesions in clinical practice.

Comparative genomic hybridization (CGH)

Comparative genomic hybridization is a fluorescent *in situ* hybridization technique capable of determining changes in DNA copy number between differentially labelled test (e.g. tumour) and reference (e.g. normal) samples. Unlike LOH analysis, which gives information at a very specific locus on a chromosomal arm, comparative genomic hybridization analysis provides information from the entire genome. This has the advantage that a single experiment can give an idea about the many changes on all the different chromosomes, data that would require hundreds of experiments using LOH analysis. Traditionally, comparative genomic hybridization has been done using competitive hybridization to normal metaphase chromosomes. This means that resolution is poor, and only capable of detecting high-level amplifications of around 2 Mb and deletions of the order of 10 Mb. Hence, there is a compromise between global information and identifying a very specific location of the change.

A large number of investigators have used comparative genomic hybridization analysis to understand the changes in DNA copy number in invasive cancer as well as precancerous lesions. As yet, specific profiles that are of prognostic significance or that predict for response to therapy have not been developed for routine use, but clearly there is hope that such a profile may be developed in time.

Expression arrays

As well as cataloguing amplifications, deletions and complex rearrangements at the genomic (DNA) level, analysis of changes in the profiles of gene expression (mRNA) may give clues to the underlying molecular events in tumorigenesis. In this method thousands of sequences of cDNA are arrayed robotically onto a glass slide. The samples to be examined are mixed and co-hybridized to the arrays in a competitive manner, and the resulting fluorescence values reveal the relative levels of each RNA transcript in the test sample compared with the reference sample. Mathematical algorithms are then used by bioinformaticians to probe differences in expression patterns between sample sets.

Expression profiles generated by cDNA arrays can reveal similarities and differences that are not necessarily evident from traditional approaches, such as morphological or immunohistochemical analysis.

The power of this technique has been elegantly demonstrated in a number of recent experiments. They first demonstrated that within the morphologically homogeneous category of large B cell lymphoma, two subtypes exist with differing patterns of gene expression. Subsequent papers have looked at other tumour types such as breast cancers and also identified subclasses of tumour not easily identified using routine microscopy.

Protein arrays

Protein molecules, rather than DNA or RNA, carry out most cellular functions. The direct measurement of protein levels and activity within the cell is likely to be the best determinant of overall cell function. Techniques are being developed to quantify the levels of all the proteins within a cell and to compare protein levels between different cell types. Proteomic analysis, consisting of two-dimensional gel electrophoresis (2D PAGE) and tandem mass spectrometry, has been used to map protein profiles in normal and tumour cells. As would be expected, the studies have highlighted differences in protein profiles between subsets of normal cells and between normal cells and tumour cells. It is unlikely that the 'proteome' is stable over time as the cell requirements are constantly changing as it adapts to its environment. Any proteomic data are therefore likely to represent only a snapshot of the 'proteome'.

At present, protein array techniques are labour intensive and require large amounts of purified samples. They are therefore not yet appropriate for use in clinical practice. However, use of this technology will undoubtedly lead to the identification of new cancer-associated proteins.

CONCLUSION

Pathological assessment of tissues has remained the linchpin of diagnostic practice for over a hundred years. It has become the core science of clinical medical practice, providing data for clinical management and a framework for future correlation of new markers and new therapies. With the current explosion of technology and data, it is important for pathologists and other clinical specialists to embrace and incorporate these changes into their training and practice. Molecular biologists will also benefit from a closer interaction with pathologists.

That brings us to the end of this section on the cellular events involved in producing the cancer cell. Of course, we have a long way to go before we have a full understanding, but our knowledge is advancing at an exciting pace, and a whole new language of tumour terminology is emerging. For the scientist, the battle is the biology; for the clinicians and students trying to understand and apply the new knowledge, it is often the terminology!

The next question we need to address, and one that will be in the forefront of the patient's mind, is how will a given tumour behave?

CHAPTER 13

The behaviour of tumours

The behaviour of a tumour can be considered under a number of headings covering how fast it will grow, whether it is likely to metastasize, which sites are affected and what symptoms and complications the patient is likely to suffer.

GROWTH OF TUMOURS

It is often assumed that tumours grow faster than normal tissues because they expand to compress the surrounding structures. However, this does not mean that the cells are dividing more often, but that there is an imbalance between production and loss. The time taken for tumour cell division varies between 20 and 60 hours, with leukaemias having shorter cell cycles than solid tumours but, in general, tumour cells take longer than their normal counterparts. Cells can be in a resting phase or in growth phase, i.e. in one of the stages of mitosis. Some normal tissues have a high turnover of cells, such as the intestine, where around 16 per cent of the cells will be in the growth fraction. In contrast, most tumours have only 2–8 per cent of their cells actively dividing. This is important therapeutically because the cells in the growth phase are most readily damaged by chemotherapy and so tumours with a large growth fraction (e.g. leukaemias, lymphomas and lung anaplastic small cell carcinoma) will respond better than tumours with few cells proliferating (e.g. colon and breast).

Can we predict how fast a tumour is growing? To some extent, yes. The number of mitotic figures present per unit area in a light microscopic section is a crude measure of how active the proliferation is within a tumour. A tumour with a large number of cells in mitosis is likely to behave aggressively and this is why a mitotic count is one of the criteria for grading tumours (page 227). However, the number of cells seen to be in mitosis is not only influenced by

the growth fraction and the cell cycle time but also by whether they get 'stuck', i.e. the tumour cell can enter mitosis but, possibly because of an irregularity in chromosome number or in the internal organization of the mitotic spindle, may fail to complete the mitosis. Thus, on the examination of a tissue section, the tumour appears to be highly proliferative but it is really 'stuck'. Tumour growth will also be influenced by factors like the blood supply and, possibly, the host's immune response (Chapter 5, page 263).

It would also be wrong to assume that every cell in a tumour behaves similarly. The daughter cells of a dividing cell are identical genetically to the parent cell and are said to be clones. However, tumour cells are also prone to develop genetic instability, which results in some cells developing further abnormalities and the formation of multiple subclones (page 252). These may have certain survival advantages; for example, they may have enhanced angiogenic, invasive or metastatic capabilities. This is referred to as tumour heterogeneity and it is important to consider when planning treatments, because it means that some tumour cells may respond differently to particular chemotherapeutic agents. This is analogous to bacterial resistance to antibiotics: just as a combination of antibiotics is most effective against an unknown organism, so a mixture of treatment modalities is often used against a tumour.

HOW DO TUMOURS SPREAD?

Just over a hundred years ago, Stephen Paget (no, not the man who described Paget's disease – that was Sir James Paget) collected post mortem records of 735 patients who had died of breast cancer and he found that the majority of the metastases were in the liver and brain. He concluded, therefore, that certain tumours were predisposed to metastasize to certain tissues. He wrote, 'When a plant

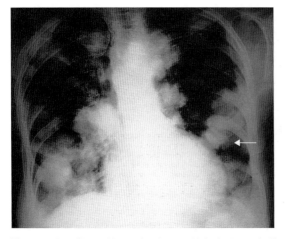

Figure 13.1 Chest X-ray showing multiple 'cannon ball' metastases

goes to seed, its seeds are carried in all directions; but they can only live and grow if they fall on congenial soil'. Not surprisingly, it came to be known as the 'seed and soil' theory.

James Ewing, 40 years later, suggested that tumours went to particular organs not because of the seed and soil effect, but rather because of the routes of the blood supply to the primary organ. Using his hypothesis, organs directly in line away from the primary site would be targets for metastatic disease.

We know now that they are both partially correct. Tumours of the colon do indeed go to the liver, which is next in line through the portal circulation, but then so do many other tumours much farther away, such as melanomas arising in the eye. We also know that organs such as the heart and skeletal muscle, despite being exposed to large volumes of blood, rarely develop metastases. In broad terms, tumour spread through lymphatics will produce metastases in the anatomically related lymph nodes, while spread through the blood is influenced more by 'seed and soil' considerations, although anatomy is still of some importance.

The main routes of spread are via:

- lymphatics
- veins
- transcoelomic cavities
- cerebrospinal fluid
- arteries.

Lymphatic spread is common in carcinomas (tumours of epithelia) and the nodes that are involved first are the nodes that drain the tumour

site. Thus a knowledge of the lymphatic anatomy is useful for predicting where the tumour will spread and is the basis for many of the staging protocols (page 229). However, lymph nodes near tumours can enlarge as part of an immune reaction that particularly results in expansion of the macrophage compartment (sinus histiocytosis). This means that the doctor must try to distinguish between soft, mobile nodes, which are likely to be reactive, and the hard, fixed nodes that contain metastatic tumour.

Venous spread will take tumours of the gastrointestinal tract to the liver and tumours from a variety of sites to the lungs. It is also the favoured route of spread for sarcomas (tumours of connective tissue). Some tumours may even grow along a vein, causing its obstruction (e.g. renal cell carcinoma in the renal vein). Arteries are not often penetrated by tumours but, in the later stages of metastatic spread, tumour nodules can start to develop almost anywhere and it is likely that this happens after pulmonary metastases enter the pulmonary vein and are then distributed through the systemic arterial system. It is easy to understand how tumours that reach the pleural or peritoneal cavities can drop into the fluid and be disseminated throughout that coelomic cavity. Similarly, the CSF (cerebrospinal fluid) provides an easy route of spread for cerebral tumours, which do not generally metastasize outside the central nervous system.

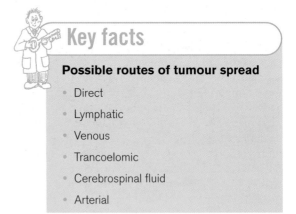

Key facts

Possible routes of tumour spread

- Direct
- Lymphatic
- Venous
- Trancoelomic
- Cerebrospinal fluid
- Arterial

One cubic centimetre of tumour can shed millions of cells into the circulation each day – so why are metastases not inevitable? Let us consider the steps required to produce a metastases.

First, the tumour has to grow at the primary site and infiltrate the surrounding connective tissue, which may necessitate breaking through a basement

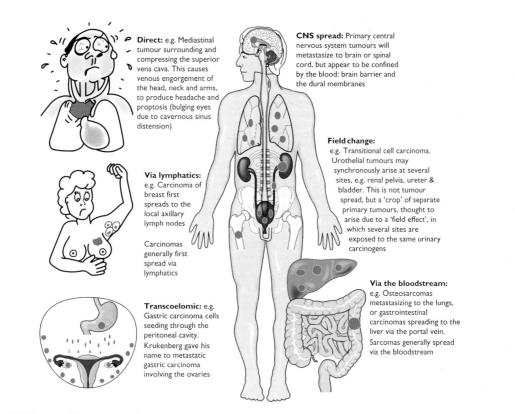

Direct: e.g. Mediastinal tumour surrounding and compressing the superior vena cava. This causes venous engorgement of the head, neck and arms, to produce headache and proptosis (bulging eyes due to cavernous sinus distension)

CNS spread: Primary central nervous system tumours will metastasize to brain or spinal cord, but appear to be confined by the blood: brain barrier and the dural membranes

Via lymphatics: e.g. Carcinoma of breast first spreads to the local axillary lymph nodes

Carcinomas generally first spread via lymphatics

Field change: e.g. Transitional cell carcinoma. Urothelial tumours may synchronously arise at several sites, e.g. renal pelvis, ureter & bladder. This is not tumour spread, but a 'crop' of separate primary tumours, thought to arise due to a 'field effect', in which several sites are exposed to the same urinary carcinogens

Transcoelomic: e.g. Gastric carcinoma cells seeding through the peritoneal cavity. Krukenberg gave his name to metastatic gastric carcinoma involving the ovaries

Via the bloodstream: e.g. Osteosarcomas metastasizing to the lungs, or gastrointestinal carcinomas spreading to the liver via the portal vein. Sarcomas generally spread via the bloodstream

Figure 13.2 Routes of tumour spread

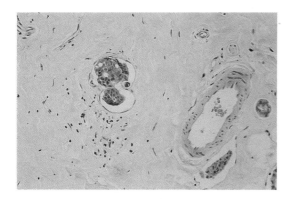

Figure 13.3 Photomicrograph of breast with lymphatic permeation by tumour

membrane and the connective tissues nearby. It may also have to overcome inhibitor substances to the enzymes it produces to break down these connective tissue proteins. Then it can reach the lymphatic and blood vascular channels, which are important routes for dissemination. It has to find a way of attaching to the endothelium and subsequently enter the channels. The vessel wall is traversed and

the tumour cells must detach to float in the blood or lymph and hope to evade any immune cells that might destroy them. Next they must lodge in the capillaries at their destination, attach to the endothelium again and penetrate the vessel wall to enter the perivascular connective tissue, where they finally proliferate to produce a tumour deposit.

What stands between the primary tumour and the vessel? First, there are a variety of extracellular matrix components to break through, for which the tumour may produce a number of enzymes. Loose connective tissue is not much of a barrier, but dense fibrous areas, such as tendons and joint capsules and cartilage, can resist tumour spread. Next is the basement membrane, for which the tumour has to be able to secrete a type IV collagenase. Tumours often have collagenases to dissolve collagen but are less able to digest elastic tissue. This may be one of the reasons why arterial walls, which contain a lot of elastic tissue, are less readily penetrated than venous walls. Alternatively, it may be because arterial walls are thicker and contain protease inhibitors. Once in the vessel lumen, tumour

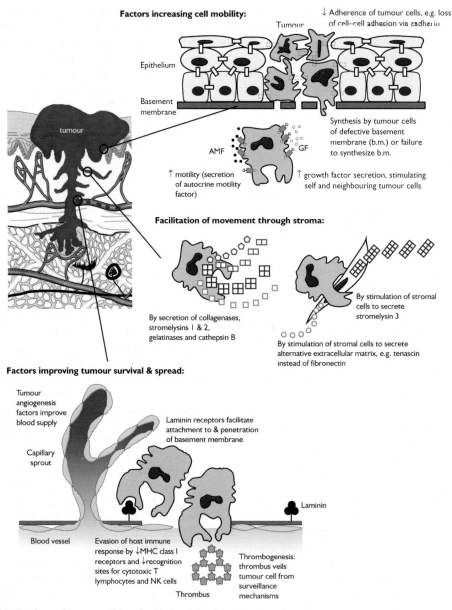

Factors increasing cell mobility:

Tumour

↓ Adherence of tumour cells, e.g. loss of cell–cell adhesion via cadherin

Epithelium

Basement membrane

AMF GF

↑ motility (secretion of autocrine motility factor)

Synthesis by tumour cells of defective basement membrane (b.m.) or failure to synthesize b.m.

↑ growth factor secretion, stimulating self and neighbouring tumour cells

tumour

Facilitation of movement through stroma:

By secretion of collagenases, stromelysins 1 & 2, gelatinases and cathepsin B

By stimulation of stromal cells to secrete stromelysin 3

By stimulation of stromal cells to secrete alternative extracellular matrix, e.g. tenascin instead of fibronectin

Factors improving tumour survival & spread:

Tumour angiogenesis factors improve blood supply

Capillary sprout

Laminin receptors facilitate attachment to & penetration of basement membrane

Laminin

Blood vessel

Evasion of host immune response by ↓MHC class I receptors and ↓recognition sites for cytotoxic T lymphocytes and NK cells

Thrombogenesis: thrombus veils tumour cell from surveillance mechanisms

Thrombus

Figure 13.4 Mechanisms of tumour cell invasion and metastasis

cells are prey to immune surveillance by the body's lymphocytes and monocytes.

Finally, the tumour must attach to the endothelium at its destination, which may involve specific adhesion molecules (addressins) that 'home' the metastatic tumour to a particular site, analogous to the 'homing' of lymphocytes (Chapter 5).

Most of our discussions about tumour cell biology have concentrated on how genetic changes enhance cell proliferation. However, we should now look at how a proliferating tumour cell differs from a proliferating normal cell. Early experiments involving *in vitro* cell cultures demonstrated that normal cells would grow to form monolayers and then stop. This was referred to as contact inhibition. If some cells from this culture were transferred to a new culture vessel (passaged), they would begin to grow again in the same way; however, normal cells would only survive about 30–50 serial passages. Cultures of proliferating tumour cells differed in that they lost contact inhibition and so could grow as disorganized multilayers and they were also immortal, i.e. although each individual cell did not last forever, the clone of cells could be passaged indefinitely. Now it is known that tumour cells may show decreased expression of E-cadherin, which normally acts as an adhesion molecule between epithelial cells, and that their increased motility may be influenced by an autocrine motility factor released by some transformed culture cells.

Tumour cells can also influence the production of stroma, so that tenascin (a high-molecular-weight extracellular matrix glycoprotein involved in cell–cell and cell–matrix interaction) may predominate, which does not bind readily to tumour cells. This sort of information suggests that it is not only changes in the tumour cells that produce local invasion and metastasis, but that interactions between tumour cells, normal cells and stroma are also important.

THE ROLE OF THE IMMUNE SYSTEM

We are all aware of the role played by the immune system in defending us against infections, so it is not surprising that questions have been raised as to whether it has any role in protection against cancer. It was Paul Ehrlich, in 1909, who postulated that without the immune system constantly removing the 'aberrant germs', human beings would inevitably die of cancer. Many attempts have been made to establish the role of the immune system in cancer and initial experiments, which involved transplanting tumours from one animal to another, appeared to support the concept. It was later realized that the destruction of these transplanted tumours was not due to immunity but to transplant rejection. Now, inbred mice can be used experimentally, thus avoiding the factor of transplant rejection.

For certain tumour types it has been shown that, if the tumour is removed from a mouse and the animal rechallenged with the tumour, the tumour is rejected. This supports the idea that immunity is involved in tumour rejection, but life is not quite so simple as we shall see.

You will recall that the cells of the immune system have to be able to distinguish between 'self' and 'non-self', by identifying specific antigens on the cell surface (page 133). Malignant tumours are derived from 'self', so if the immune system is to defend against tumours, the malignant cells must acquire antigens that differentiate them from normal cells.

These are termed tumour-specific antigens and the whole subject has been highly controversial. In humans, such tumour-associated antigens are beginning to be defined and include differentiation antigens (e.g. CD19 and CD29), growth factor receptors such as epidermal growth factor receptor (EGFR) and intracellular proteins such as the MAGE family of proteins, which are highly expressed in melanoma. These antigens have been identified by isolating tumour reactive T cells from patients with malignancies.

While tumours clearly do elicit immune responses, the degree of response does not appear to be sufficient to hold the progression of the malignancy in most cases. It is conceivable that as tumours progress, clones of cells without the antigens proliferate and escape immune destruction.

A whole new area of cancer vaccination is developing rapidly and initial trials appear encouraging. For example, vaccination with ganglioside GM2 in melanoma appears to increase survival. However, time will tell whether the effects of immunization live up to the promise suggested by initial trials.

There is also evidence from animal experiments that surface antigens are altered in some tumours induced by viruses or chemicals. Viral-induced tumours in animals can display a new surface antigen (T), which is believed to be a viral peptide associated with major histocompatibility complex (MHC). This provokes a specific cytotoxic T cell response and all tumours induced by a particular virus display the same antigen, regardless of the cell of origin. The obvious potential application for this lies in immunizing against tumours.

Chemically induced tumours in animals (e.g. by benzopyrene) may also display new surface antigens that induce a specific immune response, but these antigens are very varied, with primary tumours in the same animal exhibiting antigenic differences, so there is no cross-resistance through immunization.

Of course, the immune response need not be antigen-specific. Besides B and T lymphocytes, the body has at its disposal natural killer cells (NK cells) and macrophages. NK cells have the capacity to destroy cells without prior sensitization as well as the ability to participate in antibody-dependent cellular cytotoxicity (ADCC). Macrophages are also involved, either due to non-specific activation or in collaboration with T lymphocytes, and can participate via ADCC or by the release of cytotoxic factors, such as tumour necrosis factor (TNF), hydrogen peroxide or a cytolytic protease.

CHAPTER 14

The clinical effects of tumours

LOCAL EFFECTS

The local effects of a tumour will depend on its site, its type and its growth pattern. Some complications, such as haemorrhage, are more common in malignant tumours because of their ability to invade underlying tissues and their vessels, but it must be remembered that even a microscopic benign tumour (e.g. a meningioma on the surface of the brain) can kill the patient as a result of its local effects.

Local effects can complicate both benign and malignant tumours. They include:

- compression
- obstruction
- ulceration
- haemorrhage
- rupture
- perforation
- infarction.

Compression and obstruction

A patient with any intracranial tumour (e.g. meningioma, astrocytoma, oligodendroglioma) may present with headaches, nausea and vomiting, because the mass growing within the closed cavity of the cranium raises the intracranial pressure. If the tumour is not removed and the pressure continues to rise, the patient will die from pressure effects on the vital respiratory centres.

A more localized example of the effect of compression is when the pituitary gland enlarges in the small cup-shaped space of the sella turcica. Local pressure will cause erosion of the bony sella and compression of the optic chiasma that sits directly above. The patient will then present with visual disturbance, classically a bitemporal hemianopia.

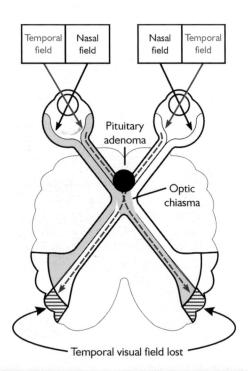

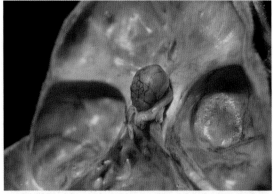

Figure 14.1 Benign tumours may have profound effects. Here, a small pituitary adenoma produced blindness in both temporal visual fields by compressing optic nerve fibres at the optic chiasma

Compression and obstruction have been included in the same section here because there is often an overlap. Compression can directly damage normal tissue, as described in the pituitary, or it may cause obstruction. This occurs, for example, when a tracheal tumour obstructs a normal oesophagus or vice versa. In the brain, compression of the brainstem structures may obstruct the flow of cerebrospinal fluid, and a large prostate (benign or malignant) may compress the prostatic urethra. Alternatively, a tumour can grow into the lumen of the gut or into an airway so that it produces obstruction directly.

Ulceration and haemorrhage

An ulcer is defined as a macroscopically apparent loss of surface epithelium, and may be benign or malignant. Ulceration of the skin will lead to a crust of dried fibrin and cells covering the area and is unlikely to produce severe haemorrhage. However, ulceration in the gastrointestinal tract, particularly the stomach and duodenum, may result in life-threatening haemorrhage or perforation. Here the absence of epithelium means the loss of an important defence mechanism, which normally protects the underlying tissue from acid and enzymes. Once the submucosa is exposed to these agents, large vessel walls can be digested, resulting in massive bleeding.

Rupture or perforation

Rupture or perforation typically affects tumours of the gastrointestinal tract and will occur if the intraluminal pressure exceeds the strength of the

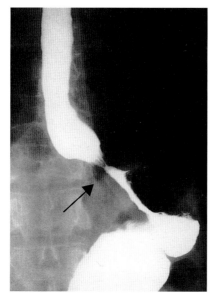

Figure 14.2 X-ray showing constriction of lower oesophagus by oesophageal carcinoma

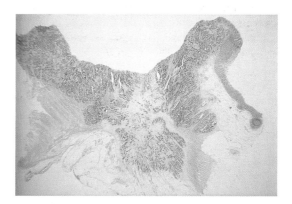

Figure 14.4 Photomicrograph showing rectal ulceration due to adenocarcinoma

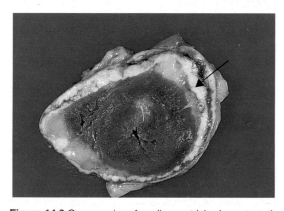

Figure 14.3 Compression of cardiac ventricles by metastatic lung carcinoma infiltrating the pericardium

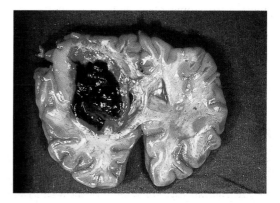

Figure 14.5 Haemorrhage within intracerebral tumour

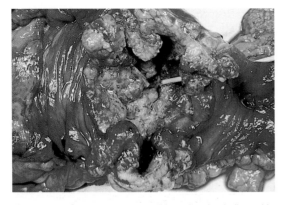

Figure 14.6 Colonic carcinoma with perforation indicated by probe

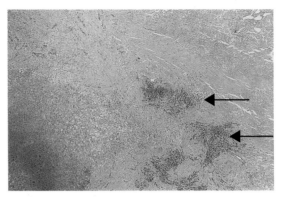

Figure 14.7 Extensive infarction in tumour, leaving small islands of viable cells

wall or if the wall is eroded or weakened by tumour, ischaemia or enzymic action, etc. Obviously, there is a risk of dilatation and rupture when part of the gut becomes obstructed as the gut contents cannot follow their normal route. Rupture may also occur in closed organs, such as the ovary, because the tumour has stretched the capsule, often because of accumulation of fluid or mucin as well as the proliferation of neoplastic cells.

Infarction

Many malignant tumours will show necrosis and infarction in their central region, which is believed to result from inadequate blood supply. In experimental models, a tumour can only expand to a diameter of 1–2 mm before it must stimulate new blood vessel formation and, in human tumours, zones of necrosis may be encountered approximately 1–2 mm from a blood vessel. Therefore, it appears that this is the maximum distance for diffusion of nutrients. Tumours attempt to solve this by secreting angiogenic factors that stimulate capillaries to grow into the neoplasm.

Local anatomy influences the likelihood of infarction related to large vessel obstruction. The bowel, ovaries and testes are particularly liable to torsion, i.e. twisting on their vascular pedicle, which occludes the vessels.

Although we often separate the complications of tumours under the headings of local tumour and metastatic tumour, a metastasis can produce any of the local effects mentioned above. In particular, lymph nodes containing metastases can cause obstruction at crucial sites, such as the porta hepatis or the hilum of the lung.

ENDOCRINE EFFECTS

Well-differentiated tumours do not only look like their tissue of origin but can also act like them. Thus tumours of endocrine organs can produce hormones that act on the same tissues as their physiological counterparts but are not under normal feedback control.

Cushing's syndrome provides an interesting example in which different endocrine tumours produce the same clinical problems. In Cushing's syndrome, the patient suffers from osteoporosis, muscle wasting, thinning of the skin with purple striae and easy bruising, truncal obesity and impaired glucose tolerance. All this is the result of excess glucocorticoids. The same picture can be produced by prolonged administration of steroids to treat diseases (e.g. chronic asthma), but in this section we are interested in the tumours that can cause it (page 220).

The adrenal produces corticosteroids when stimulated by adrenocorticotrophic hormone (ACTH) from the pituitary. The corticosteroids then provide negative feedback to the pituitary and ACTH levels drop. Cushing's syndrome can result from an adenoma in the pituitary gland, which produces ACTH, or a cortical tumour in the adrenal cortex, which secretes corticosteroids. Normal feedback does not operate as the adenoma cells behave autonomously. However, if very high doses of steroid (dexamethasone suppression test) are given, then the pituitary adenoma will reduce its ACTH production and endogenous steroid levels will fall, but excess steroid due to an adrenal adenoma will not be suppressed.

Some non-endocrine tumours can produce substances that have the same effects as hormones, so-called inappropriate production. One of the most common results is Cushing's syndrome when ACTH is produced by oat cell (anaplastic small cell) carcinoma of the bronchus, carcinoid tumours, thymomas or medullary carcinoma of the thyroid. This inappropriate and autonomous production does not suppress with high doses of dexamethasone.

PARANEOPLASTIC SYNDROMES

Symptoms in cancer patients that are not readily explained by local or metastatic disease are referred to as paraneoplastic syndromes. Endocrine effects are generally included as paraneoplastic if the production is inappropriate (as above), but not if the tumour arises from a tissue that normally produces that hormone.

Hypercalcaemia is a common, clinically important and complex problem with malignant tumours. In a patient with widespread metastases in bone, it may be explained as a local destructive effect of the tumour on bone which releases calcium. However, hypercalcaemia can also occur without metastatic bony deposits and, in some cases, it appears that a parathyroid hormone-like peptide or TGFα is secreted by the primary tumour and this is most likely with bronchial squamous cell carcinoma and adult T cell leukaemia/lymphoma.

Clubbing of the fingers and hypertrophic osteoarthropathy are also common with lung carcinoma, but can occur in non-neoplastic conditions including cyanotic heart disease and liver disease. It is not clear how it develops, nor why sectioning the vagus nerve can lead to its disappearance! Equally mysterious are the skin disorders, peripheral neuropathy and cerebellar degeneration that may also occur in association with malignant tumours.

GENERAL EFFECTS

The general effects of tumours are not classed as paraneoplastic syndromes, although they are extremely common and must not be forgotten. These include general malaise, weight loss and lethargy, which are due to a combination of metabolic and hormonal influences exacerbated by any malnutrition or infection. This results in the clinical picture known as cachexia. An important chemical factor that may play a role in cachexia is cachexin, also known as tumour necrosis factor (TNF). This molecule is not produced by the tumour cells, but by activated macrophages. Anaemia is also common and can contribute to the general malaise. This may be a direct effect of metastatic deposits in bone marrow or an indirect effect of mediators that suppress haematopoiesis.

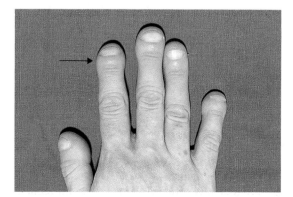

Figure 14.8 Finger clubbing

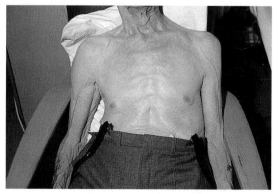

Figure 14.9 Cancer-related muscle wasting (cachexia)

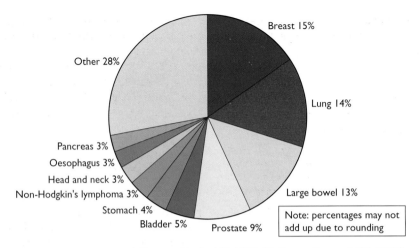

Figure 14.10 The ten most common cancers* diagnosed in the UK, 1999. (© Cancer Research UK, 2002)
* Excludes non-melanoma skin cancer

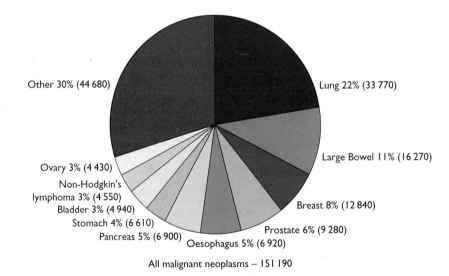

Figure 14.11 The ten most common causes of death from cancer in the UK, 2000 (© Cancer Research UK, 2002)

MANAGEMENT OF CANCER

Although we will discuss the management of cancer under individual headings, many patients receive a combination of management strategies.

Screening programmes

The concept of the multistep model of carcinogenesis has led to the idea that mortality from the tumour may be reduced if it is identified at an earlier stage or when it is still precancerous. Screening programmes have been instituted for cervical and breast cancer and there is considerable debate as to whether other tumour types such as prostate and colon should be included. The screening programme has undoubtedly reduced mortality, although not as dramatically as had been envisaged. It has also highlighted deficiencies in our knowledge of the classification and natural history of early lesions, making management of patients with these 'precancers' problematic. In order to circumvent this problem, management decisions are now made in multidisciplinary teams (comprising surgeons, physicians, oncologists, pathologists, radiologists, specialist nurses, etc.), bringing all their expertise to bear on deciding the final strategy.

Local excision

Local treatment is aimed either at achieving a cure or providing specific symptomatic relief. Cancers such as squamous and basal cell carcinomas of the skin and cancers arising within polyps in the colon can be cured by local excision. In tumours of the bowel, local excision may relieve an obstruction and provide good long-term remission of symptoms or even cure.

Radiotherapy

Radiotherapy can be given from an external source or by implanting a small radioactive source into the tissues. Delivery schedules vary from centre to centre but the general idea is to divide, or fractionate, the doses in order to get the maximum kill of tumour cells with the minimum damage to normal tissues. Implanted radioactive sources are very useful for providing high-dose local radiation and are particularly useful in cancers of the head and neck, where there are many vital structures close together.

Chemotherapy

Chemotherapy is a relatively new and rapidly evolving form of treatment. In patients suffering from haematological malignancies (e.g. leukaemia) or disseminated disease, surgery and radiation are not realistic options. You cannot excise a leukaemia and you cannot irradiate metastases which are widespread in the body!

In the 1950s, alkylating agents (e.g. busulfan) and antimetabolites (e.g. methotrexate) were introduced and proved useful in the management of disseminated cancers. The main problem with such agents is that all of the body's normal tissues are also exposed to the drug and so the challenge is to deliver enough drug to kill the tumour without killing the patient!

Endocrine-related treatment

This often involves giving a drug that inhibits tumour growth by removing an endocrine stimulus. For example, many breast carcinomas have receptors for oestrogen that stimulate tumour growth. A drug such as tamoxifen will block these receptors and reduce progression of the disease. An alternative approach would be to remove the ovaries, which produce oestrogen, much as the testes can be removed in males with prostatic adenocarcinomas to reduce the stimulus for tumour growth from androgens.

Immunotherapy

DNA recombinant technology has enabled the production of cytotoxins in sufficient quantities for therapeutic use. The interferons (IFN) and tumour necrosis factors (TNF) are of particular interest. IFNα and IFNβ have been used to treat a variety of tumours with some good effect, although it appears that they may best be used in combination with other treatments. Renal carcinomas, melanomas and myelomas have shown a 10–15 per cent response, various lymphomas show a 40 per cent response and hairy cell leukaemia and mycosis fungoides have an 80–90 per cent response rate. TNFα has been used in the treatment of melanoma, although, to date, the response has been disappointing. Lymphokine-activated killer (LAK) cells are a subset of NK cells that have been used in combination with interleukin 2 to treat renal carcinomas and some melanomas and colorectal cancers.

As mentioned previously, attempts to identify specific tumour antigens are in progress and initial trials of vaccination seem encouraging. There is also considerable interest in raising monoclonal antibodies to tumour cells. The hope is that it might be possible to attach drugs to these antibodies so that they will be delivered specifically to the tumour cell; the concept of the 'magic bullet'. A lot of questions remain unanswered but the field of immunization and targeted treatment is bound to create excitement over the next decade.

Molecular mechanism-based therapies

With our increasing understanding of the mechanisms of disease, therapies directed at specific molecular pathways are rapidly emerging. These include monoclonal antibodies and enzyme inhibitors directed at specific genetic changes.

C-erb-B2, also known as HER-2/neu, is a tyrosine kinase-associated receptor located on 17q. It is amplified in 10–34 per cent of human breast carcinomas. Recently, a humanized monoclonal antibody directed against c-erb-B2 oncogene (rhuMAB HER-2 – herceptin) has been used to treat women with metastatic breast carcinomas who have HER-2 amplification. The results have been promising and the drug has been approved by the National Institute for Clinical Excellence (NICE) in the UK.

Since the early 1990s, much effort has been put into the discovery of molecules that are able to block specific kinases. The first drug that showed promising results was STI-571, which was tailored to specifically inhibit the BCR/ABL fusion gene product. BCR/ABL results from a balanced translocation between chromosomes 9 and 22, and is found in more than 95 per cent of chronic myeloid leukaemias (CML). Patients treated with this drug showed remarkable improvement. Not unexpectedly, STI-571 is not specific for this kinase and has been shown to inhibit other oncogenic tyrosine kinases, such as c-KIT and PDGFR. STI-571 seems to have a remarkable effect on neoplasms arising as a result of mutations of these genes and in particular in patients with gastrointestinal stromal tumours (GISTs) (with c-KIT activating mutations). The era of molecular-based therapies has made a good start.

Gene therapy

Gene therapy has recently emerged as an alternative to conventional cancer treatments. The idea behind the treatment is to exploit the knowledge gained over the last few decades in our understanding of the differences between a normal and a neoplastic cell and the technological developments of gene transfer between cells. Hence it has become possible to transfer genetic material (i.e. functional tumour suppressor genes) into a cell to transiently or permanently alter its biology (i.e. to induce cell cycle arrest/apoptosis). This may be achieved by using modified virus encoding specific DNA sequences (viral vector systems).

The introduction of genes that encode tumour suppressor proteins is known as therapeutic gene transfer. There are a number of drawbacks to this type of treatment, including the specificity of the virus for neoplastic cells, the side effects of the presence of the 'new gene' in normal cells and the reaction of the host immune system. Despite the deserved enthusiasm, the clinical application of gene therapy is still in its early days.

Dictionary box

- **Viral vector system or retroviral vector system:** A system in which the genome of a given retrovirus is modified. The genome of adenoviruses (*gag*, *env* and *pol* genes and long-terminal repeats, LTRs) is manipulated and the viral sequences are replaced by a given therapeutic gene (usually a lost tumour suppressor gene), whose transcription may be under control of LTRs. One advantage of retroviral vectors is their inability to infect non-dividing cells.

- **Adenoviral vector:** The adenovirus genome encodes several proteins that interfere with cell cycle, including E1a, which binds to and neutralizes pRB, and E1b, which binds to p53 and targets it for degradation. This disruption of the cell cycle is necessary for replication of the virus. Thus, the deletion of one of these genes results in viruses that can only replicate in cells with defective p53 or pRB pathways.

- **Antisense oligonucleotides:** Oligonucleotides are molecules that are complementary to a portion of a given mRNA. Usually they are designed to be complementary to an oncogene's transcripts (mRNAs). When injected into cells, it combines with its complementary mRNA. This complex (antisense oligonucleotide/oncogene transcript) cannot be 'read' by ribosomal machinery.

Palliative treatment

The treatment of cancer has a wider role than merely providing a cure and cancer physicians are not interested in simply achieving a response to the administered treatment. Palliative treatment does not just refer to treatment that is given to patients in order to make them comfortable prior to death. It is and should be part of the oncological support given to all cancer patients and not only includes medication for the control of pain and nausea but also chemotherapy and radiotherapy for the relief of local symptoms. The term 'continuing care' is sometimes used for this multidisciplinary approach, starting with diagnosis and extending to the patient's death. The important point is that our knowledge of all modalities of treatment, including pain control, has advanced considerably in recent years and the pessimistic view that if one has cancer one must pass one's last hours either conscious, but in agony, or pain-free but unconscious is no longer justified.

cloning of genes that cause familial predisposition to malignancy. Recently, two breast cancer predisposition genes called *BRCA1* and *BRCA2* have been cloned. Both these genes are large and mutations in almost every part of the gene have been identified in patients with cancers. This has highlighted many ethical and social implications of genetic testing for cancer susceptibility. It has brought to the forefront the financial considerations as private organizations fight for patency rights for genetic sequences. Millions of pounds and dollars have been invested in the search, billions will be reaped in screening tests.

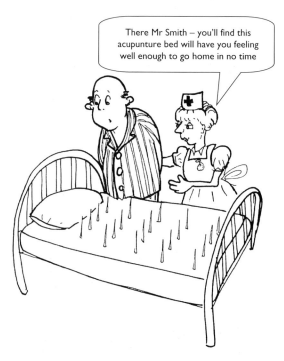

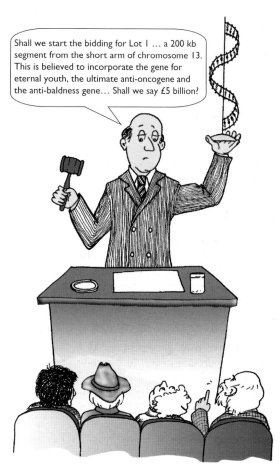

In conclusion; science, like most aspects of life, has its fashions. Much of this chapter has concentrated on our evolving understanding of the role of the genetic code in producing cancer. Current fashion lies very much with the identification and

Clinicopathological case study – cervical cancer

Clinical

A 38-year-old woman came to the surgery for a cervical smear.

She was single and had been living with her boyfriend for the last six months. She divorced her husband two years ago and since then had had a number of casual relationships. Her first sexual contact was at the age of 16.

Four years ago her smear showed warty change and the last one, a year ago again showed extensive warty change with possible dyskaryosis. The hospital had asked for a repeat smear as the epithelial cells were obscured by inflammatory debris.

She initially ignored the recall due to social problems.

The result of the repeat smear showed warty change and severe dyskaryosis and she was referred for a colposcopic biopsy.

The cervical biopsy confirmed the above findings and she was booked in to have a cervical cone biopsy.

The results of the cone biopsy came as a shock. The report read that she had extensive squamous metaplasia with wart virus change together with severe dysplasia between 3 o'clock and 5 o'clock and a focus of invasive squamous cell carcinoma which was completely excised. Invasive tumour did not involve deep tissues or invade blood vessels. The dysplastic epithelium extended to the endocervical excision margin and was therefore not completely excised.

The report was discussed with the patient and she was advised to have a hysterectomy.

The examination of the hysterectomy specimen showed residual foci of severe dysplasia but no invasive carcinoma. The excision was complete and she was discharged after an uneventful recovery.

Pathological

Carcinoma of the cervix is an important cause of death and the cervical screening programme has been instituted to try and reduce this toll. The idea is that if the disease can be picked up at an early stage, it should be possible to cure it.

The risk factors for cervical cancer include: smoking, early onset of sexual intercourse, multiple sexual partners, a sexual partner with a history of promiscuity and infection with the human papilloma virus (HPV).

Her history reveals that she had a number of risk factors including wart virus change on her previous cervical smears.

The normal routine recall for cervical smears is three years, but early recall is instituted for suspicious or abnormal smears.

Severe dyskaryosis is the cytological equivalent to severe dysplasia on histological examination.

Dysplasia is a premalignant condition in which there are cytological features of malignancy, i.e. increased nuclear:cytoplasmic ratio, nuclear pleomorphism, hyperchromatism, loss of maturation and mitotic activity. Dysplasia can be graded as mild, moderate or severe. Severe dysplasia implies a full-thickness abnormality and the feature distinguishing this from carcinoma is the presence of invasion through the basement membrane.

Metaplasia, on the other hand, is entirely benign. It is a form of adaptation to injury, where one type of epithelium is replaced by another. In the cervix, the glandular epithelium, after repeated bouts of inflammation, changes to a more resistant squamous epithelium.

The cone biopsy is a way of performing a local excision of the cervix; the tissue removed is in the form of a cone. A suture is usually put at 12 o'clock to orientate the specimen. The role of the pathologist is to map the abnormal areas, to assess the abnormality in terms of severity and to comment on completeness of excision.

She was 38, and still capable of having children. The decision to have a hysterectomy can be a difficult one, although she had very little choice.

The hysterectomy specimen did not reveal any more areas of carcinoma and the single focus of carcinoma was completely excised, so she should be cured.

QUESTIONS

Define hyperplasia, hypertrophy and atrophy and give some examples of each.

Physiological and pathological alterations in cell size and number are summarized on page 215 and in Fig. 9.4.

List five features that would help to differentiate between a benign and malignant neoplasm

Circumscription, tethering, necrosis, mitotic activity, spread to adjacent lymph nodes. See page 225 for complete list of features.

What are the risk factors for cancer?
See the key facts on page 241 and the preceding section.
Give examples of three viruses and their associated cancer.
Hepatitis B – hepatocellular carcinoma; EBV – Burkitt's lymphoma; HPV-16 – cervical cancer. For full list see Table 11.2, page 237.
List the salient differences between oncogenes and tumour suppressor genes.
See page 244 for the answer.
List the clinical effects of tumours.
Compression, obstruction, ulceration, haemorrhage, rupture, perforation and infarction.

FURTHER READING

Balmain, A. (2001) Cancer genetics: from Boveri and Mendel to microarrays. *Nature Reviews. Cancer* **1**(1), 77–82.

Cooper, G.M. (1997) Cancer. In: *The Cell. A Molecular Approach*, ch. 15. ASM Press, Washington.

Cotran, R.S., Kumar, V. and Collins, T. (1999) *Robbins Pathologic Basis of Disease*, 6th edition. W.B. Saunders, Philadelphia.

Hahn, W.C. and Weinberg, R.A. (2002) Modelling the molecular circuitry of cancer. *Nature Reviews. Cancer* **2**(5), 331–41.

Special Issue (1996) What you need to know about cancer. *Scientific American*, September.

Underwood, J.C.E. (2000) *General and Systematic Pathology*, 3rd edition. Churchill Livingstone, London.

Verma, I.M. and Somia, N. (1997) Gene therapy – promises, problems and prospects. *Nature* **389**, 239–42.

Epilogue

So what is a disease? The definition provided at the outset regarding a loss of homeostasis is, we believe, a good one. What we hope is apparent is that the mechanisms involved in maintaining the balance are incredibly intricate and complex. This is the paradox of life – complexity and simplicity existing together. To maintain homeostasis – balance – seems a simple thing to do. We hardly notice the constant adaptations that the body undergoes moment to moment as we move about our daily lives, the change in body temperature, heart rate and the flexing or relaxation of muscles as we change posture. Yet the processes that allow such a seamless transition from moment to moment are both complex and beautiful.

Imagine a cell with its 30–40 000 genes. These genes are transcribed into messages, which are then read and translated into proteins, which are modified to make yet more proteins, which in turn regulate the genes and messages. The pattern of gene expression is different from cell to cell depending on its function and its role at that time. Imagine this whole network like a three-dimensional tube/metro system buzzing within the cell, constantly adapting to fulfil its function. Now imagine this cell as one of a hundred forming a tissue and one of thousands forming an organ and one of billions forming the body. Can you imagine a billion tube/metro networks all working together in a coordinated manner?

We have to admit that we can't! It is totally mind-boggling and yet, this is exactly what must be happening every second, every minute of the day for the tissues, organs and body to maintain the homeostasis that allows us to function as part of a bigger 'organism' that we call life. This is not such a crazy concept – we know that our own homeostasis is not just to do with our own genes and proteins but also with the interaction of our bodies with the environment in which it finds itself. Cancer may be a 'genetic disorder' but we are all aware that the genes provide a 'predisposition', which, given the right lifestyle and interaction with the environment, leads to cancer. Not everyone with an inherited mutation develops cancer, but they are at increased risk, which may become manifest given the right circumstances.

The beginning of the twentieth century marked the change in the way the physicists looked at the world. The quantum theory and the theory of relativity has questioned what we mean by 'reality' and the wave-particle duality continues to show us just how simple (we all think we understand it) and complex light really is. Lest you think that this 'new' physics has nothing to do with you, the quantum physics that is used to describe light is also the same physics that applies to all atoms, including those in our DNA.

The end of the twentieth century has seen the emergence of a revolution in biology, the sequencing of the human genome and the ability to look at thousands of genes and their expression profiles in one experiment. This will undoubtedly change the way we look at disease and therefore how we decide to intervene in the process. Perhaps that is the key – disease, like education and life itself, should be viewed as a process rather than a defined thing with a beginning and an end.

> I saw a child carrying a light.
> I asked him where he had brought it from.
> He put it out, and said:
> 'Now, you tell me where it is gone.'
>
> *Hasan of Basra (d. 957)*

Appendix

FRANCIS BACON (1561–1626)

Francis Bacon was born on 22 July 1561 at York House, off The Strand, in London. He was the second son of Sir Nicholas Bacon, Lord Keeper, and his second wife, Ann Cooke.

Although recognized as an important figure in the history of thought, Bacon has not really been taken as a serious figure by philosophers. He is, of course, well known to students of literature for his sharp wisdom and clever writing. Besides literature, Bacon also wrote about law, which was his profession, and about the history of the reign of Henry VII. His main works, *The Advancement of Learning* and *Novum Organum* (a presentation of a new method of logic) are, however, philosophical, and it is from his discourse on inductive reasoning that the quote on page 86 comes.

The *Advancement of Learning* consisted of two books, published in 1605. The first is essentially about the value of knowledge, which may seem a bit strange if you are unaware of the opposition to the acquisition of knowledge that existed at the time. The opposition was both religious and social and many believed that knowledge weakened action. It is not surprising, therefore, that Bacon felt inclined to provide a defence for knowledge.

The second book is about the classification of knowledge and is a reflection of his ordered mind. In Bacon's classification, all knowledge is divided according to the faculties of Memory ('history'), Imagination ('poesy') and Reason ('philosophy'). Although he divided them into separate groups, he believed in the wholeness of knowledge. He did, however, have his own bias, as he put it, in the 'domain of philosophy and the sciences'.

It is true that Bacon has often been rejected and criticized for his lack of understanding of mathematics and the scientific advances that were being made at the time. In this there is an element of truth. What Bacon did, however, was to propagate the idea that it was possible to have a continuous growth of knowledge and that it was possible to find more knowledge. Until then, there was a preoccupation with hanging on to the old knowledge in fear that it might disappear!

In his other main work, *Novum Organum*, the teaching was in the form of aphorisms. There are a group of three ideas: the need for a new logic, the attempt to discover the 'forms' of the simple natures, e.g. heat, and the collection of a comprehensive natural history. He believed that these three were tied in with natural history at the base, the laws of physics in the middle and logic as the crown.

A great deal has been written about the philosophical and scientific works of Francis Bacon and there is considerable literature about his personal and political life. He had a strong association with the Royalty and served in Parliament as Member for Melcombe Regis in Dorset and later for Taunton and Liverpool. He fell out of favour in 1621 after admitting charges of bribery.

For those who are interested in reading more about the life of Francis Bacon, the *Encyclopedia Brittanica* is a good starting point. Oxford University Press also produce a series of 'Past Masters' and the one on Bacon has been written by Anthony Quinton.

GITANJALI (1961–1977)

Gitanjali was born in Meerut, India on 12 June 1961. She died soon after her 16th birthday on 11 August 1977. That she died of cancer is not particularly remarkable in itself, many children and many adults do. What is remarkable is that born from a realization of her own mortality she left us with a record of her fears and worries and her faith and courage.

Rabindranath Tagore (1861–1941), probably India's greatest poet, is best remembered for his poem entitled 'Gitanjali', which means 'song-offering'. The first verse of Tagore's poem is as follows:

> Thou has made me endless, such is thy pleasure. This frail vessel thou emptiest again and again, and fillest it ever with fresh life.
>
> This little flute of a reed thou has carried over the hills and dales, and hast breathed through it melodies eternally new.
>
> At the immortal touch of thy hands my little heart loses its limits in joy and gives birth to utterance ineffable.
>
> Thy infinite gifts come to me only on these very small hands of mine. Ages pass, and still thou pourest, and still there is room to fill.

Gitanjali's wish was that she might live up to her name. She did. The publication of the poems in the form of a book is remarkable in itself. Gitanjali's mother had discovered the poems hidden around the house amongst her books and clothes. She tried in vain to get them published until, having almost given up hope, she sent one to *The Illustrated Weekly of India*. They were so moved by it that they decided to publish it.

The book *Poems of Gitanjali* was published by Oriel Press in 1982.

WILLIAM HARVEY (1578–1657)

William Harvey was born in Folkestone on 1 April 1578. It may have been April Fools' day but this man provided Medicine with the boost it needed to get it out of stagnation. The value of his work is put into perspective when you realize that to be honoured as a Harveian Orator by the Royal College of Physicians is the greatest distinction that one can aspire to in Medicine.

Harvey did his medical training at Caius College, Cambridge and later at Padua, Italy. In Padua, Harvey studied with Fabricius, who had succeeded Fallopio (of Fallopian tube fame). Galileo was the Professor of Mathematics at Padua at the time but does not appear to have been influential in Harvey's development.

Harvey was elected a full fellow of the College of Physicians in 1607 and soon afterwards became Assistant Physician to St Bartholomew's Hospital. This helped to establish his private practice and, interestingly, his famous patients included James I, Charles I and the Lord Chancellor, Sir Francis Bacon!

Although Bacon is given the credit for inductive thinking, it was Harvey who applied it to his investigations of the heart. Harvey, in fact, had very little respect for Bacon and had stated that Bacon 'writes philosophy (science) like a Lord Chancellor; I have cured him of it'.

The quote at the beginning of Part 3 is the first paragraph of his famous book, *De Motu Cordis*. The movements of the heart were so fast and complicated that he often despaired at ever being able to work out the sequence of each of the movements. *De Motu Cordis* evolved in two stages: initially it was an investigation into the heart beat and the arterial pulse and only later did he include the investigation of the circulation. Together, it forms one of the most important pieces of scientific work. The book is quite small, 72 pages, and would probably fit into a white coat pocket, but the few remaining copies of the original 1628 edition would set you back a cool £200 000! That is assuming anybody is willing to sell it.

William Harvey died of a stroke on 30 June 1657.

Much has been written about Harvey and the Keynes translation of 1928 is believed to be the most accurate. Keynes has written a couple of books on Harvey: *The Personality of William Harvey*, published by Cambridge University Press in 1949 and *The Life of William Harvey*, Oxford University Press, 1966.

WERNER KARL HEISENBERG (1901–1976)

Heisenberg, who is well known for his contribution to quantum mechanics, was born on 5 December 1901 in Würzburg, Germany. He studied physics at the University of Munich. His doctoral thesis, which he presented in 1923, was on turbulence in fluid streams.

In 1927, Heisenberg published his 'uncertainty principle', which says that, in the subatomic world, it is not possible to know both the position and the momentum of a particle accurately. The better we know one variable, the less sure we can be of the other. The important point is that it is not the limitation of the technique of measurement that imposes this law, it is simply the limitation of the principle. What this means is that the uncertainty principle is a mathematical way of expressing the limitation of our classical models of looking at the world.

Our classical way of looking at the world is derived from gross appearances and we have a tendency to divide things into discrete units or, to put it another way, we perceive the world as being particulate. At the subatomic level, this particulate view is an idealization without any meaning and it is not possible to describe anything without a reference to the whole. Hence 'entities' such as position and momentum are interrelated and cannot be defined precisely at the same time, since changes in one are tied in with changes in the other. These connections are of a statistical nature, i.e. probabilities rather than certainties.

This idea of interactions led to the proposal of the concept of the 'S Matrix', which is a mathematical model for these interactions. It was this belief in the fundamental principles of a shift from objects to events that led to the quotation on page 5. Just as in the subatomic world, the various events in the body are a manifestation of the many interactions between the various processes. They are not isolated events, but interact and combine in intricate ways in any given situation.

Heisenberg is mainly known for his achievements in physics, but he was also a philosopher trying to understand the relationships that are fundamental in nature. He was awarded the Nobel Prize in 1932.

WILLIAM OSLER (1849–1919)

For many people, Sir William Osler was the greatest physician of recent times. This was not for his scientific contribution but for his ability to fascinate young students and for completely transforming medical education and clinical medical training.

Osler was born at Bond Head, Ontario, Canada. His parents were English missionaries who had migrated to Canada. He was the youngest of nine children and his initial intention was to follow his father into the church, so he started his studies at Trinity College, Toronto. He changed his mind, however, and enrolled at the Toronto Medical School in 1868. He finished his medical education at McGill University. Having qualified, he spent the next 2 years travelling around Europe, the longest period being spent with Sir John Burdon-Sanderson at University College, London.

Osler returned to Canada with the intention of entering general practice but within a few months was appointed lecturer in Medicine at McGill, teaching physiology and pathology to the medical students. The following year, he was appointed Professor. After a decade in Montreal, he went as

Professor of Medicine to Pennsylvania and, in 1888, he accepted a post at the new Johns Hopkins Hospital in Baltimore. He was the second of the famous 'Hopkins four', the others being William Welch, chief of pathology, Howard Kelley, chief of obstetrics and gynaecology and William Halstead, chief of surgery. It was with these three colleagues that Osler revolutionized the medical curriculum.

For the first 4 years at Johns Hopkins, there were no medical students and Osler used these years to write *The Principles and Practice of Medicine*, first published in 1892.

In 1904, while visiting the UK, he was offered the Regius Chair of Medicine at Oxford. This was to succeed Burdon-Sanderson. Osler accepted and started his post in 1905.

Osler's name is associated with three medical conditions: Osler's nodes (tender, red swellings on the palms and fingers in bacterial endocarditis), Osler–Vaquez disease (polycythaemia rubra vera) and the Rendu–Osler–Weber disease (recurrent haemorrhages from multiple telengectasias in skin and mucous membranes).

Osler wrote a great deal about almost everything, and especially about the relationship between the teacher and student, teacher and teacher, and teacher and patient. The quotation on page 206 is from his book *Counsels and Ideals from the Writings of Sir William Osler*, 1905.

FURTHER READING

Bamforth, J. and Osborn, G.R. (1958) Diagnosis from cells. *Journal of Clinical Pathology* ii, 473–82.

Capra, F. (1983) *The Tao of Physics*, 2nd edition. Fontana Paperbacks, Glasgow.

Harding Rains, A.J. (1974) *Edward Jenner and Vaccination*. Priory Press Ltd, London.

Nuland, S.B. (1988) *Doctors. The Biography of Medicine*. Gryphon Editions, Birmingham, Alabama.

Paget, S. (1897) *John Hunter. Man of Science and Surgeon*. T. Fisher Unwin, London.

Pickering, G. (1964) William Harvey, physician and scientist. *British Medical Journal* 2, 1615–19.

Rather, L.J. (1957) Rudolf Virchow and scientific medicine. *Archives of Internal Medicine* 100, 1007–14.

Sergerist, H.E. (1935) *Great Doctors. A Biographical History of Medicine*. George Allen & Unwin, London.

Weimerskirch, P.J. and Richter, G.W. (1979) Hunter and venereal disease. *The Lancet* 1, 503–4.

Theme maps

In this book, we have tried to integrate elements of the various pathological disciplines rather than write separate sections for each individual specialty, and we have also tried to interweave the basic science and clinical topics. This is because we believe that medical education should be as focussed as possible on patients, and patients' problems frequently cross disciplinary boundaries. However, when studying a subject as vast and complex as medicine, it is often helpful to be able to break it down into smaller areas and then build and interweave the topics as your experience and understanding grows.

Most modern health curricula adopt an integrated approach and refer to horizontal and vertical integration. Horizontal integration is the blending of disciplines that are studied within a year. Vertical integration aims to ensure that certain themes run through all the years of the course. To illustrate these approaches, we present six theme maps.

The first four maps relate to the traditional pathological disciplines of haematology, histopathology,

immunology and microbiology. In effect, we are disintegrating the horizontal integration back to some of its constituent parts. You will notice that haematology and immunology have a similar basic map structure. This is because both are based on a specific body system, i.e. the haemopoietic system and the immune system. In fact, these maps could easily be adapted to cover other systems such as respiratory or gastrointestinal.

The other two maps are 'Science and disease' and 'Patient and disease' and these are the types of theme that can run vertically through the whole length of a course. None of these themes is covered comprehensively in this book, but you are likely to need to study them at some stage in your course. We have constructed these maps by considering how authors generally present their topic in undergraduate texts and then taken a greatly simplified approach. To help you identify the topics in this book, we have tried to colour-code the chapter titles to match the theme or main branches of the maps.

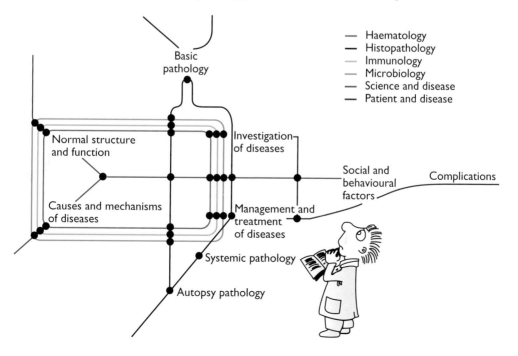

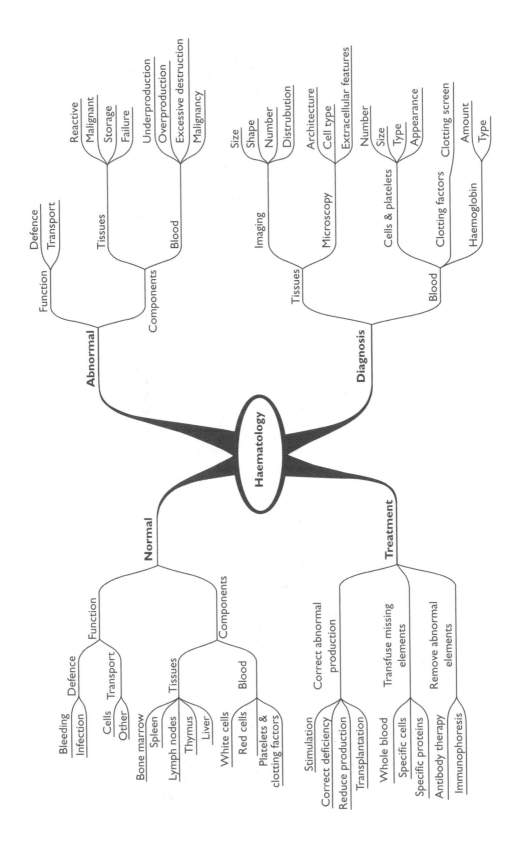

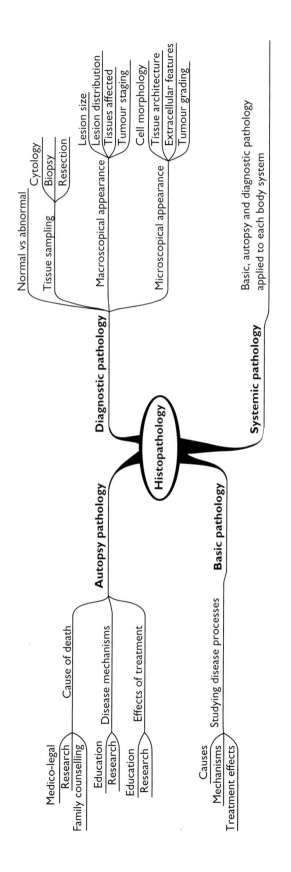

Histopathology

Diagnostic pathology

Normal vs abnormal

Tissue sampling
- Cytology
- Biopsy
- Resection

Macroscopical appearance
- Lesion size
- Lesion distribution
- Tissues affected
- Tumour staging

Microscopical appearance
- Cell morphology
- Tissue architecture
- Extracellular features
- Tumour grading

Systemic pathology

Basic, autopsy and diagnostic pathology applied to each body system

Autopsy pathology

Cause of death
- Medico-legal
- Research
- Family counselling

Disease mechanisms
- Education
- Research

Effects of treatment
- Education
- Research

Basic pathology

Studying disease processes
- Causes
- Mechanisms
- Treatment effects

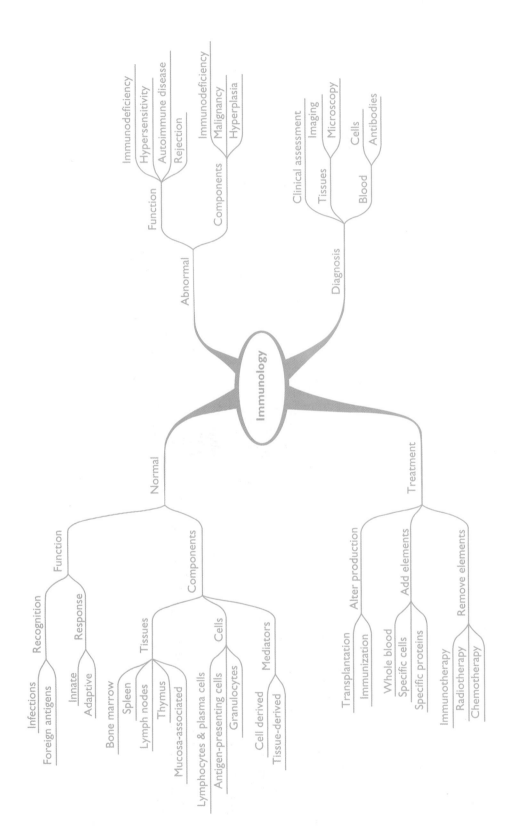

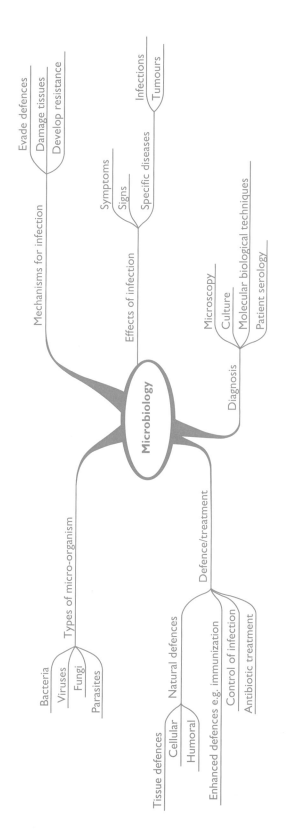

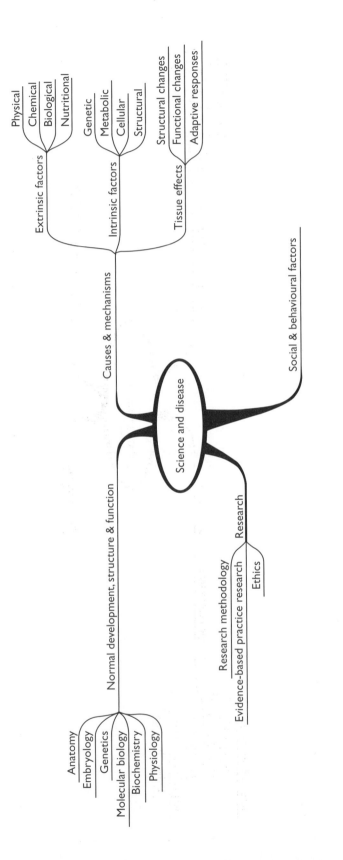

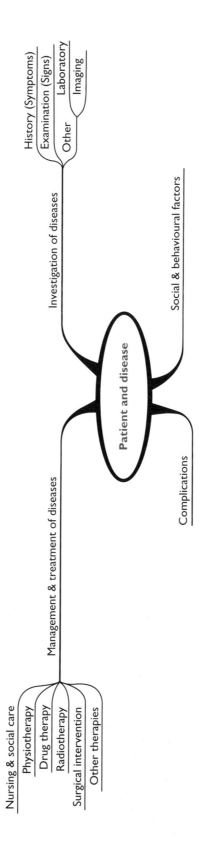

Patient and disease

Investigation of diseases
History (Symptoms)
Examination (Signs)
Other
Laboratory
Imaging

Social & behavioural factors

Complications

Management & treatment of diseases
Nursing & social care
Physiotherapy
Drug therapy
Radiotherapy
Surgical intervention
Other therapies

Index

Page numbers followed by (f) refer to pages on which figures appear; page numbers followed by (t) refer to pages on which tables appear.